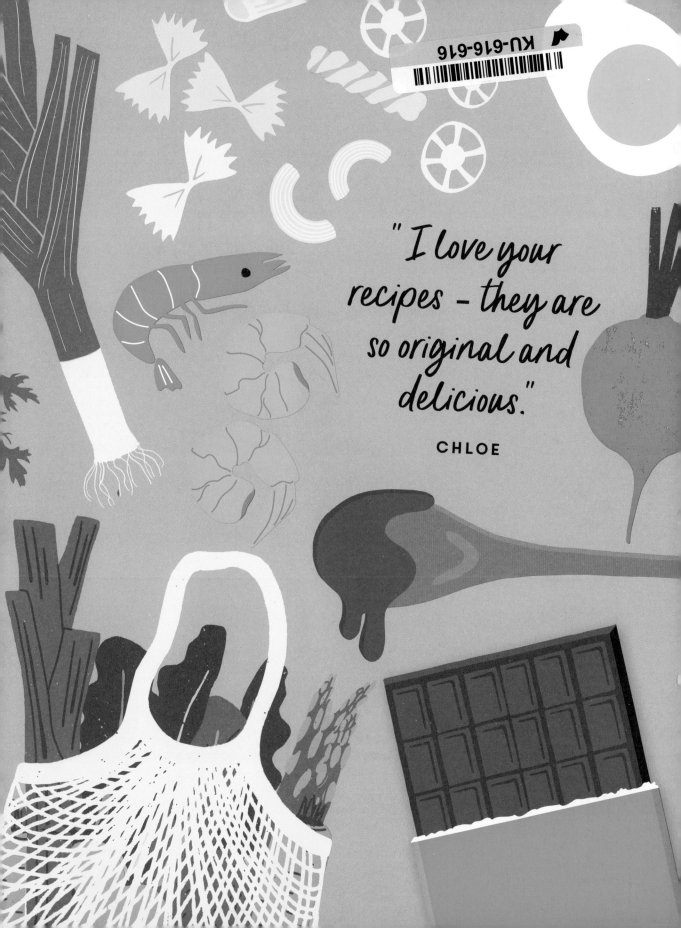

"I love your recipes – they are so original and delicious."

CHLOE

Pinch

of

Nom

COMFORT
FOOD

First published 2021 by Bluebird
an imprint of Pan Macmillan
The Smithson, 6 Briset Street, London EC1M 5NR
EU representative: Macmillan Publishers Ireland Ltd, 1st Floor,
The Liffey Trust Centre, 117–126 Sheriff Street Upper,
Dublin 1, D01 YC43

Associated companies throughout the world
www.panmacmillan.com

ISBN 978-1-5290-3501-8

1 3 5 7 9 8 6 4 2
A CIP catalogue record for this book is available from the British Library.
Printed and bound in Germany.

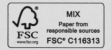

Publisher Carole Tonkinson
Project Editor Katy Denny
Project Manager Laura Nickoll
Senior Production Controller Sarah Badhan
Art Direction Nikki Dupin and Emma Wells, Nic&Lou
Design Emma Wells, Nic&Lou
Illustration Shutterstock / Emma Wells
Food Styling Kate Wesson
Prop Styling Cynthia Blackett

Visit www.panmacmillan.com to read more about all our books
and to buy them. You will also find features, author interviews and
news of any author events, and you can sign up for e-newsletters
so that you're always first to hear about our new releases.

KATE ALLINSON & KAY FEATHERSTONE

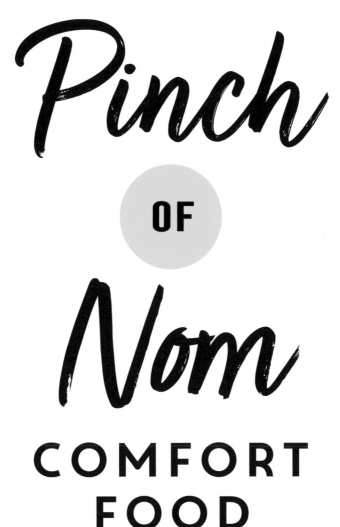

Pinch

OF

Nom

COMFORT FOOD

100 SLIMMING, SATISFYING MEALS

bluebird
books for life

Contents

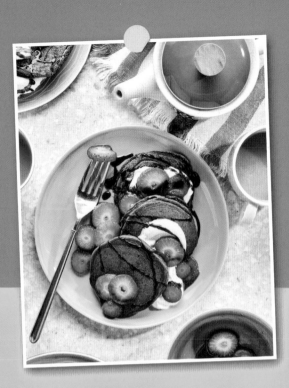

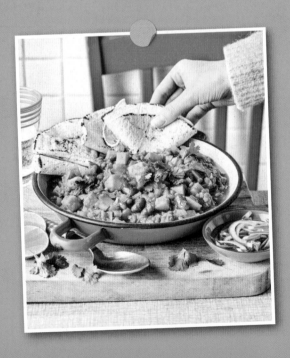

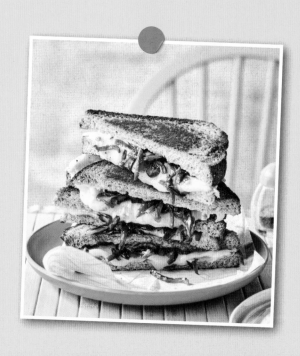

WELCOME to Pinch OF Nom

COMFORT FOOD

HELLO

Well, here we are – book four! What a whirlwind it has been, and we've loved every second of it. At the heart of every book we write is YOU, the Pinch of Nom community. When you tell us what you want to eat, and what you find challenging, we listen and get in the kitchen to come up with simple, delicious slimming-friendly recipes to help you on your journey. We've written this book during the Covid-19 pandemic and what has become clearer to us than ever – from talking to our readers – is the capacity of food to provide comfort in tough times, as well as nourishment.

SO WHAT'S COMFORT FOOD ALL ABOUT?

Satisfying, homely dishes remind so many of us of childhood and give us a sense of nostalgia. For all of us at Pinch of Nom, cooking comfort food is about sharing and getting everyone together around the table. Comfort food, the Nom way, means hearty stews that tick all the boxes, slow-cooked dishes that are wholesome yet full of flavour, roasts with all the trimmings, and healthy twists on family favourites. This book is about the kind of food you know and love, made according to our failsafe Pinch of Nom blueprint, with cheeky flavour tweaks. We've included calorie breakdowns so you know exactly where you're at (we bet you won't notice how low the calorie counts are).

All of the 100 brand-new comfort food recipes are easy to make and easy to adapt (keep an eye out for our Swap This tips). We know how much you love our fakeaways, and snacks and sides, so these get the 'comfort' makeover too. Many of you have asked us how you can convert Pinch of Nom recipes so that they can be cooked in different appliances, such as an electric pressure cooker, so for this book we've tested lots of our favourite one-pots using a variety of cooking methods, with some recipes giving the option of air fryer, slow cooker and traditional hob-top cooking so you can take your pick. You don't get more comforting than Beef Stew and Dumplings (page 162) and Sweet Potato Chilli (page 108), and don't worry – we've not forgotten Sweet Treats: with Jam Roly Poly (page 258) and our Choco Nut Lava Cakes (page 263) we've got you covered! As always, we've flagged vegan and vegetarian recipes, and for book four we've added chilli-heat icons, so you can make a beeline for the 🌶🌶 if you want a kick of heat (though you can always leave out the spice if you prefer).

Now, with every comfort food craving catered for, you can dive into these fab recipes and feel amazing. We hope you love every bite!

Kay x Kate

THE FOOD

As a classically trained chef, Kate has always looked at recipes and dishes then worked on how to improve or recreate them. That is still the case and it's how the Pinch of Nom recipes are formed. The aim for Kate and her small team is to come up with the best ideas for recipes, then get into the kitchen and throw around ingredients until the right balance is made!

It is important to the Pinch of Nom team that all of the recipes are easily accessible and that they use ingredients that can be used time and again to save on cost. Ingredients that may seem a little less common are only ever featured where they add a unique touch to the dish – you'll see that they pop up occasionally in a few deserving recipes.

We've also made sure that the recipes work for whatever cooking ability you have. We're confident that even the novice cook can tackle these recipes and end up with a decent meal without spending hours in the kitchen.

An impressive 47 of the 100 recipes in this book are vegetarian. However, by being careful with types of ingredients used (vegetarian Parmesan, for example) or by using a protein replacement of your choice, almost all of the recipes could be made veggie. We've flagged those as non-veggie for ease of reference.

KEEP THE COMFORT LOSE THE Calories

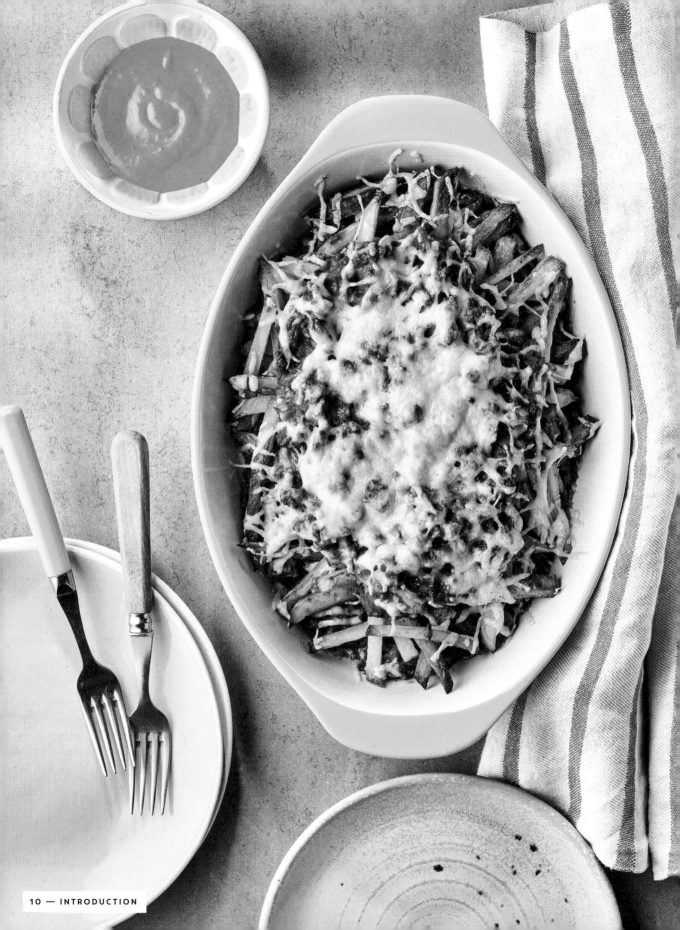

RECIPE TAGS

EVERYDAY LIGHT

These recipes can be used freely throughout the week. All the meals, including accompaniments, are under 400 calories. Or, in the case of sides, snacks and sweet treats, under 200 calories. Of course, if you're counting calories, you still need to keep an eye on the values, but these recipes should be a sure thing for staying under your allowance.

WEEKLY INDULGENCE

These recipes are still low in calories, at between 400 and 500 calories, or 200–300 for sides, snacks and sweet treats, but should be saved for once or twice a week. Mix Weekly Indulgence recipes into your meal plans alongside Everyday Light recipes for variety.

SPECIAL OCCASION

These recipes are often lower in calories than their usual full-fat counterparts, but they need to be saved for a special occasion. This tag indicates any main meals that are over 500 calories or over 300 for sides, snacks and sweet treats.

All of these calculations and dietary indicators are for guidance only and are not to be taken as complete fact without checking ingredients and product labelling yourself.

KCALS *and* CARB VALUES

All of our recipes have been worked out as complete meals, using standardised portion sizes for any accompaniments as advised by the British Nutrition Foundation. Carb values are included for those who need to measure their intake.

GLUTEN-FREE RECIPES

We have marked gluten-free recipes with a GF icon. All these recipes are either free of gluten, or we have suggested gluten-free ingredient swaps of common ingredients, such as stock cubes and Worcestershire sauce. Please check labelling to ensure the product you buy is gluten free.

FREEZABLE RECIPES

Freezer icons apply to main dishes only, not the suggested accompaniments.

OUR RECIPE ICONS

V	Veggie	**DF**	Dairy Free
VG	Vegan	**LC**	Low Carb
F	Freezable	**GF**	Gluten Free
BF	Batch Friendly	** ʃʃ **	Spice Rating

BATCH COOKING

As in our last book, we've grouped our favourite batch-cooking recipes together in their own chapter, because batch-cooking ideas are often requested by our community and batch cooking is an efficient way to prepare food in advance, for when you're short of time. These recipes have their own specific guidelines, but there are also plenty of other recipes in the book that you can batch cook with a few tweaks, such as upping the portions of Fish Chowder (page 158) and freezing some for later. It's important to store food safely, so we have included the latest NHS food-safety guidelines (correct at the time of writing).

- **Divide food into individual portions to refrigerate or freeze** so you can just reheat one portion, or four portions, or six, etc., without needing to chisel pieces off a big frozen block! It will also ensure they cool and freeze (and defrost) quicker.

- **Make sure you have enough space** in the fridge or freezer before you get cooking!

- **Use refrigerated foods within 2 days.**

- **When freezing food**, use airtight containers or freezer bags. Invest in some decent freezer- and microwave-proof storage containers. If not, your containers may crack or melt, which is not what you need when you want a quick meal. Make sure your containers are sealed properly to avoid 'freezer burn' (when the food has been damaged from air getting inside).

- **Always label food.** Use freezer-proof stickers, adding the date you made it. Nobody wants mystery food in the freezer, and it's likely it will end up going to waste if it's not labelled. Meals can be frozen for 3–6 months. Up to 3 months is ideal and beyond 6 months is still safe, but the food may not taste as good.

- **Only reheat food once.**

- **Defrost food thoroughly** in the fridge or microwave before reheating it.

- **Thoroughly defrosted food** should be reheated and eaten within 24 hours – only defrost what you need. NHS guidelines state you should reheat food until it reaches 70°C /158°F and holds that temperature for 2 minutes. Make sure it's piping hot throughout. Stir while reheating to ensure this.

- **You can freeze the sauce or meat for some recipes**, but in most cases the rice, pasta or other accompaniments will need to be cooked at the time you want to eat, as they either cannot be reheated, or they're a lot nicer cooked fresh.

- **If you are batch-cooking rice**, it's important to store it correctly before you reheat it. Cool it as quickly as possible, ideally within 1 hour. (With other foods this could be up to 2 hours.) Putting rice in a wide, shallow container will help it cool quicker. There is a risk of bacteria growing the longer it is left at room temperature. Cooked rice should only be kept in the fridge for 1 day before reheating (it can also be frozen, then defrosted thoroughly in the fridge before reheating). When you reheat rice, make sure it is piping hot all the way through. Never reheat rice more than once.

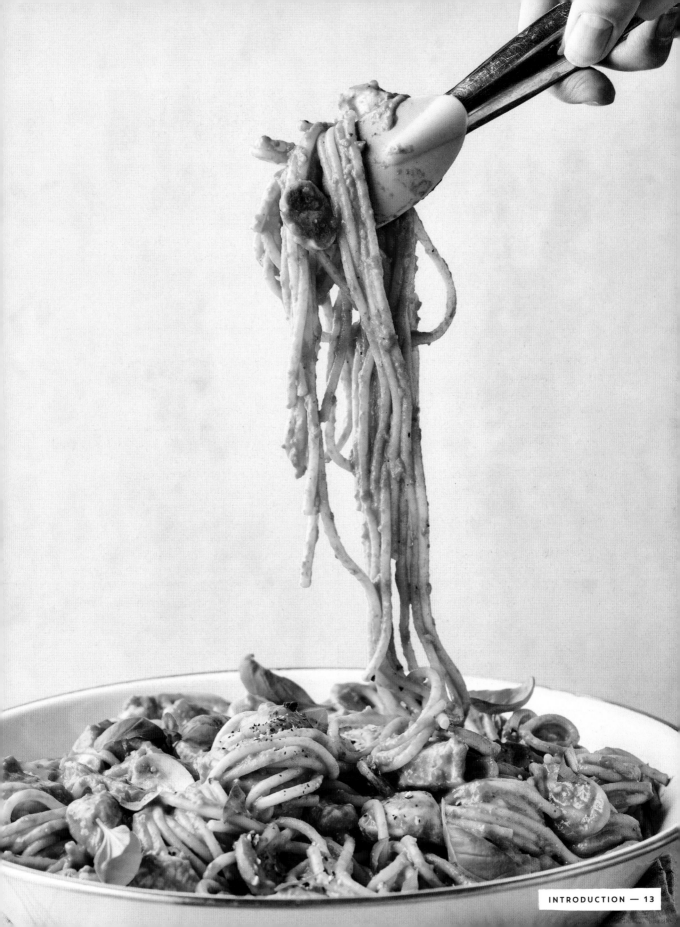

KEY INGREDIENTS

PROTEIN

Lean meats are a great source of protein, providing essential nutrients and fantastic filling power. In all cases where meat is used in this book, you will need to ensure you are using the leanest cuts and trimming off all fat. Fish is another great source of protein and naturally low in fat. Pinch of Nom's favourite phrase? If it swims, it slims! Fish provides nutrients that the body struggles to produce naturally, making it perfect for some of Pinch of Nom's super-slimming recipes. Vegetarian protein options can always be used instead of meat in all of the recipes in this book.

HERBS *and* SPICES

We love a bit of spice! One of the best ways to keep your food interesting when changing ingredients for lower fat/sugar/calorie versions is to season it well with herbs and spices. In particular, mixed spice blends, either pre-prepared or homemade, are perfect for certain recipes in this book, like our Chicken and Cheese Curry (page 74), or Steak and Chips Pie (page 187). Don't be shy with spices – not all of them burn your mouth off! We've added a spice-level icon to our recipes in this book, so you know what to expect.

STOCKS, SAUCES *and* THICKENERS

When you remove fat from a dish, flavours can dwindle. Most people simply make something spicy to counteract the lack of flavour coming from fat, but sometimes the level of acidity in a dish is more important. That's why we love vinegar, soy sauce, fish sauce and Worcestershire sauce or Henderson's relish for boosting flavour and balancing out a dish. In addition, one of Pinch of Nom's most essential ingredients is the lowly stock cube or stock pot: they add instant flavour and are so versatile. We use various flavoured cubes and pots throughout this book, but they are all interchangeable. It is worth noting that these sauces, stock cubes and pots are often high in salt, so swap for reduced-salt varieties if you prefer.

Something we get asked quite often is 'How can I thicken this...?' Pre-slimming we wouldn't think twice about using a few tablespoons of flour to thicken a soup or gravy. Now, however, we're always on the lookout for lower-calorie and gluten-free options. Reducing liquid by evaporation is a good way of thickening soups or stews without having to add anything else, and it concentrates the flavours too. Potatoes, a starchy veg, can also be used to thicken a dish, just by simmering some potato in the liquid and blitzing or mashing. This method adds extra calories (1 large potato, approx. 369g, is about 311 kcal). If you're making a tomato-based dish, like soup, tomato sauce or Bolognese, you can thicken it slightly with tomato puree. This will add about 50 kcal per 51g tbsp. You can use egg yolks or whole beaten eggs to thicken some soups and sauces. Drizzle a little of the hot liquid onto the egg, whisking vigorously, then stir the egg back into the pan and heat gently until it thickens. 1 medium (57g) egg is about 76 kcal and 1 medium (18g) egg yolk is about 55 kcal. Traditionally, flour is added to melted butter to make a roux before adding liquid, but as butter adds loads of calories, a better way is to make a slurry: just mix measured flour with a little water, then stir it into the boiling liquid and simmer for a few minutes to cook the flour. 1 level tbsp (20g) of plain flour is about 71 kcal. Cornflour is another instant thickener for soups and stews. Make a slurry with a little cold water, then add to the boiling liquid. Remove from the heat when the starchy taste has gone. 1 level tbsp (20g) of cornflour is about 69 kcal. If you're making a stew or chilli, it's tempting to sprinkle in gravy granules to thicken it and add flavour, but it can add quite a few calories if you use a heavy hand. 1 tsp (5g) of gravy granules is about 21 kcal (depending on the brand) so do account for this (and bear in mind that the gravy granules will be high in salt).

LEMONS *and* LIMES

Lemons and limes pack a punch when it comes to flavour. They're perfect for a dish such as the Creamy, Cheesy Garlic Mushroom Risotto (page 135), where it adds that extra bit of zing.

REDUCED-FAT DAIRY

Substituting some high-fat dairy products with clever alternatives can make a dish instantly lower in calories. Quark and reduced-fat soft cheese or spreadable cheese are some essentials that Pinch of Nom are always looking to substitute in for higher-fat versions.

PLANT-BASED ALTERNATIVES

We often use plant-based alternatives to dairy milk. Not only are they low in fat but they bring added flavour to a dish. Coconut dairy-free milk alternative is a great substitute for high-fat tinned coconut milk in our Caribbean Lamb Curry (page 57), and almond milk brings a nutty flavour to our Bakewell Rice Pudding (page 270).

TINS

Don't be afraid to bulk-buy tinned essentials! Beans, tomatoes, sweetcorn... You'll find many of these ingredients add texture and flavour to Pinch of Nom stews, salads and soups. They keep the cost down and make hardly any difference to the taste of these sorts of dishes in comparison with their fresh counterparts.

FROZEN FRUIT *and* VEG

Frozen fruit and veg make great filler ingredients and are perfect low-cost alternatives where fresh options aren't necessarily required (for stews, etc.). They often have the added bonus of being pre-prepared, so it's the perfect time-saver for recipes like Slow-cooker Oats (page 26) or Cherry Pie (page 272)!

PULSES, RICE *and* BEANS

High in both protein and fibre, keeping a few tins of beans and pulses in the cupboard is never going to do any harm! Rice is a fantastic filler and, flavoured with spices and/or seasoning, is a great accompaniment to many Pinch of Nom recipes.

BREAD

A great source of fibre and therefore providing that all-important filling power, wholemeal bread can be used as it is, in our Ultimate Grilled Cheese (page 232), or crumbed down to bind ingredients, such as in the Chestnut Roast (page 194). We often use gluten-free breads, as they tend to contain fewer calories and less sugar, making them an easy swap to shave off some calories.

EGGS

Eggs are protein-rich, tasty and versatile! The ultimate in slimming yet filling ingredients, the humble egg can be used as an integral ingredient in recipes such as our Chocolate Custard (page 240), or for meals where they're the starring role such as the Pizza-topped Omelette (page 37). You'll always want a box in the house.

LOW-CALORIE SPRAY

One of the best ways to cut down on oils and fats being used to cook with is to use a low-calorie cooking spray.

There is little difference to the way that most ingredients are cooked, but it can make a huge difference to the calories consumed.

READY-MADE PASTRY

We have a few recipes using pastry in this book. There's no need to become a pastry chef overnight – just buy it ready-made! Not only can you usually find a light version with reduced calories, but ain't nobody got the time to be making filo pastry for our Cheese, Onion and Potato Pie (page 200)!

TORTILLA WRAPS

Our recipes are well known for creating magic with wraps! It's amazing what you can conjure up using the humble wrap – as well as using them in a more traditional way, like Scrunchiladas (page 59), you can also use them to replace pastry (see our Cherry Pie on page 272). Wholegrain or wholewheat wraps provide fibre and filling power, too.

SWEETENER

There are so many sweeteners out there, and it can be tricky to know which is the best substitute for regular sugar, as they vary in sweetness and swapping them weight-for-weight with regular sugar can give you different results. In our recipes, we use granulated sweetener, not powdered sweetener, as it has larger 'crystals' and can be used weight-for-weight as a sugar substitute.

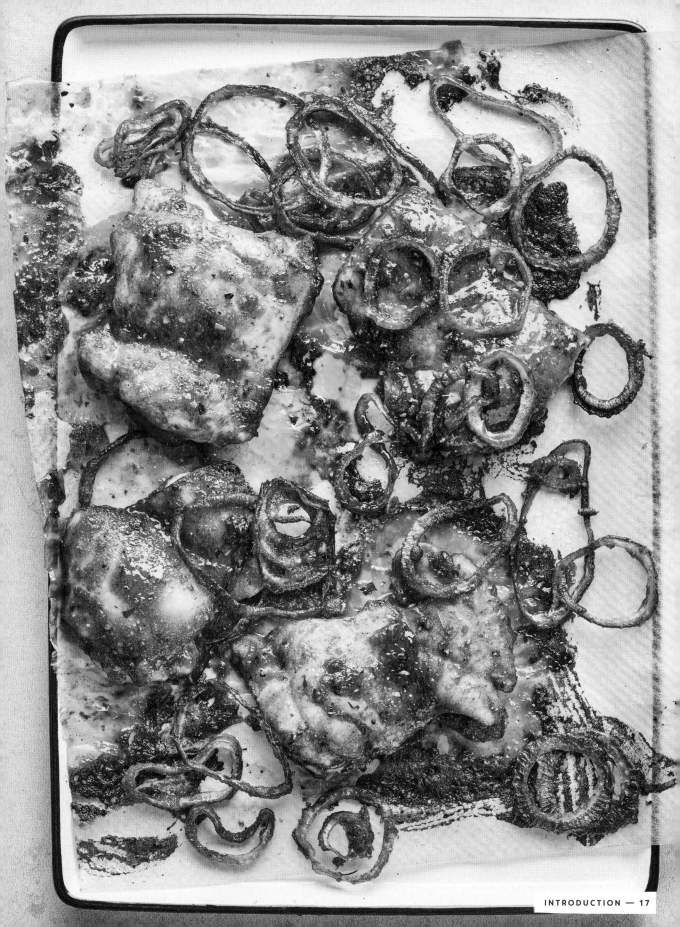

ESSENTIAL KIT

NON-STICK PANS

If there's one bit of kit that Pinch of Nom would advise as an investment kitchen piece, it would be a decent set of non-stick pans. The better the non-stick quality of your pans, the fewer cooking oils and fats you will need to avoid food sticking to your pan and burning. Keep your pans in good health too – clean them properly and gently with soapy water. We recommend a good set of saucepans, a small and large frying pan and a griddle pan if you can – a few of our recipes call for a griddle pan, but you can use a frying pan if you can't get your hands on one.

MIXING BOWLS

Large and small. Something that you'll find more useful than you believed possible in the kitchen are a couple of mixing bowls. We recommend getting a smaller one and a larger one: a small one will give you more control when whisking etc., and a large one will give you room to mix ingredients.

KITCHEN KNIVES

Every kitchen needs a set of knives. But more so, every kitchen needs a *good* set of knives. We would strongly advise you invest a little bit and get some super-sharp knives. Blunt knives are actually more dangerous than a sharp knife, as they have a habit of 'bouncing' off the food. Be careful with sharp ones too, of course, but you won't believe the difference of having knives that glide through veg when you're chopping.

KNIFE SHARPENER

There is nothing worse than trying to chop up a butternut squash with a spoon, so why would you recreate the experience with your knives? Keep those babies sharp! It will save you so much time and effort.

POTATO MASHER

Used in a number of recipes, you'll need a decent masher to ensure you're not straining muscles every time you want a bit of mash!

SLOW COOKER

We are big fans of the slow cooker. Throw in some ingredients, go off and enjoy your day and return to a home-cooked meal, ready and waiting. They are also a relatively inexpensive bit of kit that will save you a lot of time. We use a 3.5-litre slow cooker. Don't attempt to make dishes in a slow cooker that is any smaller than this.

FOOD PROCESSOR / BLENDER / STICK BLENDER

These are essential pieces of kit for a lot of Pinch of Nom recipes. As quite a few of the recipes involve making sauces from scratch, a decent blender or food processor will be a godsend! A stick blender can also be used on most occasions if you're looking for something a bit cheaper or more compact. It's worth the cost of this equipment for all those flavourful and handmade sauces.

TUPPERWARE *and* PLASTIC TUBS

Most of the Pinch of Nom recipes in this book are freezable and ideal for batch cooking. Planning ahead is so much easier when you can cook ahead too. So invest in some decent freezer-proof tubs – they don't have to be plastic. For a more eco-friendly solution, glass storage containers are also available. Just be sure to check they are freezer-proof.

Note on plastic: We have made a conscious effort to reduce the amount of non-reusable plastic such as cling film when making our recipes. There are great alternatives to cling film now available, such as silicone stretch lids, beeswax food wraps, elasticated food covers, fabric food covers, and biodegradable food and freezer bags.

RAMEKIN DISHES

One of the best ways to handle portion control on sweet treats or desserts is to do exactly what 'portion control' suggests: create controllable portions. By making dishes in small ramekins, you've already given yourself a set portion, which not only makes calorie-counting much easier, but also, if we're honest, makes the food look faaaancy!

OVENWARE

Used in a high percentage of Pinch of Nom dishes, oven trays, roasting tins and oven dishes are an essential bit of kit – keep them in good condition for longer by using disposable baking paper or foil to line them before cooking. We recommend some baking trays, square and round cake tins, a loaf tin, a large heavy-based casserole dish with a lid and a pie dish and lasagne dish as essentials. If a specific size of dish is required and essential to the success of the dish, we've listed this as 'Special Equipment'.

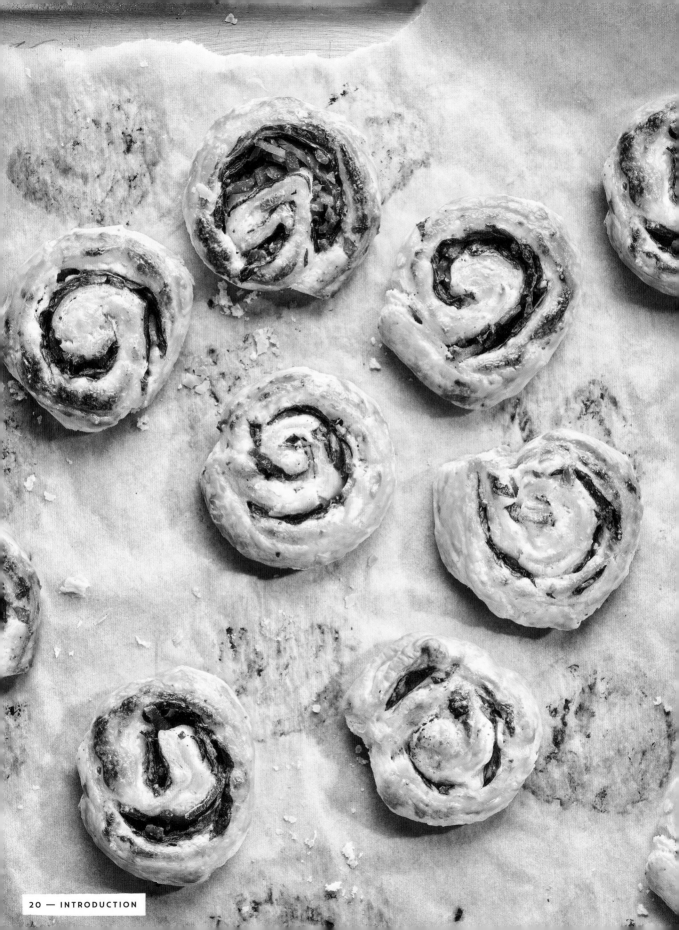

HOB

We cook on an induction hob. If you have a ceramic/hot-plate hob, you may have to cook dishes for a little longer.

FINE GRATER

Using a fine grater is one of those surprising revelations. You won't believe the difference in grating cheese with a fine grater versus a standard grater. 45g of cheese, for example, can easily cover an oven dish when using a fine grater. We also use the fine grater for citrus zest and for garlic and ginger. It helps a little go a long way.

ELECTRIC PRESSURE COOKER

A pressure cooker is such a good investment, saving valuable time. The high-pressure cooking also creates perfectly tender meat and it will seem like stews have been bubbling away for hours after just a short time in the cooker. We recommend electric models for safety and ease of use.

AIR FRYER

An air fryer has become a slimming staple in recent years. Being able to get crispy, deep-fried textures and tastes, without plunging your food into fattening oils, is the ultimate in guilt-free deliciousness! And there's the added bonus that excess oil drains away rather than food sitting in it. It's the ideal appliance for chips, breaded meats and much more. If your air fryer doesn't have a preheat function, heat it at cooking temperature for a few minutes before air-frying your food.

SET OF MEASURING SPOONS

Want to make sure you're not putting a tablespoon of chilli in your dish, rather than half a teaspoon? This is one of the most essential items of kitchenware you'll ever require. Especially if you've ever made the aforementioned mistake, as Pinch of Nom has never done. Not ever.

ELECTRIC HAND WHISK

Have you ever tried to make meringue or whip cream with a hand whisk? I can still feel the arm throb! Of course, if working out while you cook is good for you, then just get a good-old balloon whisk. However, we recommend using an electric whisk – they're relatively inexpensive and much less effort!

HEATPROOF JUG

A measuring jug is essential for measuring out wet ingredients. We recommend getting a heatproof version that you can stick in the microwave when needed.

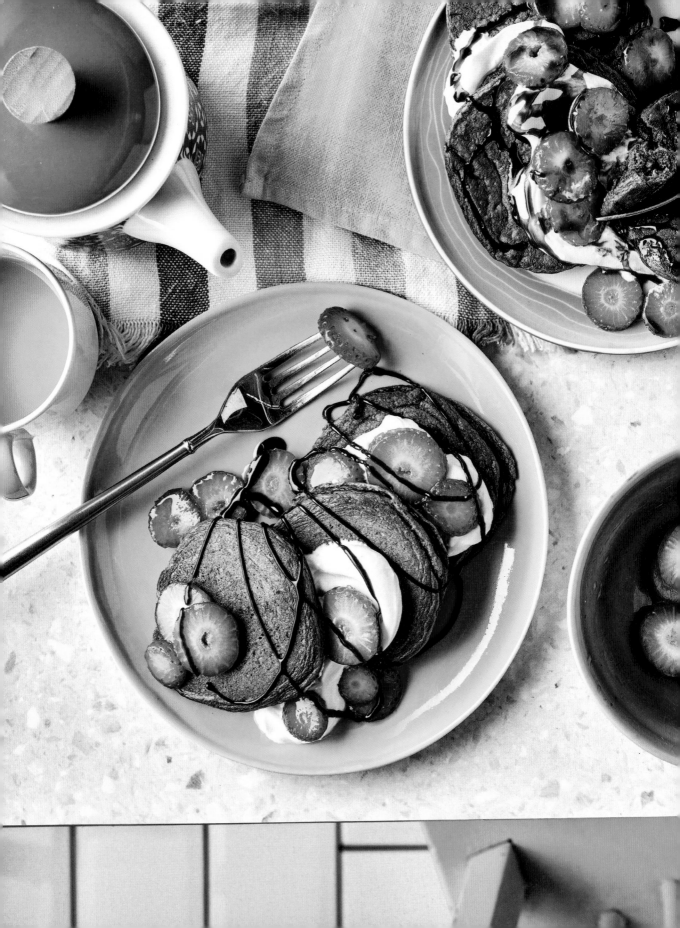

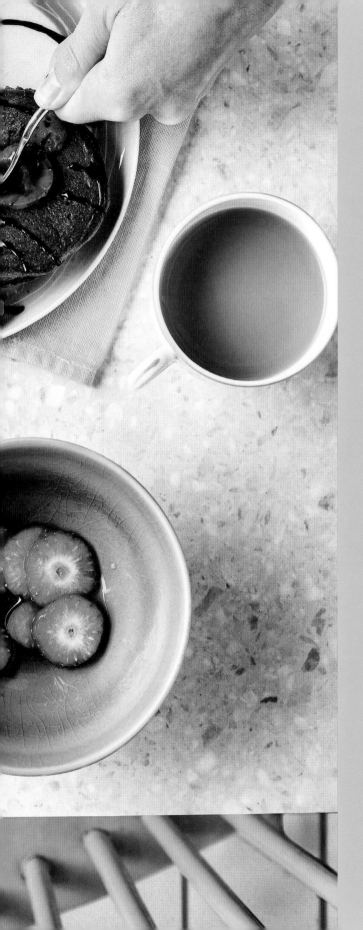

Breakfast

MARMITE MUSHROOMS
on TOAST

🕐 **5 MINS** 　🍲 **8 MINS** 　✕ **SERVES 1**

PER SERVING:
187 KCAL / 20G CARBS

low-calorie cooking spray
100g mushrooms, halved or
　quartered, depending on size
1 tsp Marmite
1 slice wholemeal bread
40g reduced-fat cream cheese
a few chopped chives,
　to garnish (optional)

There is nothing subtle about the flavours here, with intense umami from the Marmite, meaty mushrooms and a rich, creamy sauce to mop up with wholemeal toast. Even better, it's on the table in less than 15 minutes. Love it or hate it, here's a quick and easy breakfast dish that will wake you up with a bang!

Everyday Light ————————————

Spray a frying pan with low-calorie cooking spray and place over a medium heat. Add the mushrooms and sauté for 5–6 minutes until soft, then remove from the heat and add 2 tablespoons of water and the Marmite. Stir well – the residual heat in the pan will help the Marmite dissolve.

Pop the bread in the toaster and return the pan to the hob over a low heat. Stir in the cream cheese until well combined and heated through.

Serve the mushrooms on the toast, sprinkled with chopped chives if desired.

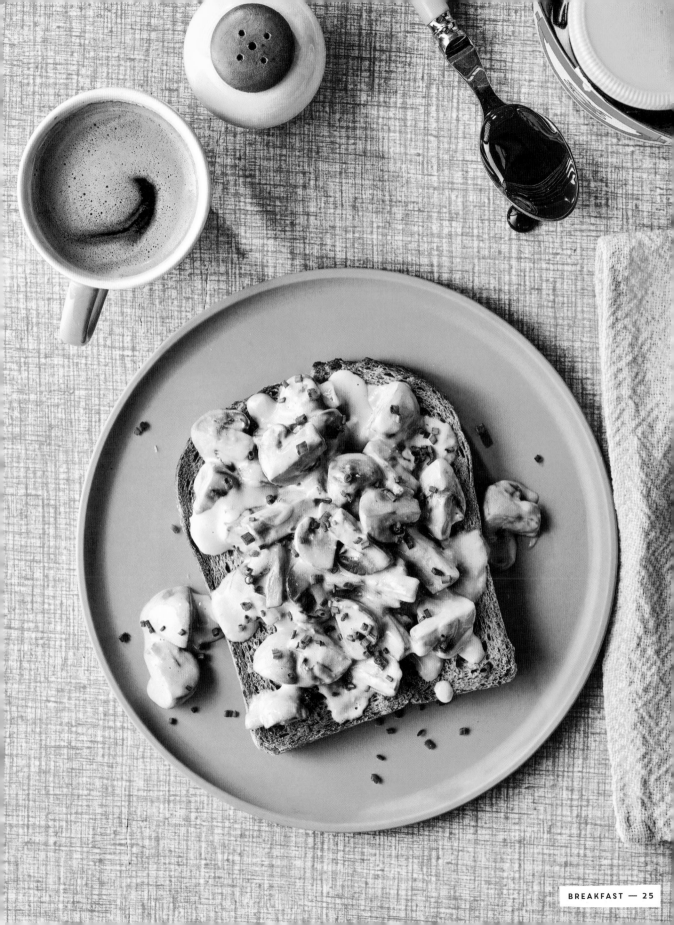

SLOW-COOKER OATS
with TWO TOPPINGS

🕐 **5 MINS**　　🍲 **4–8 HOURS***　　✕ **SERVES 4**

***PLUS 15 MINS FOR THE COMPOTE OR 5 MINS
FOR THE PEANUT BUTTER AND BANANA TOPPING**

Use GF oats

V　GF

PER SERVING FOR OATS (WITHOUT TOPPINGS):

109 KCAL /17G CARBS

*Oats with compote:
169 kcal /30g carbs
Oats with peanut and banana:
267 kcal /37g carbs*

SPECIAL EQUIPMENT

Slow cooker, heatproof bowl, jug or dish (minimum 1-litre capacity) that fits inside the slow-cooker bowl.

80g porridge oats
350ml skimmed milk
350ml water
a pinch of salt

FOR BLUEBERRY AND APPLE COMPOTE TOPPING

2 small dessert apples, peeled and cut into 1cm (½in) dice
200g frozen blueberries
juice of ½ lemon
1 tbsp granulated sweetener or caster sugar
½ tsp ground cinnamon
1 tbsp water

FOR PEANUT BUTTER AND BANANA TOPPING

2 tbsp peanut butter powder
2 tsp granulated sweetener or caster sugar
2 bananas, peeled and sliced
6 pecan halves, chopped
4 tsp maple syrup

Enjoy waking up to a warming bowl of porridge fresh from the slow cooker! We've used a water-bath method to cook them overnight. All you'll need, other than a slow cooker, is a large heatproof jug, bowl or dish. We've suggested two of our favourite toppings, but it's just as good served straight up with a little sugar or sweetener, if you like. Make the compote the day before and chill overnight, then just spoon it over your porridge in the morning.

Everyday Light ───────────────

FOR THE SLOW-COOKED OATS

Put all the ingredients for the oats into the heatproof bowl, jug or dish and stir well. Place the bowl in the slow-cooker bowl and fill the slow-cooker insert with enough water to come halfway up the bowl. Put the lid on the slow cooker and cook overnight on low. It will be ready to eat after 4–5 hours but will happily sit for 7 or even 8 hours until everyone has woken up! Serve with your own topping or one of our delicious topping recipes.

FOR THE COMPOTE

Put all the ingredients in a small saucepan, place over a medium-high heat and stir until it begins to bubble. Reduce the heat and simmer for 10–15 minutes until the apples soften. Remove from the heat, leave to cool, cover and store in the fridge overnight. In the morning, divide the oats among bowls, top with the compote and serve!

FOR THE PEANUT BUTTER AND BANANA

Stir the peanut butter powder and sweetener or sugar into the oats until well combined. Spoon into bowls and top with the sliced bananas and chopped pecans, then drizzle with maple syrup.

TIP: If you have any leftover compote, stir it through fat-free Greek-style yoghurt for a tasty, sweet snack.

SWAP THIS: Try 1 tablespoon of smooth peanut butter instead of peanut butter powder, or swap the blueberries for blackberries.

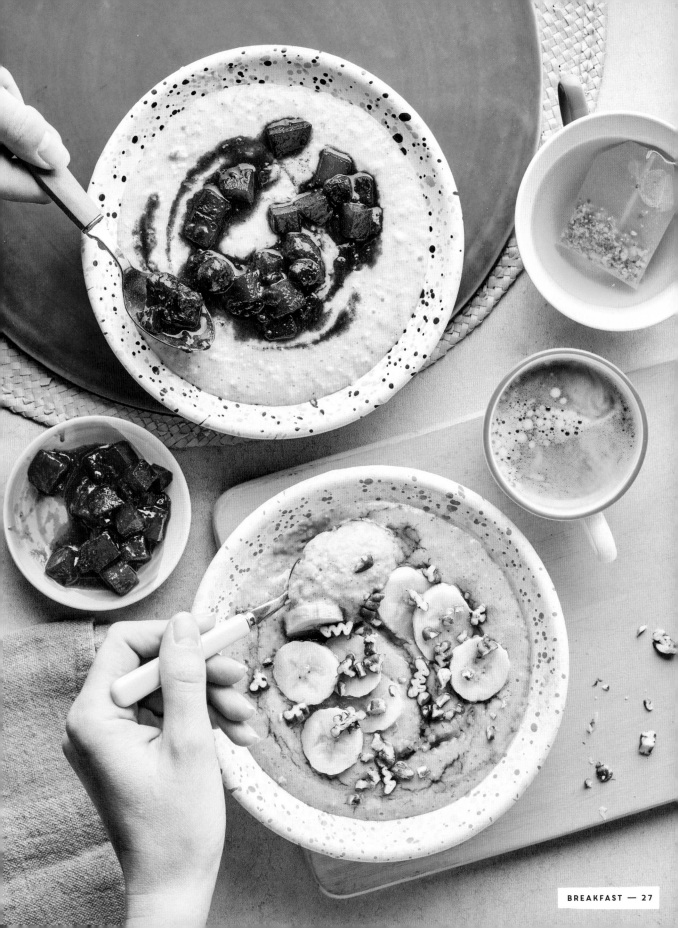

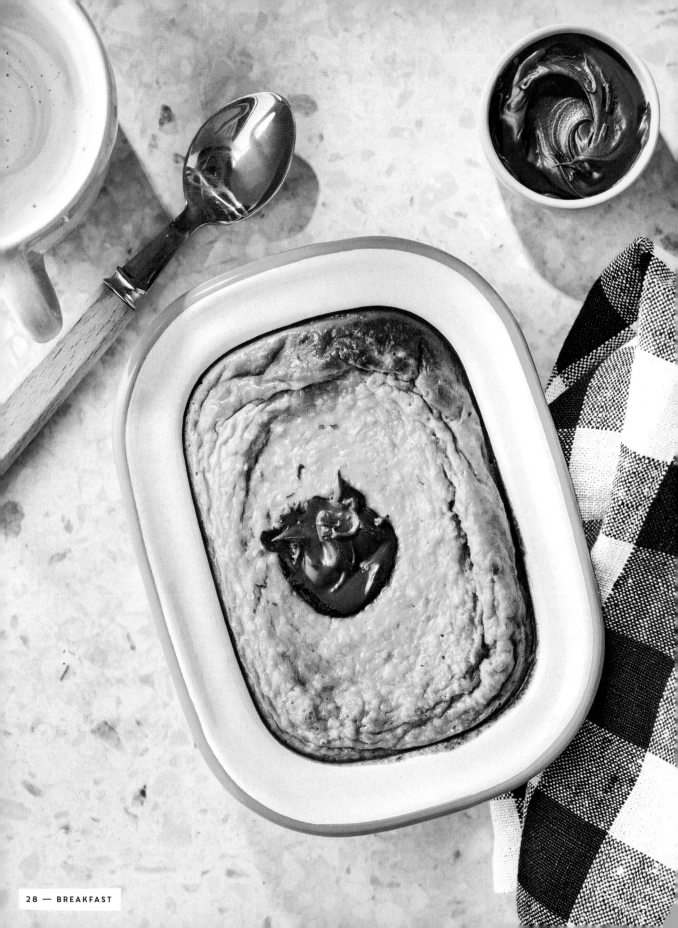

NUTELLA BAKED OATS

🕐 **5 MINS** 🍲 **35 MINS** ✗ **SERVES 1**

PER SERVING:
542 KCAL / 65G CARBS

SPECIAL EQUIPMENT
**Small ovenproof dish
(about 15cm/6in)**

40g rolled oats
175g fat-free natural yoghurt
1 tsp vanilla extract
3 tsp granulated sweetener
2 eggs
2 tsp Nutella

The perfect chocolatey treat, these baked oats feel much naughtier than they are, and they have a cake-like texture! Who wouldn't want cake for breakfast? You can also serve them as a dessert with a swirl of low-fat aerosol cream or with a dollop of your favourite yoghurt. Try making some up in advance, too: they freeze and reheat really well, which means they're fab for those busier mornings. If you want to scale it up to serve more people, adjust the cooking time as well as the ingredient quantities, and use a bigger dish.

Special Occasion

Preheat the oven to 200°C (fan 180°C/gas mark 6).

Mix the oats, yoghurt, vanilla, sweetener, eggs and just 1 teaspoon of the Nutella in a bowl until combined. Pour into an ovenproof dish and put the remaining Nutella in the centre. Bake in the oven for 30–35 minutes until set and golden. Remove from the oven and enjoy while it's warm, or leave it to cool, freeze and reheat when needed.

CHOCOLATE PANCAKES

🕐 **5 MINS***   🗑 **6 MINS**   ✕ **SERVES 2**

***PLUS 15 MINS RESTING TIME**

Use GF oats and baking powder ↗

V **GF**

PER SERVING:
289 KCAL / 34G CARBS

FOR THE PANCAKES
40g rolled porridge oats
2 medium eggs
75g fat-free Greek-style
  yoghurt
1 tbsp cocoa powder
½ tsp baking powder
1 tbsp granulated sweetener
  or sugar
low-calorie cooking spray

FOR THE TOPPING
100g strawberries, sliced
1 tsp granulated sweetener
  or sugar
75g fat-free Greek-style
  yoghurt
2 tsp low-calorie chocolate
  syrup

Chocolate for breakfast? Yes please! Mix it up with filling oats and fresh strawberries and you have a healthy breakfast that will set you up for the day ahead.

Weekly Indulgence

Sprinkle the strawberries with the teaspoon of sweetener or sugar and leave them to macerate while you prepare the pancakes.

Blitz the oats in a food processor until they resemble a coarse flour (alternatively you can use 40g of instant oat cereal). Beat the eggs and Greek-style yoghurt in a bowl until well combined.

Place the blitzed oats in a separate mixing bowl and stir in the cocoa powder, baking powder and sweetener or sugar. Make a well in the mixture and whisk in the egg and yoghurt mixture to produce a smooth batter. Cover the bowl and allow it to rest for 15 minutes.

Spray a large non-stick frying pan with low-calorie cooking spray and place over a medium-high heat. When the pan is hot, use half of the mixture to spoon three equal-sized amounts of mixture into the pan. After a minute and a half, small bubbles should have risen to the top of the pancakes and the top should be beginning to set. Using a fish slice or spatula, carefully flip the pancakes over and cook for another minute and a half.

When cooked, remove from the pan and cover to keep warm while you cook the remaining three pancakes.

Stack the pancakes onto two plates, divide the remaining yoghurt and the macerated strawberries between the plates, drizzle with the chocolate syrup and serve!

SWAP THIS: Raspberries make a great alternative to strawberries in this recipe. If you like, swap the Greek-style yoghurt for fat-free natural yoghurt.

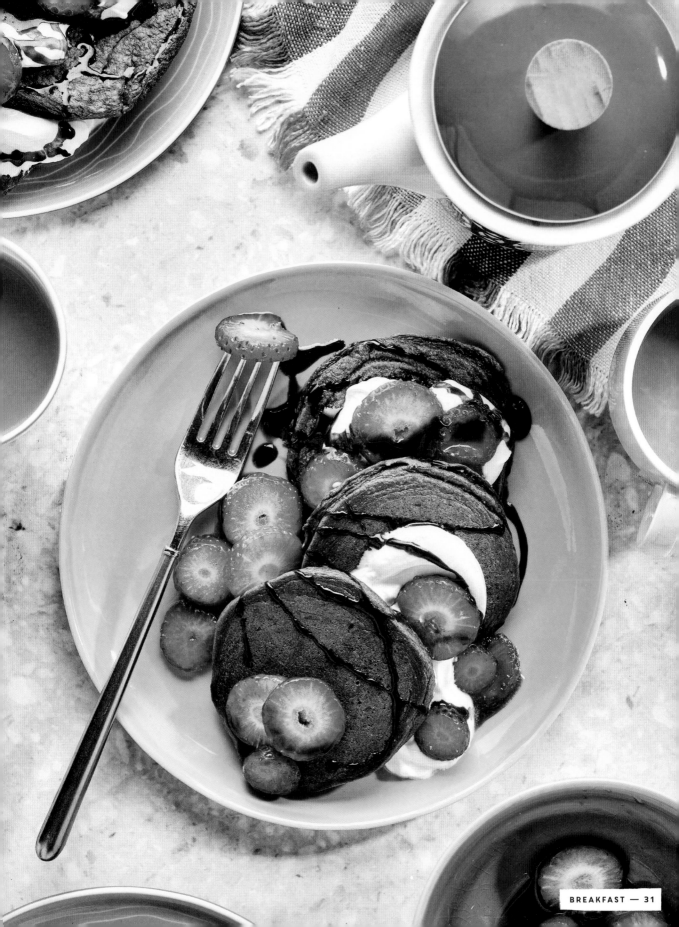

BREAKFAST CALZONES

🕐 **10 MINS**   📦 **VARIABLE** (SEE BELOW)   ✕ **SERVES 4**

PER SERVING:
173 KCAL / 19G CARBS

SPECIAL EQUIPMENT
Small ovenproof dish

low-calorie cooking spray
1 vegetarian sausage
2 low-calorie soft tortilla wraps
1 egg, beaten
½ x 410g tin baked beans
  (about 210g)
40g reduced-fat Cheddar
  (choose your favourite –
  we like to use mature),
  finely grated

TO ACCOMPANY *(optional)*
2 tbsp tomato ketchup
  (+ 15 kcal per tbsp)

TIP: Try not to overfill the calzones or they may be difficult to seal.

SWAP THIS: We've used veggie sausages in this dish, but you can use meat sausages or even bacon if you'd prefer – just remember to cook them first before adding them to the calzones!

If you're a fan of the popular cheese, sausage and bean melts from a certain well-known bakery, then this is the recipe for you! Baking the tortilla wraps in this way gives them the taste and texture of crispy pastry, but keeps the recipe low in calories, which means that you can enjoy them any day of the week.

Everyday Light _____

OVEN METHOD
🍽 **15 MINS**

Preheat the oven to 220°C (fan 200°C/gas mark 7).

Spray a frying pan with low-calorie cooking spray and place over a medium heat. Add the sausage and cook for 5 minutes, or until cooked through, then set aside.

Slice the tortilla wraps in half and brush some of the beaten egg over the wrap halves.

Cut the cooked sausage into small dice.

Spoon some of the baked beans and sausage pieces onto each half of the wrap. Sprinkle with a little grated cheese, leaving a 1cm (½in) gap around the edge, and repeat until all four halves are done.

Fold the wraps over to create four triangles and press down around the open sides. Crimp the edges using the back of a fork, then place on a baking tray sprayed with plenty of low-calorie cooking spray. Brush the top of the calzones with more beaten egg, and place in the oven to cook for 5 minutes, or until the tops are golden brown. Gently flip the calzones, brush with more beaten egg, and cook for a further 5 minutes or until golden brown and serve, with a dollop of ketchup if you like.

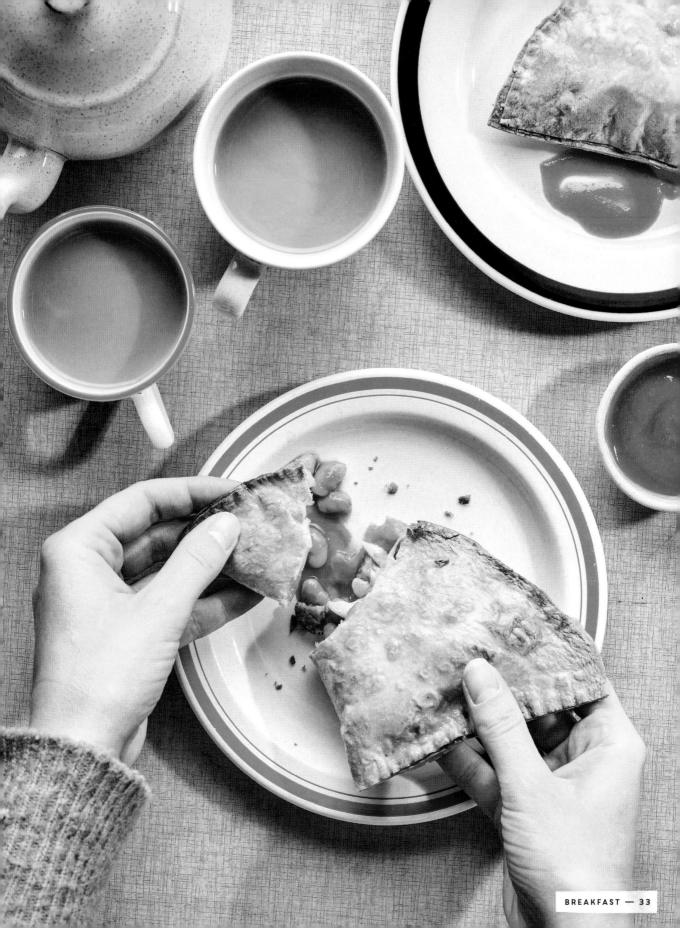

AIR-FRYER METHOD
🔥 13 MINS

SPECIAL EQUIPMENT
Air fryer

Preheat the air fryer to 180°C.

Spray a frying pan with low-calorie cooking spray and place over a medium heat. Add the sausage and cook for 5 minutes, or until cooked through, then set aside.

Slice the tortilla wraps in half and brush some of the beaten egg over the wrap halves.

Cut the cooked sausage into small dice.

Spoon some of the baked beans and sausage pieces onto each half of the wrap. Sprinkle with a little grated cheese, leaving a 1cm (½in) gap around the edge, and repeat until all four halves are done.

Fold the wraps over to create four triangles and press down around the open sides. Crimp the edges using the back of a fork, and brush the top of the calzones with more beaten egg. Place in the air fryer and cook for 5–8 minutes, flipping them halfway through cooking and brushing them with more beaten egg, until the tops are golden brown. Depending on the size and model of your air fryer you may need to cook them in batches.

"

"Thank you, Pinch of Nom, for motivating me with your delicious recipes."

—— VICKI

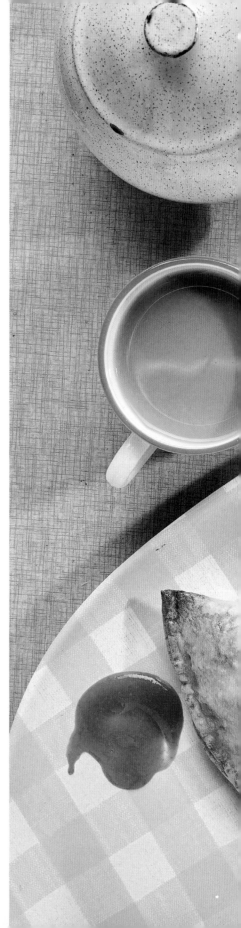

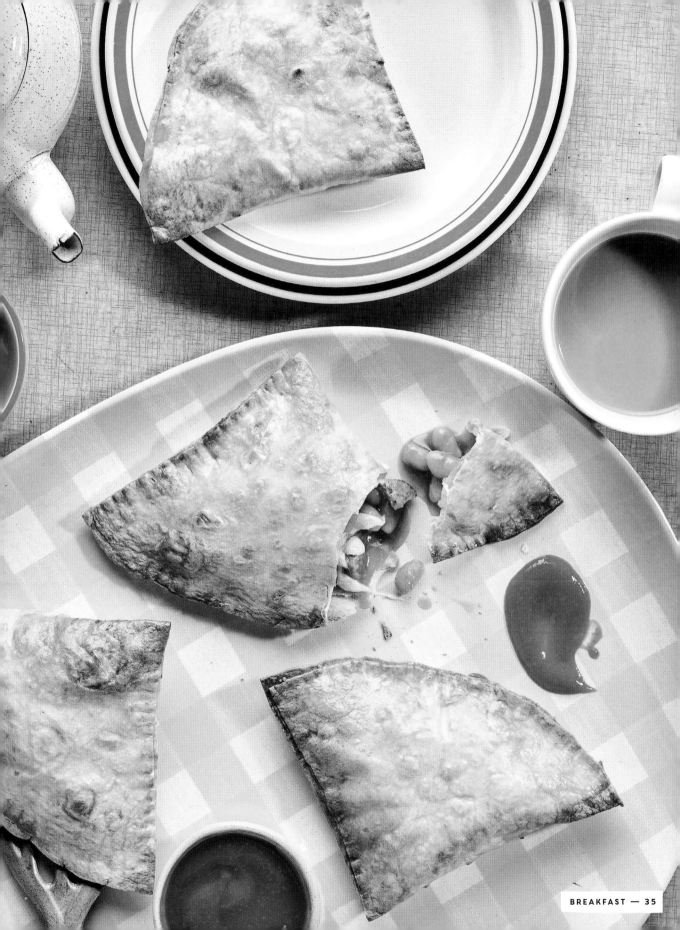

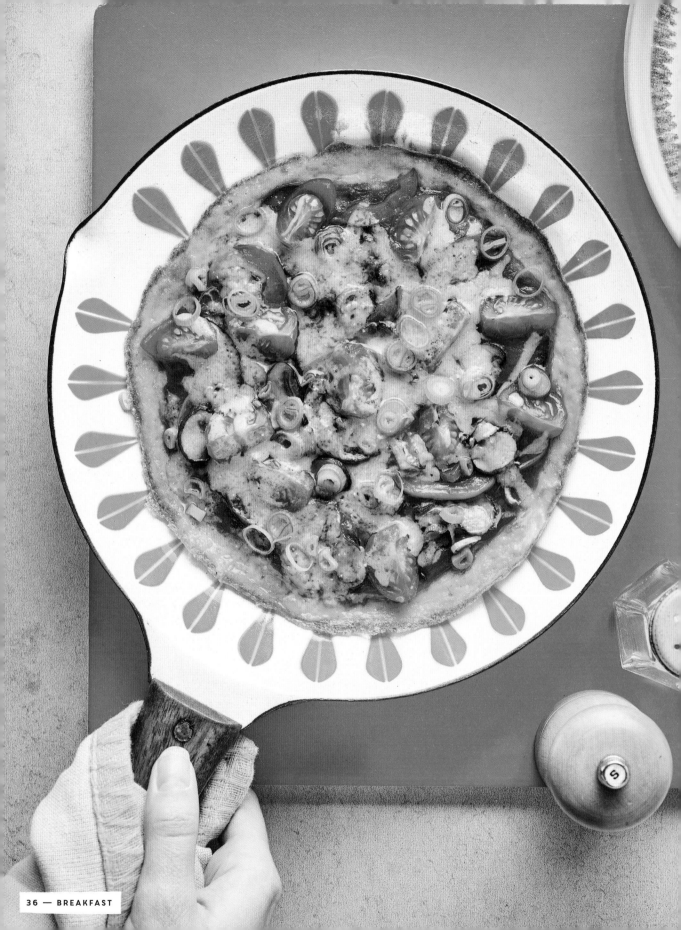

PIZZA-TOPPED OMELETTE

🕐 **5 MINS** 🍲 **10 MINS** ✕ **SERVES 1**

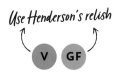

Use Henderson's relish

V GF

PER SERVING:
370 KCAL / 18G CARBS

1 tbsp tomato puree
2 tbsp passata
¼ tsp dried mixed herbs
¼ tsp garlic granules
¼ tsp Henderson's relish or
  Worcestershire sauce
low-calorie cooking spray
¼ pepper (about 40g) – we
  used a mixture of colours –
  deseeded and thinly sliced
4 mushrooms, thinly sliced
2 medium eggs
3 cherry tomatoes, quartered
30g reduced-fat mature
  Cheddar, finely grated
1 spring onion, trimmed
  and thinly sliced
sea salt and freshly ground
  black pepper

TIP: You can experiment with extra pizza toppings: why not try adding sweetcorn, sliced ham or pepperoni.

SWAP THIS: For a dairy-free pizza, swap the Cheddar for a dairy-free alternative.

Pizza for breakfast, anyone? Transform a simple omelette into your favourite pizza: use classic toppings like we have, or add in other veggies and whatever leftovers you have in the fridge. The only limit is your imagination! Prepped and cooked in less than 20 minutes, you can start your day with minimal effort and amazing taste and flavour.

Everyday Light

Combine the tomato puree, passata, dried mixed herbs, garlic granules and Henderson's relish or Worcestershire sauce in a small saucepan and heat over a low heat for 2 minutes.

Spray a frying pan with low-calorie cooking spray and set over a medium heat. Add the pepper and mushrooms and cook for 2 minutes until they are just starting to go soft, then remove from the pan and set to one side. Preheat the grill.

Whisk the eggs with 3 tablespoons of water in a mixing bowl or jug until combined, and season with salt and pepper. Spray the frying pan again and set back over a low-medium heat.

Pour the whisked eggs into the pan and swirl. Use a spatula to push the eggs around the pan, allowing the egg mixture to run into the gaps, and continue to move the eggs around the pan until there is no runny egg left and you have a solid omelette.

Add the tomato mixture to the top of the omelette and spread it out to cover the surface. Arrange the peppers, mushrooms and cherry tomatoes on top of the omelette base and top with the grated Cheddar. Place the pan under the preheated grill for 3 minutes until the cheese is bubbly and golden. Remove from the grill, sprinkle the spring onion on top and serve.

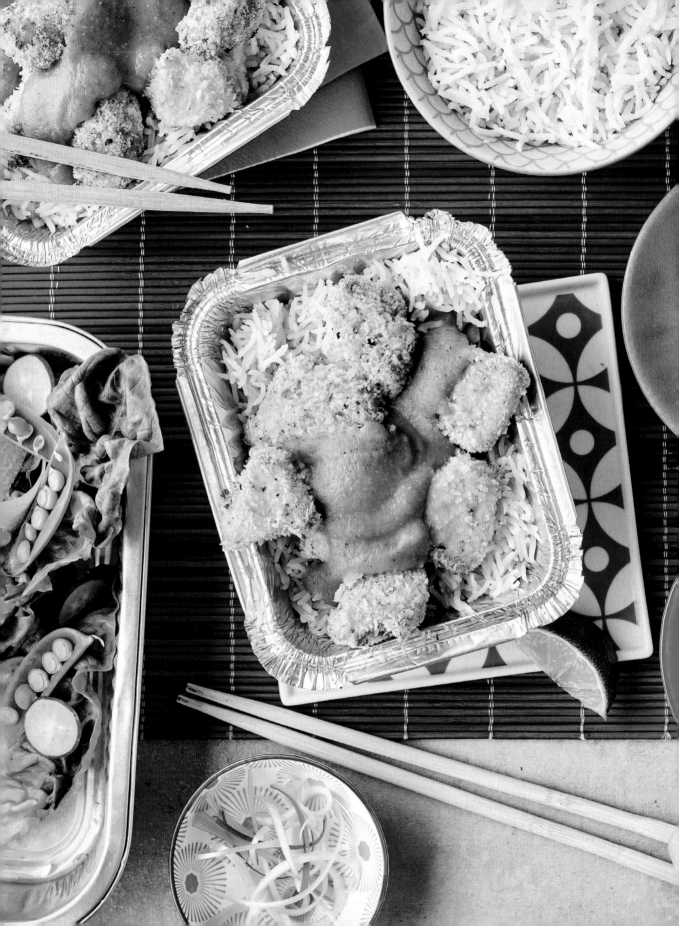

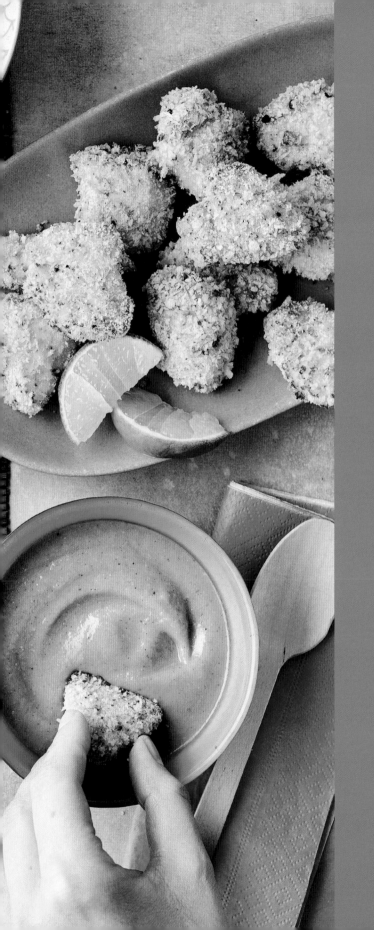

FAKEAWAYS

VODKA PASTA

🕐 **10 MINS**   🗑 **18 MINS**   ✕ **SERVES 4**

PER SERVING:
512 KCAL / 84G CARBS

400g dried fusilli pasta (or
   pasta of your choice)
low-calorie cooking spray
2 onions, peeled and finely
   chopped
4 garlic cloves, peeled
   and crushed
¼ tsp dried chilli flakes
1 tsp Italian mixed herbs
2 tbsp tomato puree
50ml vodka
1 x 400g tin chopped tomatoes
200ml vegetable stock
   (1 vegetable stock cube
   dissolved in 200ml
   boiling water)
120g low-fat cream cheese
a few basil leaves, to garnish

We tried this dish for the first time on a trip to Canada and couldn't believe there was vodka in it! The vodka increases the depth of flavour without adding a strong taste; it also mellows the acidity of the tomatoes for a perfectly balanced pasta dish. It's best to pick a good bottle of vodka – after all, someone will be drinking the rest!

Special Occasion

Cook the pasta according to the packet instructions, then drain it well.

While the pasta is cooking, spray a frying pan with low-calorie cooking spray and place over a medium heat. Add the onions and sauté for 5 minutes until they have started to soften, then stir in the garlic, chilli flakes and Italian mixed herbs and cook for a further 5 minutes. Add the tomato puree and vodka, stir and cook for a further 3 minutes.

Add the chopped tomatoes, vegetable stock and cream cheese, stir, reduce the heat and simmer for 5 minutes – the mixture should still be bubbling.

Remove the sauce from the heat and mix the pasta into the sauce. Serve, scattered with basil leaves, and enjoy!

TIP: Before you serve, you can sprinkle with grated cheese if you wish, but please remember to count the additional calories.

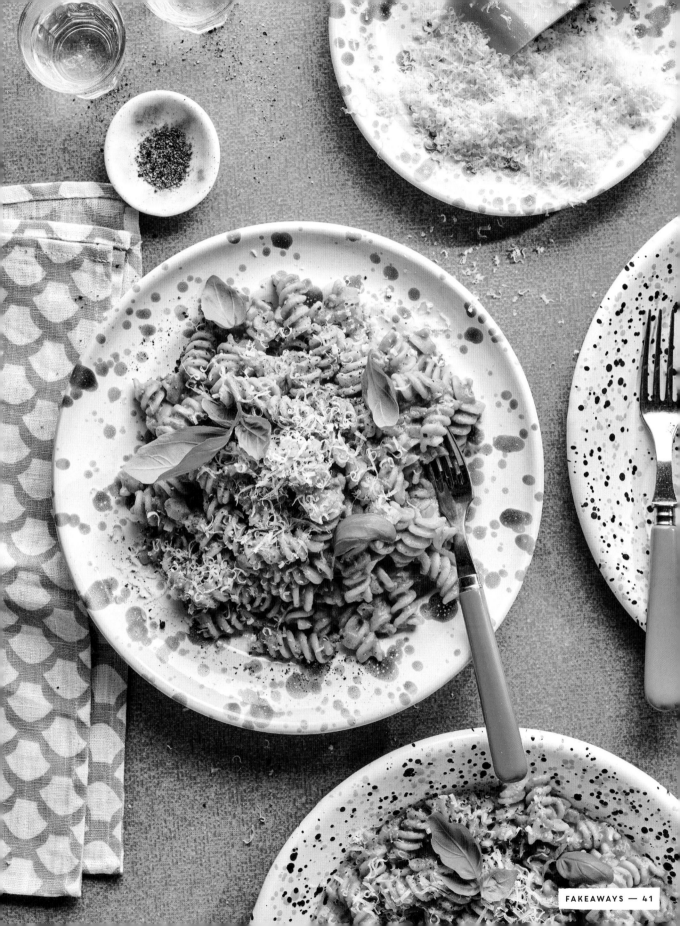

HALLOUMI COUSCOUS BURGERS *with* SALSA

🕐 **15 MINS**   🍲 **15 MINS**   ✕ **SERVES 4**

PER SERVING:
401 KCAL / 57G CARBS

150g dried couscous
1 carrot, peeled and finely grated
130ml boiling vegetable stock
   (1 very low-salt vegetable
   stock cube dissolved in
   130ml boiling water)
low-calorie cooking spray
90g reduced-fat halloumi, cut
   into 1cm (½in)-thick slices
2 tbsp chopped fresh mint
2 medium eggs

FOR THE SALSA
1 small red onion, peeled
   and finely diced
2 large tomatoes, finely diced
1 red chilli, deseeded and
   finely diced
2 tbsp chopped fresh coriander
½ tsp salt
1 tsp apple cider vinegar or
   white wine vinegar

TO ACCOMPANY *(optional)*
75g mixed salad (+ 15 kcal
   per serving) and 50g
   gluten-free ciabatta rolls
   (+ 110 kcal per roll)

Who says the best burgers at a BBQ have to be meat? These veggie-friendly patties are so easy to make and can elevate burger night to the next level! They're crispy on the outside and fluffy and cheesy on the inside, and served with a refreshingly zingy salsa. Enjoy in a bun or flatbread, with 2 tablespoons of fat-free Greek-style yoghurt (if you like), alongside a mixed green salad for a taste of summer any time of the year!

Weekly Indulgence

Put the couscous and carrot in a large bowl. Pour over the boiling stock, stir, cover and leave to sit for 15 minutes.

Meanwhile, spray a frying pan with low-calorie cooking spray and place over a high heat. Add the halloumi slices and cook the cheese for 3 minutes on each side until golden. Remove from the pan, cut into 1cm (½in) dice and set aside.

Now make the salsa. Put all the salsa ingredients in a bowl and leave to one side for the flavours to develop.

Uncover the couscous and fluff it up with a fork, then add the halloumi, mint and eggs. Mix well and form into four burgers.

Spray the frying pan with low-calorie cooking spray again and, over a low heat, fry the burgers for about 7 minutes on each side until golden.

Serve with your choice of accompaniment.

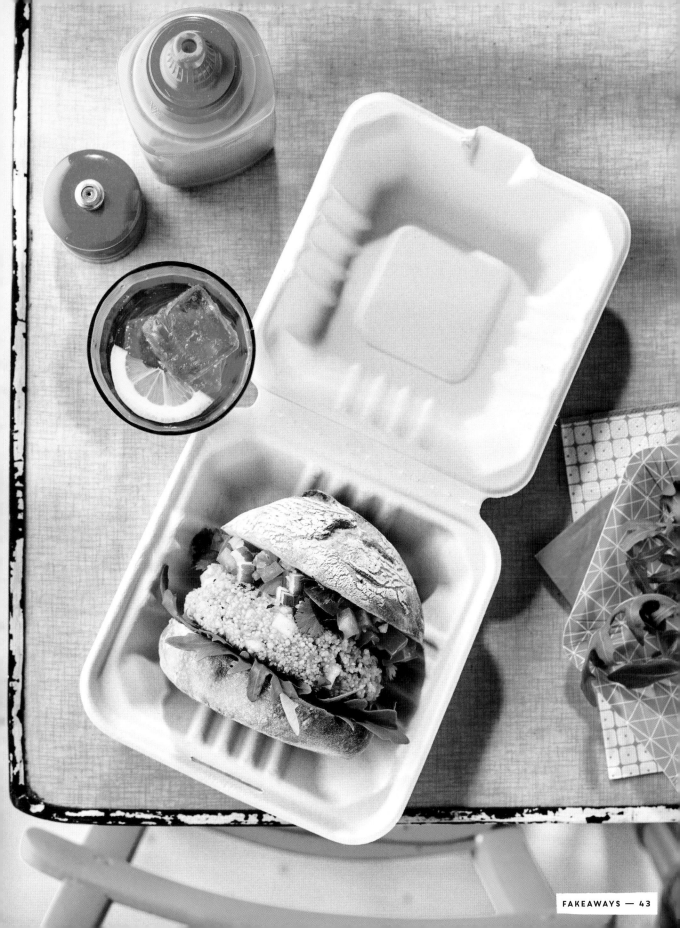

OVEN-BAKED PASANDA CURRY

🕐 **5 MINS**   🍲 **45 MINS**   ✕ **SERVES 4**

Use GF stock pot ↴

PER SERVING:
191 KCAL / 4G CARBS

500g diced chicken breast
1 tsp mild curry powder
1 tsp ground coriander
½ tsp ground cumin
½ tsp granulated sweetener
2 tbsp ground almonds
120g red onion, peeled and
   thinly sliced
250ml chicken stock (1 chicken
   stock pot dissolved in
   250ml boiling water)
2 tbsp low-fat cream cheese
1 tbsp flaked almonds

TO ACCOMPANY *(optional)*
50g uncooked basmati rice,
   per portion, cooked
   according to packet
   instructions (+ 173 kcal per
   125g cooked serving)

Pasanda curry is one of our favourite Indian dishes, and our slimming version is a one-pot recipe so you won't need to worry about heaps of washing up! You can use whichever light cream cheese you have on hand for this dish, and serve it with freshly boiled rice and extra veggies for a tasty, fuss-free fakeaway!

Everyday Light

Preheat the oven to 200°C (fan 180°C/gas mark 6).

Put the chicken, spices, sweetener and ground almonds in an ovenproof dish and mix to ensure the chicken is coated evenly in the spices and almonds. Scatter over the sliced onion, pour over the stock and bake in the preheated oven for 40 minutes.

Remove from the oven and carefully stir in the cream cheese. Sprinkle the flaked almonds over the top and pop back in the oven for another 5 minutes, until the almonds have started to become golden.

Remove from the oven and leave to stand for 5 minutes. Serve with your choice of accompaniment.

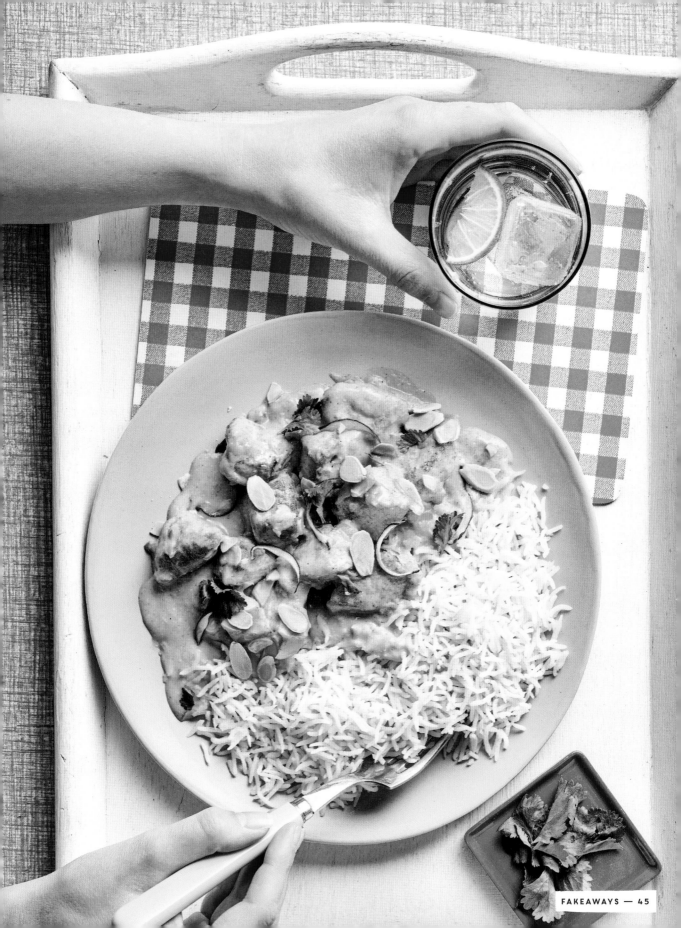

CREAMY LEMON CHICKEN

🕐 **5 MINS**   🍲 **35 MINS**   ✕ **SERVES 4**

Use GF stock cube ↘

 F **LC** **GF**

PER SERVING:
192 KCAL / 2.3G CARBS

low-calorie cooking spray
4 skinless chicken breasts,
   about 150g each
1 small onion, peeled and
   finely chopped
300ml chicken stock (1 chicken
   stock cube dissolved in
   300ml boiling water)
juice of ½ lemon
75g low-fat cream cheese
50g spinach
freshly ground black pepper

If you're craving something creamy, rich and ready on the table within 40 minutes, then this recipe is just what you're looking for! Instead of high-calorie double cream, we've used low-fat cream cheese. You get the same delicious indulgent flavour, but you won't believe the calorie saving. Spinach adds an extra vitamin boost and a burst of colour, so this dinner looks just as good as it tastes!

Everyday Light ──────────────────────

Spray a frying pan with low-calorie cooking spray and place over a medium heat. When the pan is hot, add the chicken breasts and cook for 2 minutes each side to seal and colour. Transfer to a plate and set to one side.

Give the pan another spray with low-calorie cooking spray then add the onion and sauté for 5 minutes until soft. Pour in the stock and lemon juice and bring to a simmer, then stir in the low-fat cream cheese and return the chicken to the pan. Simmer for 10–15 minutes, stirring occasionally until the chicken is cooked through.

The sauce should have reduced and thickened slightly, but if it is too runny turn up the heat and allow it to bubble until it has the consistency of single cream. Stir in the spinach and cook for a couple more minutes until it has wilted.

Season with a little black pepper and serve with your choice of accompaniment.

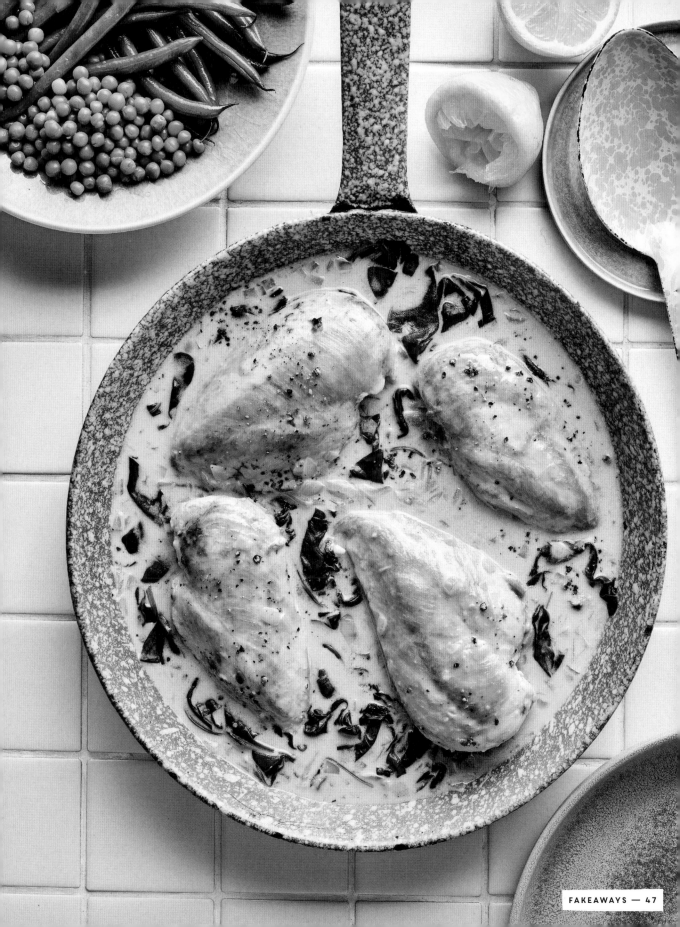

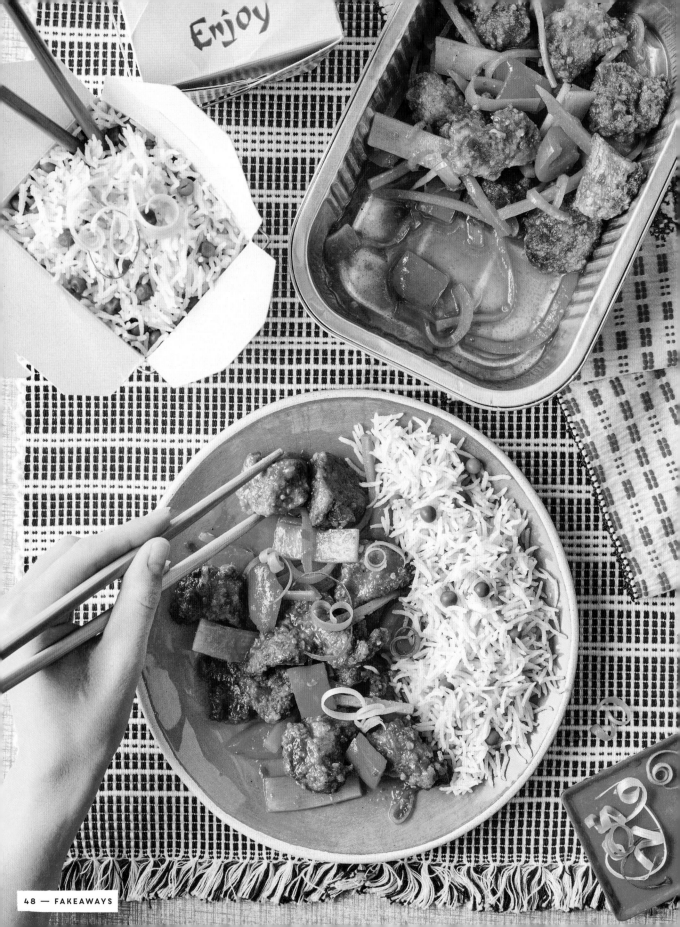

KUNG PAO PORK

⏲ **10 MINS**   🍲 **35 MINS**   ✕ **SERVES 4**

Use GF soy sauce ↗

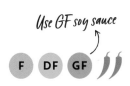

(F) (DF) (GF) 〞

PER SERVING:
298 KCAL / 38G CARBS

400g lean diced pork
2 tbsp cornflour
1 tsp Chinese 5-spice
1 tsp toasted sesame oil
2 spring onions, trimmed and
   thinly sliced, to garnish

FOR THE SAUCE
low-calorie cooking spray
60g onion, peeled and
   thinly sliced
160g red pepper, deseeded
   and cut into 2cm (¾in) dice
60g carrot, peeled and cut
   into 3mm-thick batons
2 garlic cloves, peeled
   and crushed
1 x 225g tin bamboo
   shoots, drained
1 tbsp light or dark brown sugar
3 tbsp granulated sweetener
60ml cider vinegar
1 tbsp runny honey
2 tsp dried chilli flakes
2 tbsp tomato puree
1 tbsp dark soy sauce

TO ACCOMPANY *(optional)*
50g uncooked basmati rice
   per portion, cooked
   according to packet
   instructions (+ 173 kcal per
   125g cooked serving)

This Chinese-inspired dish has the perfect balance of sweetness, saltiness and spice: it's one of our favourite takeaway options so we had to add a Nom twist! We've used baked pork instead of fried, and a few clever ingredient swaps to create a dish that's low on calories without sacrificing flavour – and it's ready to eat faster than the takeaway could deliver!

Weekly Indulgence

Preheat the oven to 200°C (fan 180°C/gas mark 6) and line a baking tray with baking parchment.

Place the pork, cornflour, Chinese 5-spice and sesame oil in a sandwich bag and shake until the pork is completely coated in the cornflour mix. Spread the coated pork out on the lined baking tray and bake in the oven for 35 minutes, turning the pieces of pork after 20 minutes.

While the pork is cooking, make the sauce. Spray a frying pan with a little low-calorie cooking spray and place over a low heat. Add the onion, red pepper and carrot and sauté for 6–7 minutes until they start to soften, then add the garlic and bamboo shoots and cook for a further 2 minutes, stirring frequently. Add all of the remaining sauce ingredients, mix well to combine and simmer over a low heat for 10–15 minutes until the sauce has thickened and reduced.

Once the pork has cooked and is crisp and golden, add it to the sauce and stir. Serve immediately with your choice of accompaniment, and garnish with the sliced spring onions.

TIPS: Don't worry if you can't find bamboo shoots – swap them for a sliced pepper, for crunch. Add a handful of cooked peas to the cooked rice, if you like.

SWEET *and* SPICY MEATBALLS

🕐 **15 MINS**   🍲 **20 MINS**   ✕ **SERVES 4**

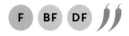

PER SERVING:
315 KCAL / 28G CARBS

low-calorie cooking spray
1 spring onion, trimmed and
  thinly sliced, to serve

FOR THE MEATBALLS
500g 5%-fat minced pork
½ tsp garlic granules
½ tsp onion granules
½ tsp ground ginger
¼ tsp salt
½ tsp freshly ground black pepper
1 medium egg, beaten

FOR THE SAUCE
½ red pepper, deseeded and diced
½ green pepper, deseeded
  and diced
2 garlic cloves, peeled and crushed
5cm (2in) piece of root ginger,
  peeled and finely grated
½ tsp garlic granules
1 tsp ground ginger
3 tbsp rice vinegar
3 tbsp low-sodium light soy sauce
3 tbsp hoisin sauce
3 tbsp honey
3 tbsp orange juice
2 tbsp reduced-sugar ketchup
2 tbsp sriracha sauce
1 tsp chilli powder

TO ACCOMPANY *(optional)*
50g uncooked basmati rice per
  portion, cooked according to
  packet instructions (+ 173 kcal
  per 125g cooked serving)

These Sweet and Spicy Meatballs are made using 5%-fat pork mince and served in a deliciously sticky sauce. At first glance, this recipe might seem like it has a lot of ingredients but we promise it's worth it, as all of the spices and sauces combine perfectly to create a dish that's ideal for a Friday night fakeaway! This is a moderately spicy recipe, but if you like your food hotter then just add an extra tablespoon of sriracha sauce or teaspoon of chilli powder.

Weekly Indulgence ————————

Preheat the oven to 200°C (fan 180°C/gas mark 6) and spray a baking tray with low-calorie cooking spray.

Combine the meatball ingredients in a mixing bowl, then take small amounts of the mixture in your hands and roll into twenty even-sized meatballs. Place the balls on the greased baking tray and bake in the oven for 15 minutes until they are slightly browned.

While the meatballs are cooking, spray a frying pan with low-calorie cooking spray and place over a medium heat. Add the diced peppers and cook for 3 minutes until they begin to soften, then add the fresh garlic and ginger and cook for a further 2 minutes.

Combine the rest of the sauce ingredients in a small bowl and add to the pan with the peppers. Reduce the heat to low and simmer for 5 minutes until the sauce is starting to thicken. Add the baked meatballs to the pan and continue to heat for 5 minutes until the sauce is thickened and the meatballs are coated.

Serve sprinkled with sliced spring onion and your choice of accompaniment.

SWAP THIS: Swap the pork mince for beef, turkey or chicken mince.

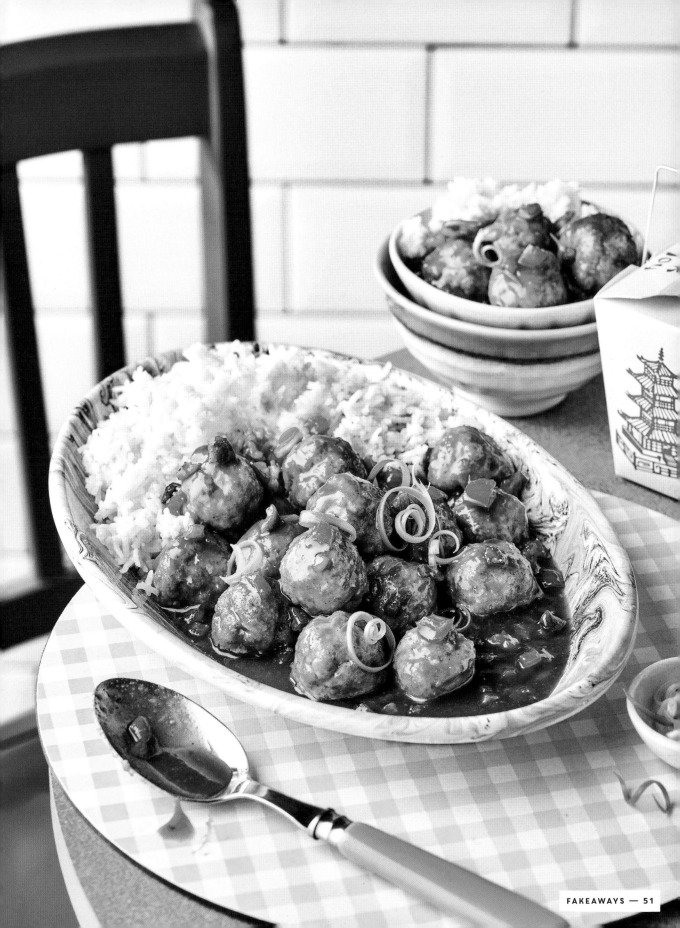

MARGHERITA CHICKEN

🕐 **5 MINS**　　🍲 **45 MINS**　　✕ **SERVES 4**

Use GF stock cube ↗

F　**LC**　**GF**

PER SERVING:
241 KCAL / 6.1G CARBS

SPECIAL EQUIPMENT
Oblong ovenproof dish about 24 x 20 x 5cm (9½ x 8 x 2in)

low-calorie cooking spray
1 small onion, peeled and
　finely diced
1 x 400g tin chopped tomatoes
1 tsp garlic granules
200ml chicken stock
　(1 chicken stock cube
　dissolved in 200ml
　boiling water)
4 skinless chicken breasts
　(visible fat removed),
　about 150g each
handful of fresh basil leaves,
　roughly chopped, and a few
　extra leaves to garnish
140g reduced-fat mozzarella
freshly ground black pepper

Sometimes the simple things in life are the best! This Margherita Chicken is the perfect flavour combo of basil and tomato, topped with delicious, melty mozzarella cheese. We've taken all of the flavours of a classic Margherita pizza, but instead of dough we've loaded the toppings onto tender, succulent chicken. It's perfect for those days when you're craving pizza but prefer something a little lighter.

Everyday Light

Preheat the oven to 200°C (fan 180°C/gas mark 6).

Spray a saucepan with low-calorie cooking spray and place over a medium-high heat. Add the onion and sauté for 5–6 minutes until golden brown, then add the tinned tomatoes, garlic granules and stock, stir and bring to the boil. Reduce the heat and simmer for 15 minutes.

While the Margherita sauce simmers, spray a non-stick frying pan with low-calorie cooking spray and place over a medium-high heat. Add the chicken breasts and seal for about 2 minutes each side, until golden, then arrange them in the ovenproof dish.

After the sauce has been simmering for 15 minutes, stir in the chopped basil and season with pepper. Spoon the sauce over the chicken breasts in the ovenproof dish. Tear the mozzarella into pieces and scatter it over the top, then bake in the preheated oven for 25 minutes, until the chicken is cooked through and the cheese is melted and golden.

Remove from the oven, scatter a few basil leaves on top and serve with your choice of accompaniment.

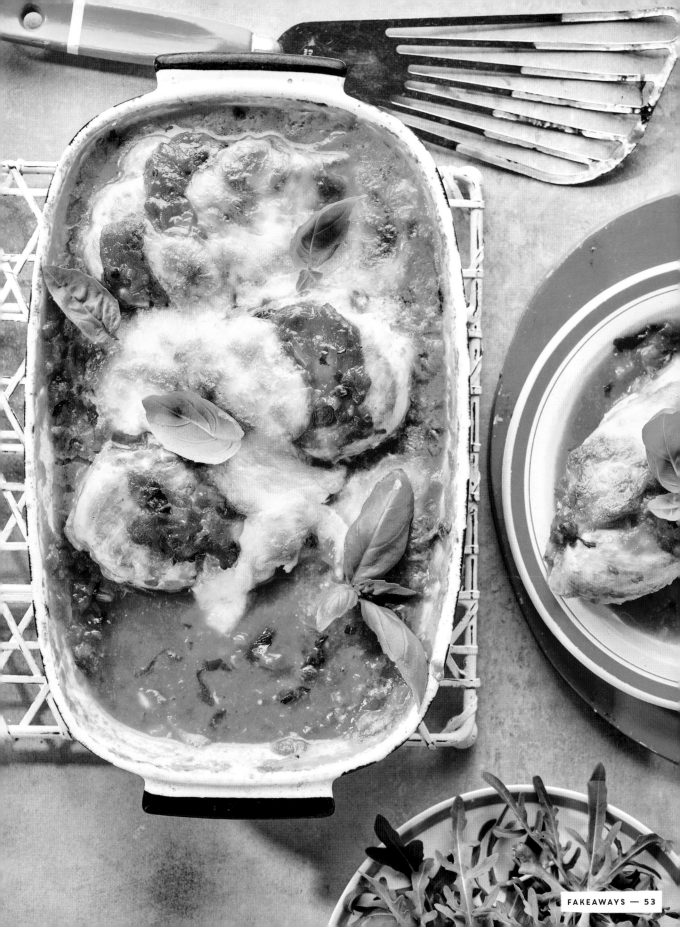

PEANUT BUTTER CHICKEN CURRY

🕐 **10 MINS**   🍲 **VARIABLE** (SEE BELOW)   ✕ **SERVES 4**

Use GF soy sauce and Henderson's relish

  (F) (DF) (GF) 🌶

PER SERVING:
342 KCAL / 18G CARBS

low-calorie cooking spray
600g skinless chicken breasts (visible fat removed), cut into 3cm (1¼in) chunks
2 garlic cloves, peeled and crushed
5cm (2in) piece of root ginger, peeled and finely grated
1 tsp garam masala
1 tsp turmeric
½ tsp ground cumin
300ml coconut dairy-free milk alternative
1 tbsp tomato puree
1 tsp sriracha sauce
1 tbsp light soy sauce
1 x 400g tin chopped tomatoes
1 medium carrot, peeled and finely diced
4 tbsp peanut butter powder
1 tbsp Henderson's relish or Worcestershire sauce
100g courgette, diced
100g spinach, washed
juice of 1 lime

TO ACCOMPANY *(optional)*
50g uncooked basmati rice per portion, cooked according to packet instructions (+ 173 kcal per 125g cooked serving)

We guarantee this will be a new family favourite! It's really easy to make and uses a lot of ingredients you will already have in your cupboards and is all cooked in one pot so there's less washing up, which is a win for us! It has a rich and creamy sauce with a lovely nutty flavour and is a really comforting and low-calorie alternative to ringing for a takeaway.

Special Occasion

HOB-TOP METHOD
🍲 **45 MINS**

Spray a frying pan with low-calorie cooking spray and place over a medium heat. Add the chicken and brown on all sides for 4 minutes, then add the garlic and ginger and fry for a further minute. Stir all the spices into the pan and cook for 1 minute, then add the coconut milk drink, tomato puree, sriracha sauce, soy sauce, chopped tomatoes and carrot.

In a small bowl, combine the peanut butter powder with 3 tablespoons of water and stir until smooth. Add to the pan with the Henderson's relish or Worcestershire sauce, give everything a good stir and allow to come to a rapid bubble. Reduce the heat to a simmer – you should see it still bubbling slowly. Cook for 20 minutes, then add in the diced courgette and spinach and cook for a further 15 minutes.

Remove from the heat, stir through the lime juice and serve with your choice of accompaniment.

SLOW-COOKER METHOD
🍲 **HIGH: 3 HOURS 5 MINS**

SPECIAL EQUIPMENT
Slow cooker

Spray a frying pan with low-calorie cooking spray and place over a medium heat. Add the chicken and brown on all sides for 4 minutes, then add the garlic and ginger and fry for a further minute.

Add the contents of the pan to the slow cooker along with all of the spices, the coconut milk drink, tomato puree, sriracha sauce, soy sauce, chopped tomatoes and carrot. In a small bowl, combine the peanut butter powder with 3 tablespoons of water and stir until smooth. Add to the slow cooker with the Henderson's relish or Worcestershire sauce and give everything a good stir.

Set the slow cooker to high and cook for 2½ hours.

After 2½ hours, add the courgette and spinach to the cooker and cook for a further 30 minutes. Stir through the lime juice and serve with rice or your choice of accompaniment.

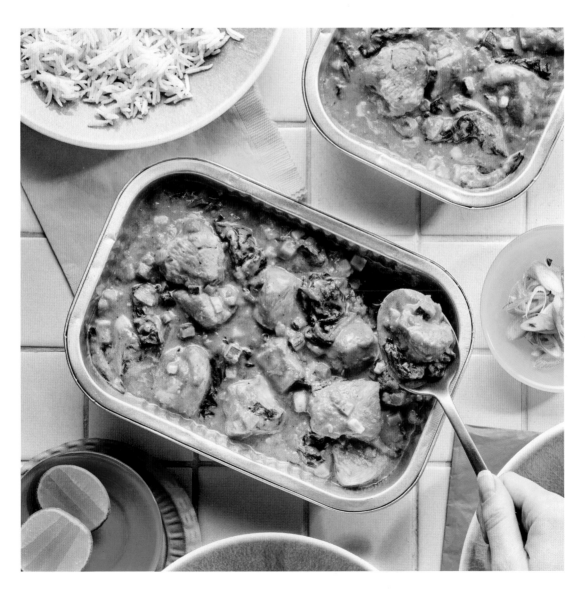

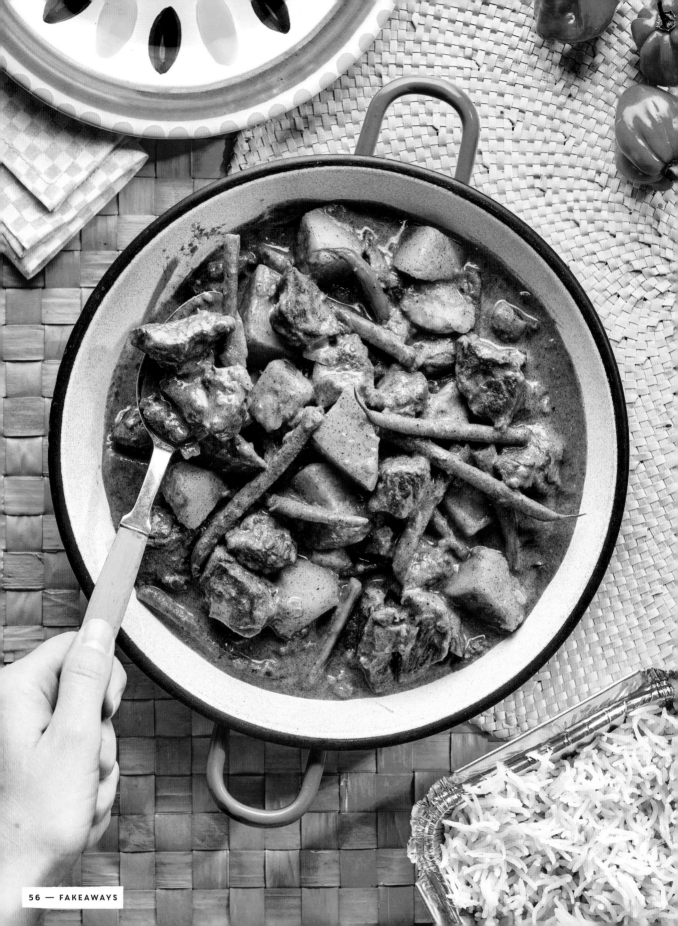

CARIBBEAN LAMB CURRY

Use GF stock cube and Henderson's relish

🕐 **15 MINS**   🍲 **VARIABLE** (SEE BELOW)   ✕ **SERVES 4**

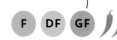 (F) (DF) (GF) "

PER SERVING:
321 KCAL / 25G CARBS

low-calorie cooking spray
400g lean, diced leg of lamb
2 onions, peeled and diced
2 garlic cloves, peeled
  and crushed
1 red chilli, deseeded and
  finely chopped
4 tsp garam masala
1 tsp ground allspice
500ml chicken stock
  (1 chicken stock cube
  dissolved in 500ml
  boiling water)
1 x 200ml tin light coconut milk
350g potatoes, peeled and cut
  into 2.5cm (1in) dice
  (prepared weight)
100g fine green beans,
  cut in half
2 tbsp Henderson's relish or
  Worcestershire sauce
sea salt and freshly ground
  black pepper

TO ACCOMPANY
50g uncooked basmati rice
  per portion, cooked
  according to packet
  instructions (+ 173 kcal per
  125g cooked serving)

This Caribbean Lamb Curry is inspired by the goat curries that are a staple in Jamaica. We've swapped the goat out for more readily available lamb, cooked it low and slow so that it melts in the mouth, and added some green beans for extra veggie goodness. This is quite a spicy dish but you can easily adjust it to suit your spice preference. If you like your food milder, you can omit the chilli, or if you love a really fiery kick then simply leave the chilli seeds in – or even add an entire extra chilli if you want!

Weekly Indulgence

HOB-TOP METHOD
🍲 **2 HOURS 40 MINS**

Spray a large heavy-based saucepan with low-calorie cooking spray and place over a medium-high heat. When the pan is hot, add the lamb and onions and cook for 5–10 minutes until the meat is sealed and the onions have begun to soften. Add the garlic, chilli and spices and cook for a further minute until fragrant. Add the stock and coconut milk and bring to the boil. Reduce the heat to low and cover with a tight-fitting lid. Allow to gently cook for 1 hour.

Remove the lid after 1 hour, add the potatoes but do not replace the lid. Continue to simmer for another hour, checking occasionally to make sure it doesn't dry out (if it does, add a little extra water).

Stir in the fine green beans and Henderson's relish or Worcestershire sauce and simmer for another 30 minutes until the green beans are cooked and the sauce is thick and glossy.

Taste and season with salt and pepper to taste, if required.

Serve!

SWAP THIS: Swap the lamb for diced stewing beef if you prefer.

SLOW-COOKER METHOD
🍲 LOW: 7 HOURS

SPECIAL EQUIPMENT
Slow cooker

Spray a large frying pan with low-calorie cooking spray and place over a medium-high heat. When the pan is hot, add the lamb and onions and cook for 5–10 minutes until the meat is sealed. Add the garlic, chilli and spices and cook for a minute or two until fragrant, then place in the slow-cooker bowl along with all the ingredients apart from the green beans and Henderson's relish or Worcestershire sauce.

Cook on low for 6–7 hours. Half an hour before serving, stir in the Henderson's relish or Worcestershire sauce and green beans. Replace the lid.

When the green beans are cooked, taste and season with salt and pepper if required. Serve!

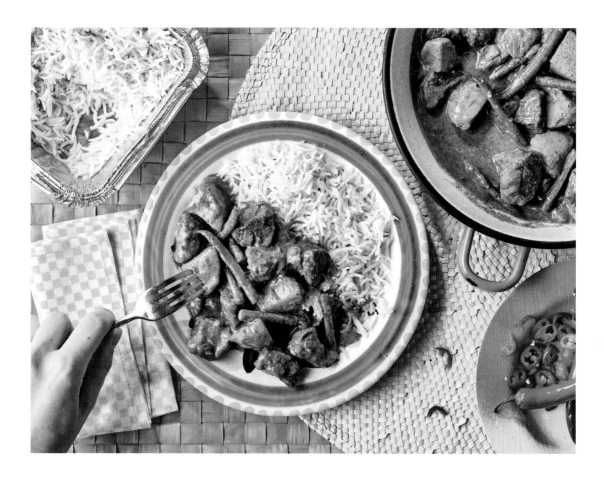

SCRUNCHILADAS

Use GF wraps, stock cube and Henderson's relish

🕐 **15 MINS**   🍲 **VARIABLE** (SEE BELOW)   ✕ **SERVES 6**

(F) (GF)

PER SERVING:
318 KCAL / 36G CARBS

FOR THE SEASONING
1 tsp garlic granules or powder
1 tsp sweet smoked paprika
1 tsp dried oregano
1 tsp ground coriander
½ tsp salt
pinch of freshly ground
  black pepper
pinch of dried chilli flakes

FOR THE SCRUNCHILADAS
400g skinless, boneless
  chicken thighs (visible
  fat removed), cut into
  bite-size chunks
low-calorie cooking spray
2 onions, peeled and sliced
1 tbsp Worcestershire sauce
  or Henderson's relish
1 x 400g tin chopped tomatoes
1 very low-salt chicken stock
  cube, crumbled
2 tbsp buffalo hot sauce
2 tbsp BBQ sauce
2 peppers (any colour),
  deseeded and sliced
1 x 400g tin kidney beans,
  drained and rinsed
5 low-calorie soft tortilla wraps
40g reduced-fat Cheddar,
  grated
40g reduced-fat mozzarella,
  grated

TO ACCOMPANY *(optional)*
75g mixed salad (+ 15 kcal
  per serving)

Life's too short to spend ages trying to roll the perfect taco, or enchilada, so why not scrunch instead? Focus on the fillings without the faff by loading up soft tortilla wraps, and finish by topping with melty cheese! You don't need to be too neat as that's part of the fun!

Everyday Light

HOB-TOP METHOD
🍲 **35 MINS**

Preheat the oven to 200°C (fan 180°C/gas mark 6).

Combine the seasoning ingredients in a large bowl, put the chicken in the bowl and gently toss it in the seasoning, making sure it is fully coated. Spray a large frying pan with low-calorie cooking spray and place over a medium heat. Add the onions and fry for 4 minutes until they start to colour, then add the seasoned chicken and fry for 3–5 minutes – the chicken will start to catch a little, which is fine, but don't let it burn.

Add the Worcestershire sauce or Henderson's relish and 1 tablespoon of water and scrape the bottom of the pan with a wooden spoon to lift the caught bits. Add the chopped tomatoes, stock cube, buffalo hot sauce and BBQ sauce and give everything a good stir. Reduce the heat and simmer for 10 minutes, stirring often.

Add the sliced peppers and the kidney beans and simmer for a further 5 minutes, then check that the chicken is cooked throughout and all pinkness has gone. Remove the pan from the heat and set aside.

Pour half the sauce into the bottom of an ovenproof dish. Take a wrap and scrunch it in up in your hands until you get a scrunched pasty shape. Place it widthways on top of the sauce. Do the same with all of the wraps until the sauce is completely covered. Pour the rest of the sauce over the wraps and sprinkle over the grated Cheddar and mozzarella. Place in the preheated oven and cook for 10 minutes until the cheese has melted.

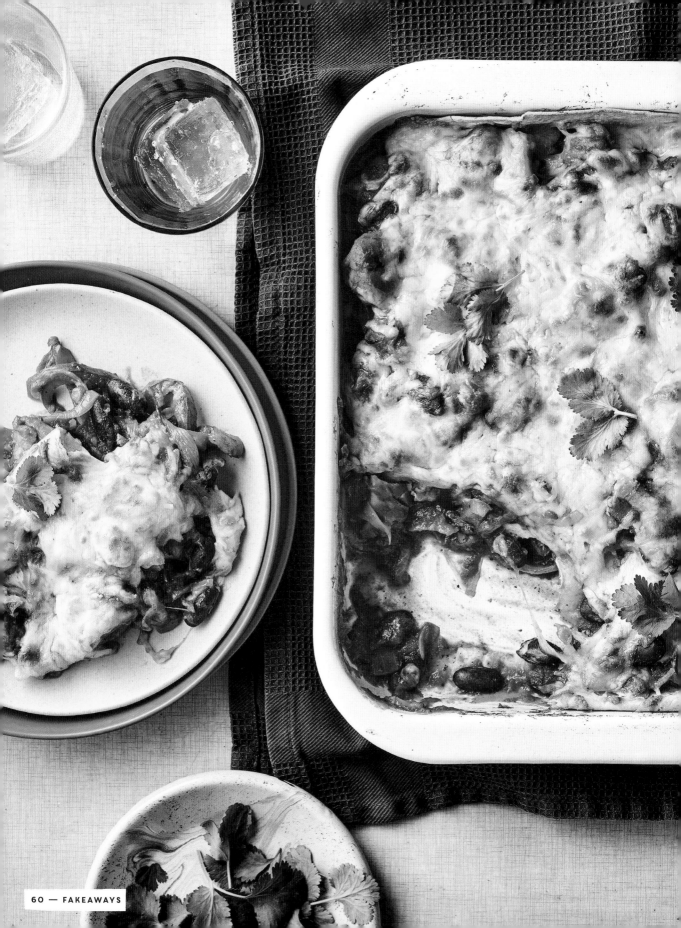

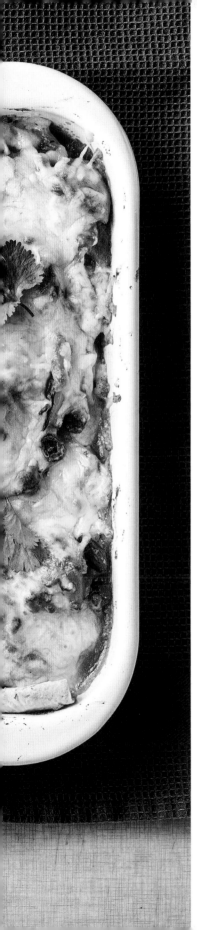

SLOW-COOKER METHOD
🍲 **HIGH: 4 HOURS LOW: 6 HOURS**

SPECIAL EQUIPMENT
Slow cooker

Combine the seasoning ingredients in a large bowl, put the chicken in the bowl and gently toss it in the seasoning, making sure it is fully coated.

Transfer the chicken to the slow cooker and add the onions, peppers, chopped tomatoes and kidney beans.

Add the stock cube, BBQ sauce, buffalo hot sauce, Worcestershire sauce or Henderson's relish and 1 tablespoon of water. Cover with the lid and cook on high for 4 hours or on low for 6 hours.

Preheat the oven to 200°C (fan 180°C/gas mark 6).

Pour half of the cooked sauce from the slow cooker into an ovenproof dish. Take a wrap and scrunch it in up in your hands until you get a scrunched pasty shape. Place it widthways on top of the sauce. Do the same with all of the wraps until the sauce is completely covered. Pour the rest of the sauce over the wraps and sprinkle over the grated Cheddar and mozzarella. Place in the preheated oven and cook for 10 minutes until the cheese has melted.

"Pinch of Nom has made it so easy to have yummy meals that don't make you feel like you're on a diet."

HARRI ⎯⎯

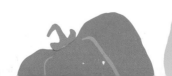

RAINBOW SOUP

🕐 **15 MINS**   🗑 **10 MINS**   ✕ **SERVES 4**

Use Henderson's relish

Use GF stock cube, stock pot, soy sauce and Henderson's relish

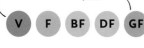

V F BF DF GF

PER SERVING:
69 KCAL /10G CARBS

500ml vegetable stock
  (1 vegetable stock pot and
  1 very low-salt vegetable
  stock cube dissolved in
  500ml boiling water)
2 garlic cloves, peeled and
  thinly sliced
60g tinned sweetcorn, drained,
  or baby corn, thinly sliced
50g sugar snap peas,
  thinly sliced
100g carrot, peeled and cut
  into thin strips
3 spring onions, trimmed
  and thinly sliced
1 tbsp low-sodium light
  soy sauce
1 tbsp rice vinegar
½ tsp hot pepper sauce
½ red pepper, deseeded
  and thinly sliced
½ green pepper, deseeded
  and thinly sliced
60g red cabbage, thinly sliced
5g cornflour
1 tbsp Henderson's relish or
  Worcestershire sauce

We adore rainbows, so why not enjoy the same spectrum of colours in a soup? Sadly you'll find no pots of gold lurking at the bottom, but you will find a bowl of sheer comfort that will cheer you up in seconds! So colourful, so tasty and if you add a tiny bit of chilli then it'd be the perfect cure for a cold!

Everyday Light

Pour the stock into a large saucepan, add the garlic and place over a medium heat. Bring to the boil, then reduce the heat and simmer for 2–3 minutes – the stock should still be bubbling slowly. Add three-quarters of the sweetcorn or baby corn, sugar snap peas, carrot and spring onions. Bring the stock back to the boil, add the soy sauce, rice vinegar and hot pepper sauce and again reduce the heat and simmer for another 2 minutes.

Add the remaining sweetcorn or baby corn, carrot and sugar snap peas, along with the peppers and cabbage, reserving a little of the vegetables for a garnish. Simmer the soup for another minute.

Mix the cornflour with 1 tablespoon of water, add it to the soup and simmer for 1 more minute, then stir in the Henderson's relish or Worcestershire sauce and serve with the reserved vegetable garnish.

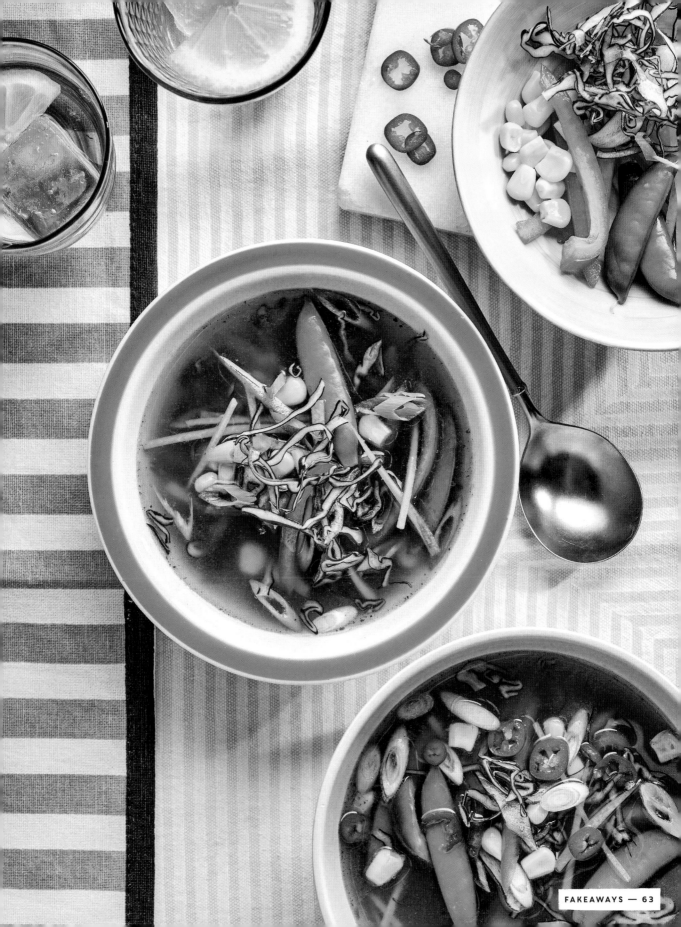

TANDOORI CHICKEN

⏱ **5 MINS***   🍲 **VARIABLE** (SEE BELOW)   ✕ **SERVES 10**

*PLUS A FEW HOURS/OVERNIGHT MARINATING

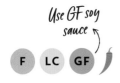

Use GF soy sauce ↘

F **LC** **GF** 🌶

PER SERVING:
233 KCAL / 4.4G CARBS

FOR THE CHICKEN
½ lemon
1 whole chicken (about 1.5kg)
2 onions, peeled and each cut
   into 3 thick slices

FOR THE MARINADE
2 tsp ground ginger
2 tsp ground cumin
2 tsp ground coriander
2 tsp paprika
2 tsp ground turmeric
1 tsp cayenne pepper
   (leave out if you like
   your tandoori mild)
1 tsp salt
1 garlic clove, peeled and
   finely grated
5cm (2in) piece of root ginger,
   peeled and grated
1 tsp dark soy sauce
a few drops of red food
   colouring (optional)
250g fat-free Greek-style
   yoghurt

TO ACCOMPANY *(optional)*
Garlic Mushroom Biryani (page
   72), Cheese and Onion Mash
   (page 218) or Balsamic
   Roasted Onions (page 222)

Tandoori is one of our favourite Indian flavours. Why not try this for an alternative Sunday roast? Serve it with a portion of Garlic Mushroom Biryani and raita (page 72) or Balsamic Roasted Onions (page 222) for a bright and colourful lunch that breaks from tradition in the best way!

Special Occasion —————————————————

OVEN METHOD
🍲 **1 HOUR 20 MINS**

Preheat the oven to 220°C (fan 200°C/gas mark 7).

Juice the half lemon into a bowl, then place the squeezed lemon half inside the chicken cavity.

To make the marinade, mix all of the spices together with the salt in a large non-metallic bowl (big enough to contain the chicken). Add the garlic, ginger, lemon juice, soy sauce, red food colouring (if using) and yoghurt and mix well.

Place the chicken in the bowl and coat it with the mix. Loosen the skin around the breast by sliding your fingers between the skin and the meat, and rub the marinade onto the chicken under the skin. Cover and leave to marinate in the fridge for a few hours or overnight.

Place the sliced onion pieces on a baking tray. Place the marinated chicken on the baking tray on top of the onions, cover with foil and roast in the preheated oven for 50 minutes, then remove the foil and cook for a further 30 minutes. Check the chicken is thoroughly cooked by sliding a knife into the thickest part of the leg. Your chicken is cooked when the juices run clear.

> **TIP:** We based our cooking time on a 1.5kg chicken, allowing 40 minutes per kilo, plus an extra 20 minutes. If you have a different-sized chicken, use the same formula or check the package instructions for guidance.

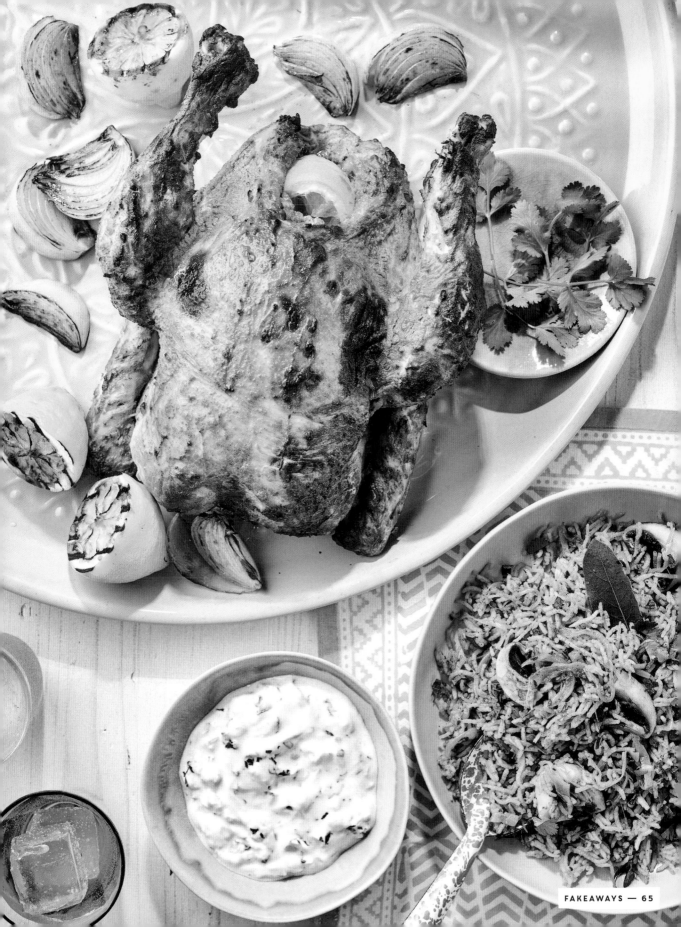

SLOW-COOKER METHOD
🍲 HIGH: 4½ HOURS LOW: 9 HOURS

SPECIAL EQUIPMENT
Slow cooker

Juice the half lemon into a bowl, then place the squeezed lemon half inside the chicken cavity.

To make the marinade, mix all of the spices together with the salt in a large non-metallic bowl (big enough to contain the chicken). Add the garlic, ginger, lemon juice, soy sauce, red food colouring (if using) and yoghurt and mix well.

Place the chicken in the bowl and coat it with the mix. Loosen the skin around the breast by sliding your fingers between the skin and the meat, and rub the marinade onto the chicken under the skin. Cover and leave to marinate in the fridge for a few hours or overnight.

Put the sliced onion at the bottom of the slow cooker. Place the chicken on top of the onions in the slow cooker and put the lid on. Cook on high for 4½ hours or 9 hours on low.

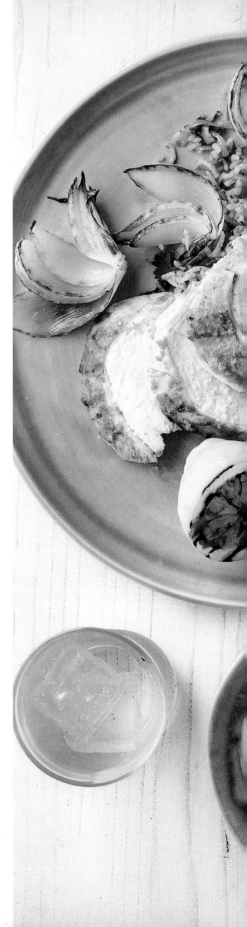

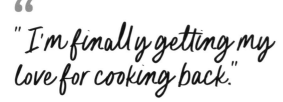

" *I'm finally getting my love for cooking back.*"

—— SAM

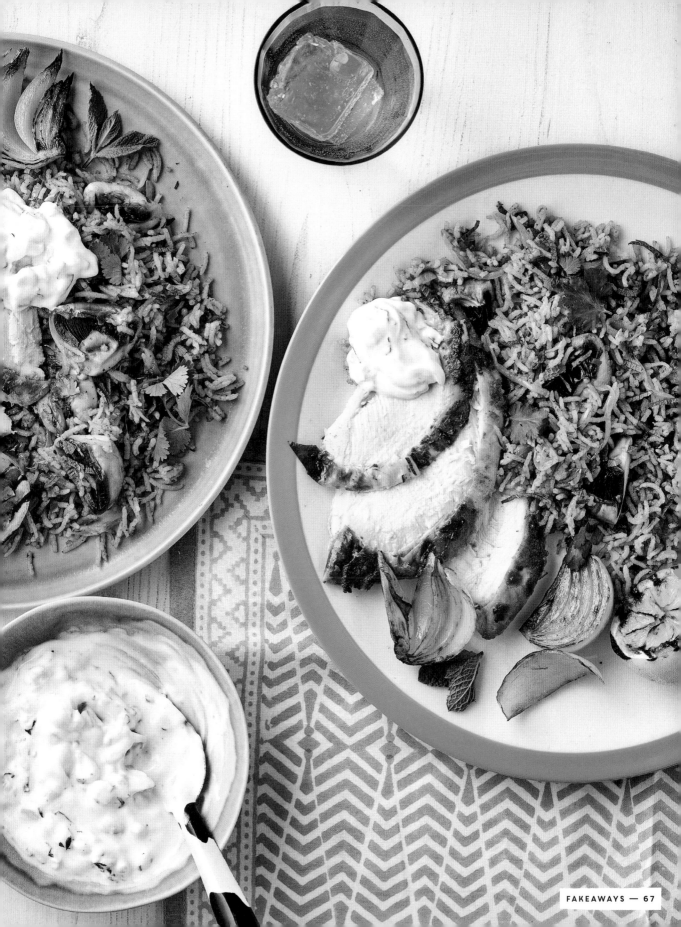

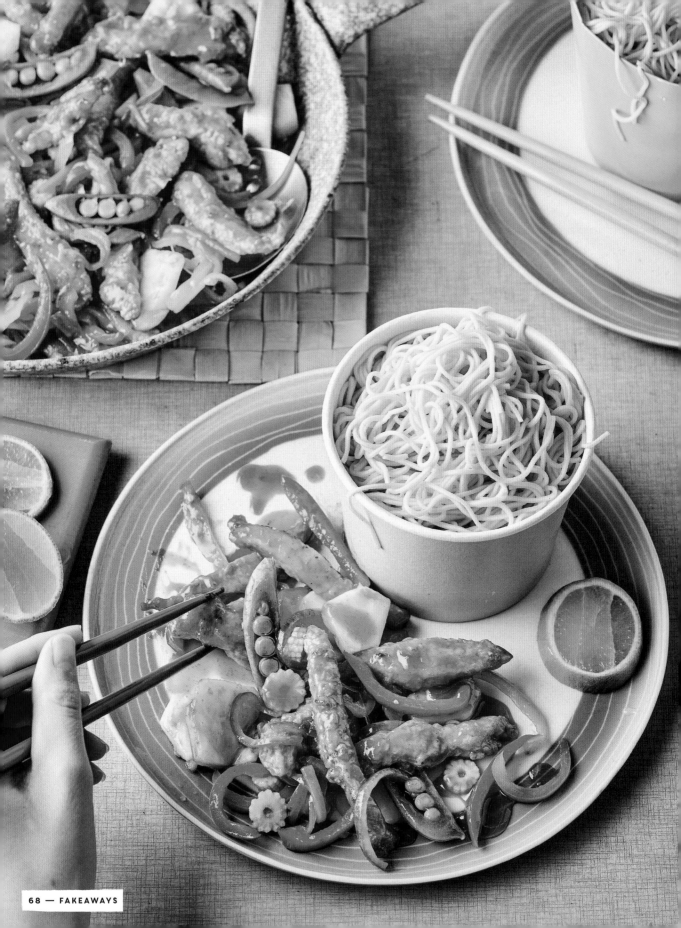

CRISPY CHICKEN *with* SWEET *and* SOUR SAUCE

⏱ **20 MINS**   🍲 **30 MINS**   ✕ **SERVES 4**

PER SERVING:
345 KCAL / 36G CARBS

500g chicken breast strips
sea salt and black pepper
1 medium egg, beaten
3 tbsp self-raising flour
4 spring onions, thinly sliced

FOR THE SWEET AND SOUR SAUCE
low-calorie cooking spray
1 white onion, peeled and sliced
120g baby corn, sliced widthways
100g sugar snap peas, halved
1 garlic clove, peeled and crushed
5cm (2in) fresh ginger, grated
2 carrots, cut into thin strips
1 green pepper, thinly sliced
1 red pepper, thinly sliced
1 small red onion, thinly sliced
juice of 1 lime
2 tsp light soy sauce
2 tbsp rice vinegar
1 tbsp Henderson's relish
½ tsp sriracha or hot sauce
100ml chicken stock
  (1 very low-salt chicken
  stock cube dissolved in
  100ml boiling water)
1 tsp honey
160g peeled pineapple, diced
5g cornflour

TO ACCOMPANY
50g nest of dried egg noodles
  per portion, cooked according
  to packet instructions
  (+ 171 kcal per serving)

Crispy chicken is one of our favourite foods from the Chinese takeaway, especially when it's slathered in a sticky sweet and sour sauce! Our version lends itself equally well to beef, turkey or even prawns, and we think it's even better than the original version without the extra calories.

Special Occasion

Preheat the oven to 220°C (fan 200°C/gas mark 7) and line a baking tray with baking parchment or greaseproof paper.

Season the chicken strips with salt and pepper, then dip them one by one into the beaten egg, then coat with the flour. Place the coated strips on the lined baking tray and cook for 10–12 minutes in the preheated oven until golden.

While the chicken is cooking, spray a large frying pan or wok with low-calorie cooking spray and place over a medium heat. Add the white onion and cook for about 5 minutes until starting to soften and colour slightly, then add the corn, sugar snaps, garlic and ginger and cook for a further 5 minutes. Add the carrots, peppers and red onion and cook for 4 minutes, then add the lime juice, soy sauce, rice vinegar, Henderson's relish and sriracha or hot sauce and give everything a stir. Add the stock and honey, bring to the boil, reduce the heat and simmer for 10 minutes.

Add the pineapple chunks to the sauce and cook for 1 more minute to heat the pineapple. Mix the cornflour with 1 tablespoon of water then stir it into the sauce and cook for another minute. Add the crispy chicken to the pan and stir to coat it in the sauce.

Serve the crispy chicken sprinkled with spring onion and your choice of accompaniment. We think it's great with noodles!

TIP: The chicken can be cooked in an air fryer. Preheat the air fryer to 200°C and cook for 8–9 minutes. If you freeze this recipe, the chicken will not be as crispy when reheated.

STICKY CHICKEN *and* PINEAPPLE SALAD

🕐 **15 MINS*** 🍲 **13 MINS** ✕ **SERVES 2**

*PLUS 2 HOURS MARINATING

Use GF soy sauce ↗

DF **GF** 〃

PER SERVING:
320 KCAL / 28G CARBS

FOR THE MARINADE
1 tbsp runny honey
2 tsp light soy sauce
1 tsp tomato puree
½ tsp garlic granules
juice of ½ lime
1 red chilli, thinly sliced
  (optional, keep the seeds
  in for extra heat)

FOR THE SALAD
300g skinless chicken breasts,
  cut into 2cm (¾in)-thick strips
1 tsp sesame seeds
low-calorie cooking spray
150g fresh peeled pineapple,
  cut into 2cm (¾in) chunks
80g (about ½ head) Chinese
  leaves, shredded
1 carrot, peeled and cut into
  matchsticks (julienne)
½ red pepper, deseeded
  and thinly sliced
1 small red onion, peeled
  and thinly sliced
1 tsp soy sauce
1 tsp lime juice
freshly ground black pepper
a small handful of fresh
  coriander leaves
lime wedges, to serve

Comfort food can include salad, too! A fresh, crisp salad that's packed with sunshine flavours can be just what you need on a warm summer's day. Lime juice, honey and soy sauce create a tangy, sticky glaze that make this protein-packed salad irresistible.

Everyday Light ——————————————

Mix the marinade ingredients together in a small bowl, then add the chicken strips and coat well. Cover and refrigerate for up to 2 hours.

Place a frying pan over a medium-high heat, add the sesame seeds and toast for 2–3 minutes, until golden brown, stirring to ensure they brown evenly and to prevent them catching. Remove from the pan and set to one side.

When the chicken has marinated, spray the frying pan with low-calorie cooking spray and place over a medium-high heat. Once it's hot, pour the chicken and marinade into the pan and stir-fry for about 6 minutes, then add the pineapple chunks. Cook for a further 2–4 minutes, until the marinade has reduced into a sticky glaze that coats the chicken and pineapple and the chicken is cooked through.

Mix the Chinese leaves, carrot, pepper and onion together in a bowl, sprinkle over the teaspoon of soy sauce, teaspoon of lime juice and a pinch of black pepper and toss. Divide between two plates. Top with the chicken and pineapple and sprinkle over the toasted sesame seeds and coriander leaves, and serve with lime wedges.

TIP: You can serve this with the chicken hot or cold.

SWAP THIS: Swap the Chinese leaves for iceberg lettuce, or the fresh pineapple for tinned pineapple (in juice).

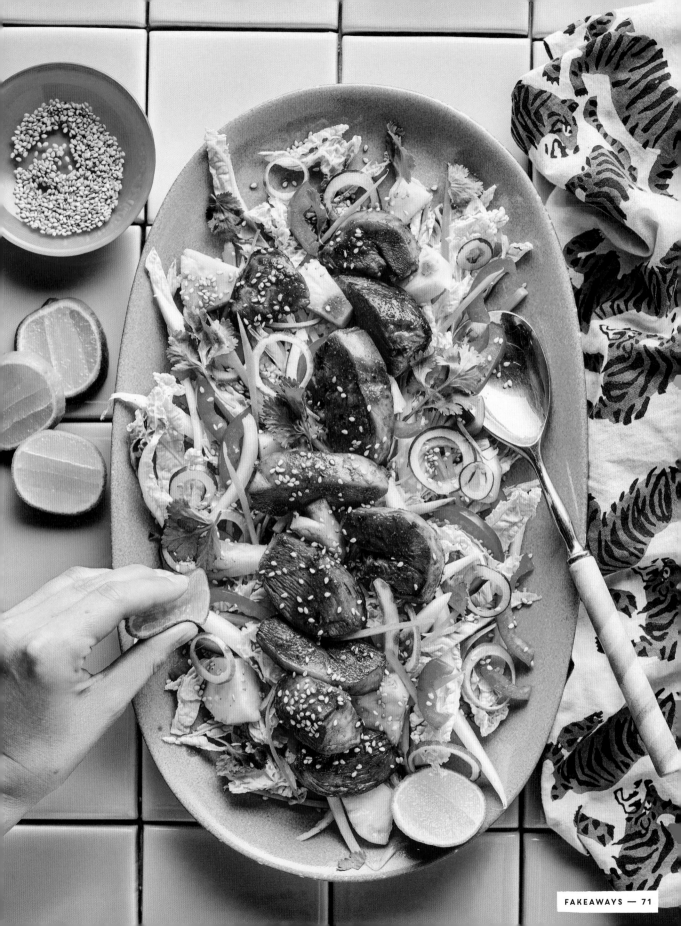

GARLIC MUSHROOM BIRYANI

⏱ **15 MINS**   🍲 **50 MINS**   ✕ **SERVES 4**

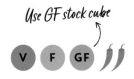

Use GF stock cube

V **F** **GF** ''

PER SERVING:
404 KCAL / 78G CARBS

low-calorie cooking spray
2 onions, peeled and thinly sliced
6 garlic cloves, peeled and crushed
4cm (1½in) piece of root
  ginger, peeled and grated
1 chilli (any colour), deseeded
  and finely chopped
2 tsp garam masala
1 tsp ground coriander
½ tsp ground cinnamon
2 tbsp tomato puree
200ml coconut dairy-free
  milk alternative
juice of ½ lemon
450g white mushrooms, quartered
a handful of fresh coriander
  leaves, chopped
a handful of fresh mint leaves,
  chopped
300g basmati rice
8 cloves
8 green cardamom pods
2 bay leaves
1 cinnamon stick
600ml vegetable stock (1
  vegetable stock cube dissolved
  in 600ml boiling water)
¼ tsp ground turmeric
a good pinch of salt
1 lemon, cut into wedges, to serve

FOR THE RAITA
150g fat-free natural yoghurt
½ cucumber, peeled, deseeded
  and finely diced
10 mint leaves, finely chopped
1 tsp granulated sweetener

A traditional biryani is a complex and time-consuming dish, involving soaking and cooking rice, veggies and meat separately before layering up. We don't always have the time to start from scratch, so we've simplified the process and created a delicious one-pot dish that couldn't be easier!

Weekly Indulgence ————————————

First mix the raita ingredients in a small bowl, cover and refrigerate until later.

Spray a large, heavy pan with a tight-fitting lid (a deep casserole dish is ideal) with low-calorie cooking spray and place over a medium heat. Add the onions and sauté for 8–10 minutes, until softened and lightly browned. Add the garlic, ginger, chilli, garam masala, ground coriander and cinnamon and cook for a further minute until fragrant, then stir in the tomato puree, coconut milk alternative and lemon juice. Add the mushrooms and cook for 3–4 minutes, then stir in half of the chopped coriander and mint. Reduce the heat to low.

Give the rice a quick rinse, then add it to the pan on top of the mushrooms in an even layer. Do not stir.

Scatter the cloves, cardamom, bay leaves and cinnamon stick on top of the rice, then pour over the stock. Sprinkle the turmeric over the rice and add the salt, then cover and cook over the lowest heat for 25 minutes. After 25 minutes most of the liquid should have been absorbed and the rice should be fluffy.

Leave to stand, covered, for 10 minutes, then remove the lid and sprinkle the remaining mint and coriander over the top.

Spoon into bowls, digging down deep to the bottom layer of mushrooms, and serve topped with raita and lemon wedges.

█ **SWAP THIS:** If you don't have garam masala, you can use regular curry powder instead.

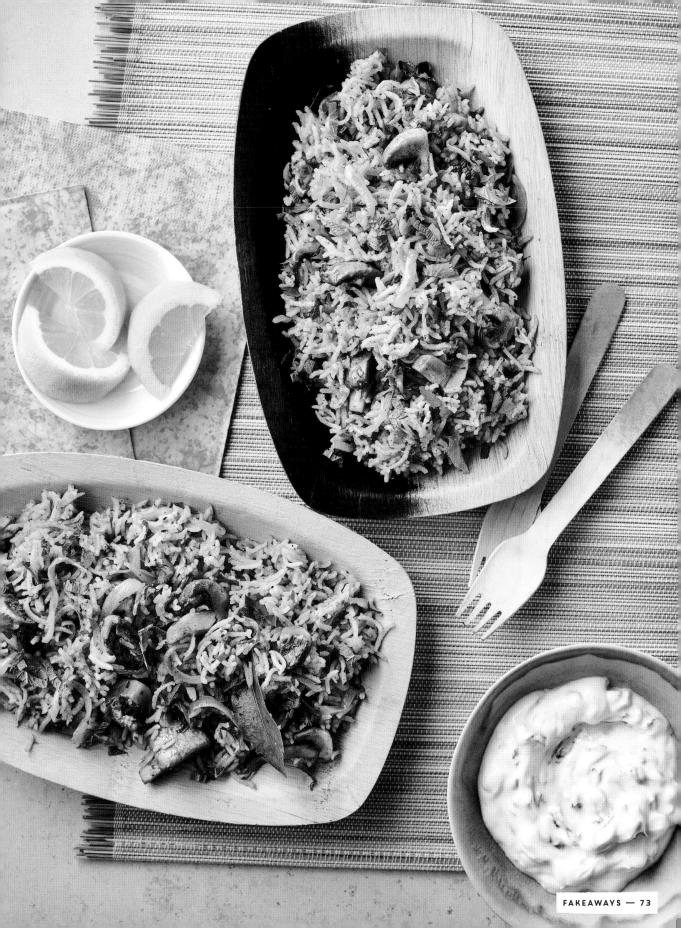

CHICKEN *and* CHEESE CURRY

🕐 **25 MINS***   🍲 **1 HOUR**   ✕ **SERVES 4**

*PLUS 1 HOUR MARINATING

Without the grated cheese ↖

(F) (BF) (GF) 🌶

PER SERVING:
353 KCAL /12G CARBS

FOR THE CHICKEN TIKKA
2 tsp paprika
1 tsp ground coriander
1 tsp ground cumin
1 tsp garam masala
½ tsp ground turmeric
½ tsp ground ginger
½ tsp garlic granules
pinch of cayenne pepper
½ tsp salt
pinch of ground black pepper
3 tbsp fat-free Greek-style
  yoghurt
2 tbsp fresh lemon juice
650g diced chicken breast

FOR THE CURRY SAUCE
low-calorie cooking spray
1 medium onion, peeled
  and finely chopped
1 medium carrot, peeled
  and finely chopped
1 garlic clove, peeled
  and crushed
1 tbsp mild curry powder
400ml coconut dairy-free
  milk alternative
1 tbsp white wine vinegar
150g fat-free Greek-style
  yoghurt
sea salt and freshly ground
  black pepper

FOR THE TOP
100g reduced-fat mature
  Cheddar, finely grated

You may be surprised to see cheese in a curry, but believe us, it works! Clever ingredient swaps keep the calories low while giving you a creamy, rich, medium-spiced sauce that's full of flavour. Our favourite bit is the cheese sprinkled on top, which melts into the curry and makes it extra tasty. Try it for yourself, and you may find you stop reaching for the takeaway menu!

Special Occasion

First, mix the tikka marinade spices. Put the ground spices, garlic granules, salt and pepper in a bowl and mix well. Put the diced chicken in a non-metallic bowl with the 3 tablespoons of yoghurt and the lemon juice and stir to coat, then add the spices and mix to coat the chicken in the marinade. Cover and marinate in the fridge for 1 hour.

While the chicken is marinating, make the sauce. Spray a medium saucepan with low-calorie cooking spray and place over a medium heat. Add the onion and carrot and cook, stirring, for 10 minutes until starting to soften. Add the garlic and curry powder and cook, stirring, for 1–2 minutes, then reduce the heat and stir in the coconut dairy-free milk alternative and vinegar. Cover and simmer gently over the lowest heat for about 20 minutes, until the onion and carrot are just tender.

Preheat the oven to 220°C (fan 200°C/gas mark 7).

Blitz the onion and carrot mixture with a stick blender or in a food processor until smooth and return to the saucepan. Cover with a lid and set aside.

To cook the chicken tikka, spray a large frying pan with low-calorie cooking spray and place over a high heat. When the frying pan is hot, add the marinated chicken and fry for 3–4 minutes to seal on all sides. Transfer the sealed chicken to a medium ovenproof dish and cook in the preheated oven for 15 minutes or until the juices run clear and there is no sign of pinkness.

TO ACCOMPANY

50g uncooked basmati rice per portion, cooked according to packet instructions (+ 173 kcal per 125g cooked serving)

MAKE IT VEGGIE:
For a vegetarian curry, swap the chicken for Quorn fillets.

Tip the cooked chicken into the saucepan of curry sauce and stir. Place over a low heat and simmer gently for about 5 minutes to heat it through.

Remove from the heat and stir in the Greek-style yoghurt until completely combined. Season to taste with salt and pepper. Sprinkle the cheese over the curry just before serving. The cheese should be melting on top when served.

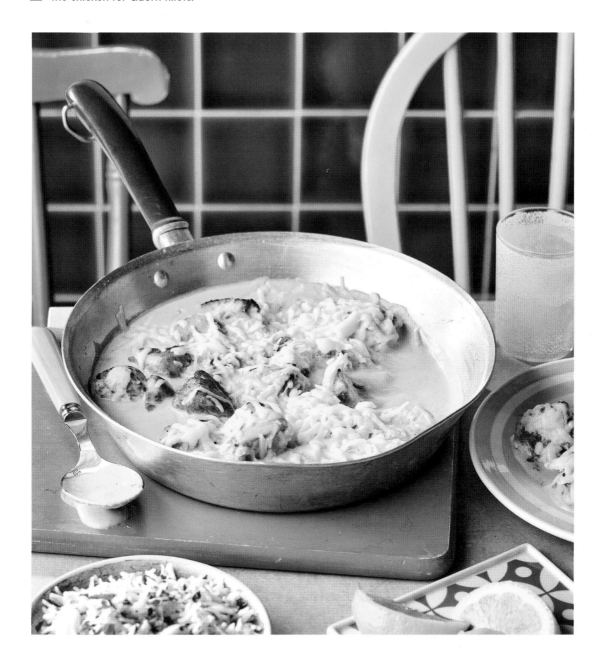

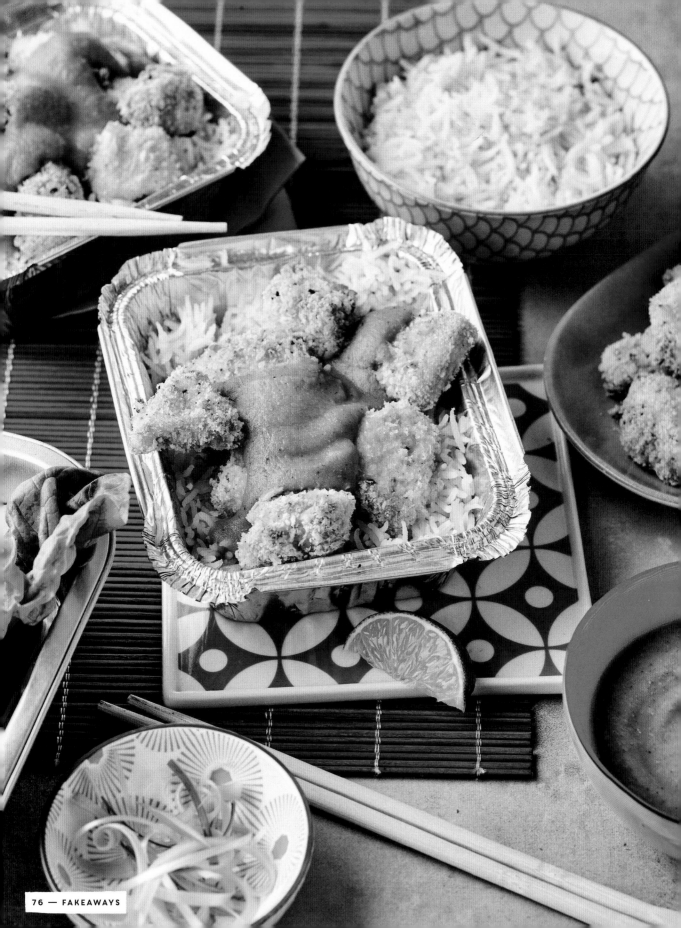

KATSU CHICKEN NUGGETS *and* CURRY DIP

Freeze sauce and cooked nuggets separately

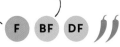

F · BF · DF

PER SERVING:
299 KCAL / 27G CARBS

low-calorie cooking spray

FOR THE CURRY DIP
1 onion, peeled and
   roughly sliced
3 garlic cloves, peeled
   and crushed
3 medium carrots, about
   200g, peeled and cut into
   1cm (½in)-thick rounds
1 small potato, about 136g,
   peeled and quartered
500ml chicken stock
   (1 very low-salt chicken
   stock cube dissolved in
   500ml boiling water)
2 tbsp curry powder, mild or
   hot depending on taste
2 tsp garam masala
2 tsp onion granules
1 tbsp reduced-sodium soy
   sauce (dark or light)
1 tsp granulated sweetener

FOR THE NUGGETS
3 large skinless chicken
   breasts (visible fat removed),
   about 510g in total
50g panko breadcrumbs
½ tsp garlic granules
sea salt and freshly ground
   black pepper
1 medium egg, beaten

⏱ **15 MINS**　　🍲 **40 MINS**　　✕ **SERVES 4**

Our Katsu twist on a classic chicken nugget that's made for dipping! We've coated succulent chicken in a crispy coating and paired it with a fragrant, mildly spiced sauce that's packed with flavour and completely customisable. If you prefer more of a kick, simply up the chilli!

Everyday Light ─────────────────────

FOR THE CURRY DIP

Preheat the oven to 220°C (fan 200°C/gas mark 7), if you're oven-baking the nuggets.

First, make the curry dip. Spray a saucepan with low-calorie cooking spray and place over a medium heat. Add the onion and garlic and fry gently for a few minutes until beginning to soften, then add the carrots, potato, stock, curry powder, garam masala, onion granules, soy sauce and sweetener and bring to the boil. Reduce the heat to a simmer, cover and cook for 35–40 minutes, stirring occasionally, until the carrots and potato are fully cooked and soft. Add more water if the liquid level reduces too much.

Once the potato and carrot for the sauce have cooked through, blend the sauce in the pan with a stick blender (or in a food processor) until smooth. A top tip is to blend twice as long as you think – you want the sauce to be super smooth! If the sauce seems too thick at this point, add some more water a little at a time until you reach the consistency you want. If it seems a little thin, reduce it over a low heat. This is all down to personal preference, so don't worry about getting it wrong!

While your sauce is cooking, prepare and cook the nuggets.

TIP: The dipping sauce's heat comes from the curry powder: if you want less heat, use a mild curry powder!

SWAP THIS: Swap the panko for normal breadcrumbs, finely crushed cornflakes or tortilla chips.

OVEN METHOD FOR THE NUGGETS

Line a baking tray with non-stick baking paper and spray it with low-calorie cooking spray.

Slice the chicken breasts into 1cm (½in)-thick slices. If some from the middle section of the chicken breast are quite large you can cut them in half. You should have roughly 40 nuggets, so there will be about 10 per serving.

Mix the panko breadcrumbs with the garlic granules, season with salt and pepper and tip onto a plate.

Make sure your chicken pieces are dry. You can use a little paper towel to dab them. Dip a piece of chicken into the beaten egg, letting any excess drip off, then lightly place the chicken piece on top of the panko mix, turn over and coat the other side. Gently shake to let any excess fall back onto the plate. You are looking for a really light coating, so do this delicately – use too much coating and you won't have enough for all the chicken! Once coated, place on the lined tray and repeat until all the chicken is done.

Spray the tops of the chicken with low-calorie cooking spray and bake in the oven for 30–35 minutes, gently flipping the nuggets halfway through. Once the chicken is white throughout (you can cut one in half to check), and the breadcrumbs are golden brown, they are ready. Serve with the dip and a side of your choice.

AIR-FRYER METHOD FOR THE NUGGETS

SPECIAL EQUIPMENT
Air fryer

Cut the chicken breasts into 1cm (½in)-thick slices. If some from the middle section of the chicken breast are quite large you can cut them in half. You should have roughly 40 nuggets, so there will be about 10 per serving.

Mix the panko breadcrumbs with the garlic granules, season with salt and pepper and tip onto a plate.

Make sure your chicken pieces are dry. You can use a little paper towel to dab them. Preheat your air fryer to 180°C.

Dip a piece of chicken into the beaten egg, letting any excess drip off, then lightly place the chicken piece on top of the panko mix, turn over and coat the other side. Gently shake to let any excess fall back onto the plate. You are looking for a really light coating, so do this delicately – use too much coating and you won't have enough for all the chicken! Once coated, place in the bottom of your air fryer in a single layer and repeat until all the chicken is done.

Spray the tops of the chicken with low-calorie cooking spray and cook for 20 minutes, gently flipping the nuggets halfway through. Depending on the size of your air fryer you may need to cook the nuggets in batches.

Once the chicken is white throughout (you can cut one in half to check) and the breadcrumbs are golden brown, they are ready. Serve with the dip and a side of your choice.

TIP: You can batch-cook this in advance and freeze portions of sauce and chicken (separately), so you always have some ready. Once defrosted, reheat the sauce according to the instructions on p12 and reheat the chicken in the oven at 210°C (fan 190°C/gas mark 6) for 10–15 minutes, until piping hot.

CHEESY CHIPS *and* GRAVY

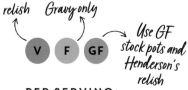

Use vegetarian stock pots and Henderson's relish

Gravy only

Use GF stock pots and Henderson's relish

🕐 **10 MINS**   🍲 **VARIABLE (SEE BELOW)**   🍴 **SERVES 4**

PER SERVING:
228 KCAL / 34G CARBS

FOR THE CHEESY CHIPS
500g potatoes, peeled and
  cut into 1cm (½in)-thick chips
low-calorie cooking spray
¼ tsp onion salt
40g reduced-fat
  Cheddar, grated
70g reduced-fat
  mozzarella, grated

FOR THE GRAVY
½ onion, peeled and
  roughly chopped
1 small carrot, peeled
  and roughly chopped
1 small potato, peeled
  and roughly chopped
2 low-salt beef stock pots
a dash of Henderson's relish
  or Worcestershire sauce
a few drops of gravy
  browning (optional)

This dish is a staple of chip shops across the north of the UK and one of our all-time favourite comfort foods. It may sound like an odd pairing at first but it works wonderfully. Try this tasty combo of piping hot gravy, gooey cheese and crispy chips for a cheap and easy Fakeaway that's just as good as the chippy!

Everyday Light

OVEN METHOD
🍲 **40–45 MINS**

Preheat the oven to 200°C (fan 180°C/gas mark 6).

Spray the potato chips with low-calorie cooking spray and toss them in the onion salt.

Scatter them on a baking sheet and cook in the preheated oven for 40–45 minutes, turning them halfway through, until the centre of the chips are soft and they're crisp and golden on the outside.

Meanwhile, make the gravy. Put all of the ingredients (except the gravy browning) in a saucepan, add 600ml of water and bring to the boil. Reduce the heat and simmer for 25 minutes until the carrots and potatoes are soft.

Remove the pan from the heat and blitz the mixture with a hand blender. Add a couple of drops of gravy browning if required. If the gravy is too thick, add a little water until it reaches a consistency you are happy with. Keep the gravy hot until the chips are cooked.

Mix the grated Cheddar and mozzarella together.

When the chips are cooked, divide them between two warmed bowls. Sprinkle half the cheese mix over, smother with the hot gravy, then sprinkle over the rest of the cheese. The heat from the gravy will melt the cheese.

Serve and enjoy!

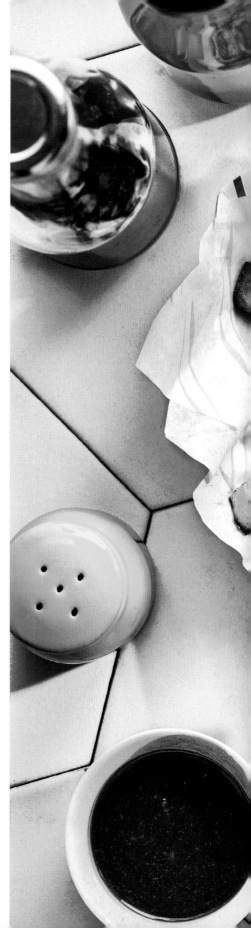

AIR-FRYER METHOD
🍲 25 MINS

SPECIAL EQUIPMENT
Air fryer

First, make the gravy. Put all of the ingredients (except the gravy browning) in a saucepan, add 600ml of water and bring to the boil. Reduce the heat and simmer for 25 minutes until the carrots and potatoes are soft.

Remove the pan from the heat and blitz the mixture with a hand blender. Add a couple of drops of gravy browning if required. If the gravy is too thick, add a little water until it reaches a consistency you are happy with.

While the gravy cooks, preheat the air fryer to 180°C. Spray the potatoes with low-calorie cooking spray and sprinkle on the onion salt. Place in the air fryer basket and cook for about 20 minutes, shaking the chips halfway through to ensure even cooking.

Mix the grated Cheddar and mozzarella together.

When the chips are cooked, divide between two warmed bowls. Sprinkle over half the cheese mix, smother in hot gravy and then sprinkle on the remaining cheese. The heat from the gravy will melt the cheese.

Serve and enjoy!

"
"Pinch of Nom has been a lifesaver when it comes to recipes and inspiration."

—— REBECCA

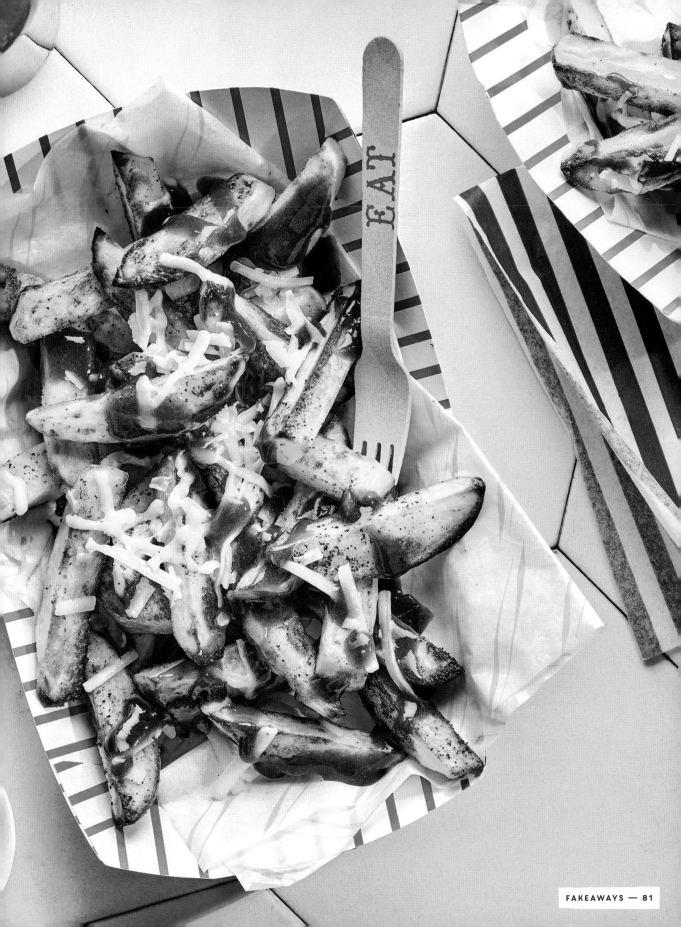

TAMARIND *and* COCONUT FISH

Use GF flour and GF stock cube

DF **GF**

🕐 **10 MINS**   🍲 **22 MINS**   ✕ **SERVES 4**

PER SERVING:
295 KCAL / 21G CARBS

FOR THE FISH
juice of 1 lime
1 garlic clove, peeled and crushed
4 sea bass fillets (120g each)
   or other skinless white fish
2 tbsp plain flour

FOR THE SAUCE
low-calorie cooking spray
2 onions, finely chopped
2cm (¾in) fresh ginger, grated
1 chilli, deseeded and finely
   chopped
6 garlic cloves, peeled
   and crushed
1 tsp sweet smoked paprika
2 tsp tamarind paste
1 tsp fish sauce
pinch of ground black pepper
pinch of chilli powder
1 fish stock cube
100g green beans, halved
4 baby corn, sliced
4 spring onions, chopped
1 x 400g tin light coconut milk
handful of fresh coriander
   leaves, chopped

TO ACCOMPANY
50g uncooked basmati rice
   per portion, cooked according
   to packet instructions (+ 173
   kcal per 125g cooked serving),
   or 50g nest of dried egg
   noodles per portion, cooked
   according to packet instructions
   (+ 171 kcal per serving)

Once upon a time, we were asked to prepare this dish for a very famous person. We can't reveal who the person was, but this recipe is so fresh and tasty, it simply can't be kept a secret! Any white fish would work with this, just be sure to check the cooking times for thicker fillets.

Weekly Indulgence ───────────────

Preheat the oven to 220°C (fan 200°C/gas mark 7) and spray a baking tray with low-calorie cooking spray.

Put the lime juice and garlic in a bowl, give it a stir and add the fish. Leave for 5 minutes to marinate.

Remove the fish from the marinade, add the flour to the fish and shake the fish to coat it lightly. Transfer the fish to the greased baking sheet and cook in the oven for 15 minutes.

While the fish is cooking, spray a frying pan with low-calorie cooking spray and place over a medium heat. Add the onions and sauté for 5 minutes until they start to soften and turn brown, then add the ginger, chilli and garlic and cook for a further minute until you start to smell their aroma. Add the smoked paprika, tamarind paste, fish sauce, black pepper and chilli powder, and crumble the stock cube over the top. Cook for 2 minutes, stirring well. Add the green beans, baby corn, spring onions and coconut milk, bring to a simmer and cook for 10 minutes.

Remove from the heat and stir through the coriander.

Serve the fish on a plate with the sauce.

TIP: Adjust the cooking time according to the type of white fish you use. Sea bass fillets are relatively thin, but if you are cooking with thicker fillets, you will need to increase the cooking time. Stir 1 tbsp of peanut butter into the finished sauce for an extra bit of umph! It will also thicken the sauce a little more. Add 28 kcal per serving.

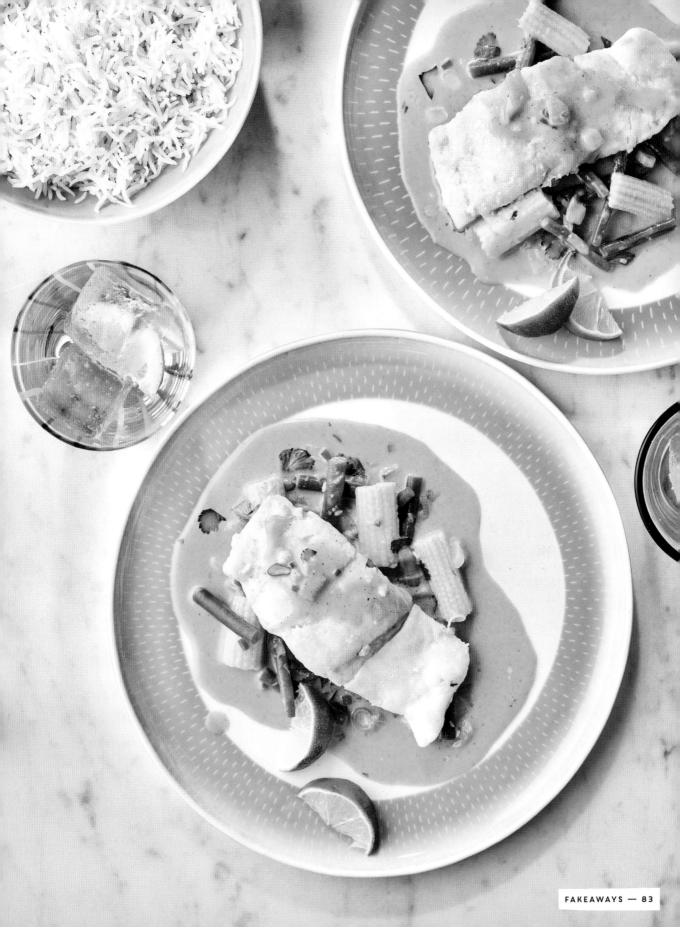

SPAGHETTI CARBONARA

🕐 **10 MINS**　📦 **20 MINS**　✕ **SERVES 2**

GF

PER SERVING:
516 KCAL / 47G CARBS

1 onion, peeled and finely diced
250g button mushrooms,
　thinly sliced
1 x 125g gammon steak,
　cut into 5mm (¼in) dice
120g dried spaghetti
low-calorie cooking spray
300ml vegetable stock
　(1 low-salt vegetable stock
　cube dissolved in 300ml
　boiling water)
1 medium egg and 1 egg yolk
1 tsp freshly ground
　black pepper
2 tbsp quark
½ tsp English mustard powder
30g Pecorino, grated, plus
　a little extra to serve
handful of fresh parsley
　leaves, chopped

Restaurant-quality food, in the comfort of your own kitchen! We've used super-simple, easy-to-find ingredients and combined them to create this decadent pasta dish that's ready to serve in 30 minutes. The key to a good carbonara is adding the egg mix when the pan is off the heat; this way you'll get glossy pasta and the egg will cook perfectly without scrambling!

Special Occasion

Boil the kettle and, while you're waiting for it to boil, prepare the onion, mushrooms and gammon.

Cook the pasta according to the packet instructions.

While the pasta's cooking, spray a large frying pan with a few sprays of low-calorie cooking spray and place over a medium heat. Add the onions and fry for 5 minutes until softened, then add the mushrooms and gammon and cook for 5 minutes until slightly browned.

Add the vegetable stock to the frying pan, increase the heat to high and cook, stirring frequently, for 7–10 minutes until it reduces by half.

Meanwhile, whisk the egg and egg yolk, black pepper, quark and mustard in a bowl. Set aside.

Drain the cooked pasta and tip it into a big bowl. Add the cooked onion, mushrooms, reduced stock and gammon and stir well. Slowly add the whisked eggs, Pecorino and quark, stirring constantly. DO NOT do this over the heat otherwise you'll end up with scrambled egg!

Once it's all stirred through, add the chopped parsley. Plate up and sprinkle with a little more Pecorino. Enjoy!

TIP: We don't recommend freezing this recipe as the sauce can end up splitting.

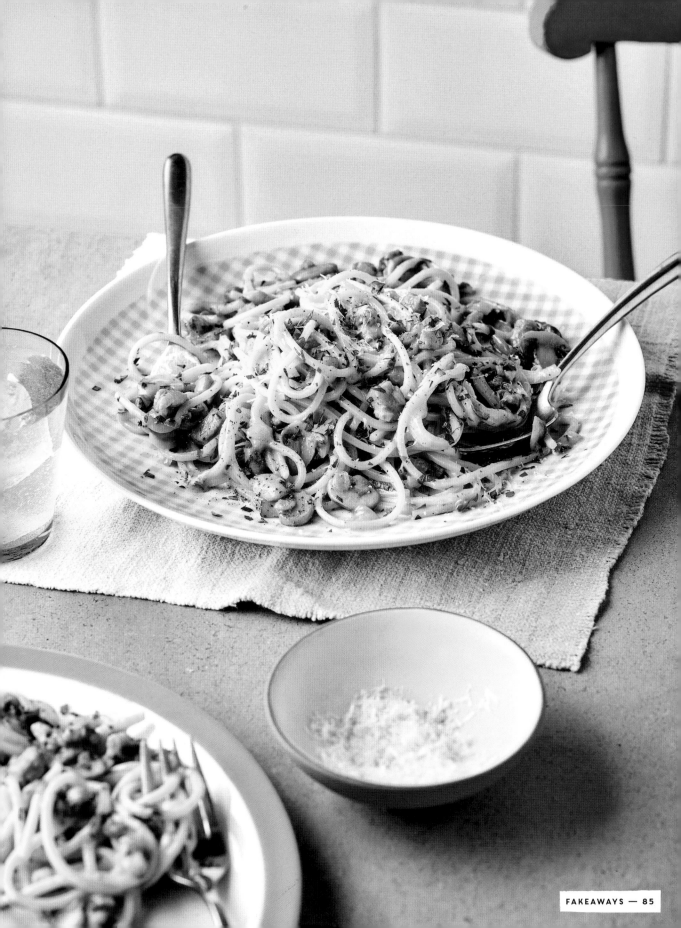

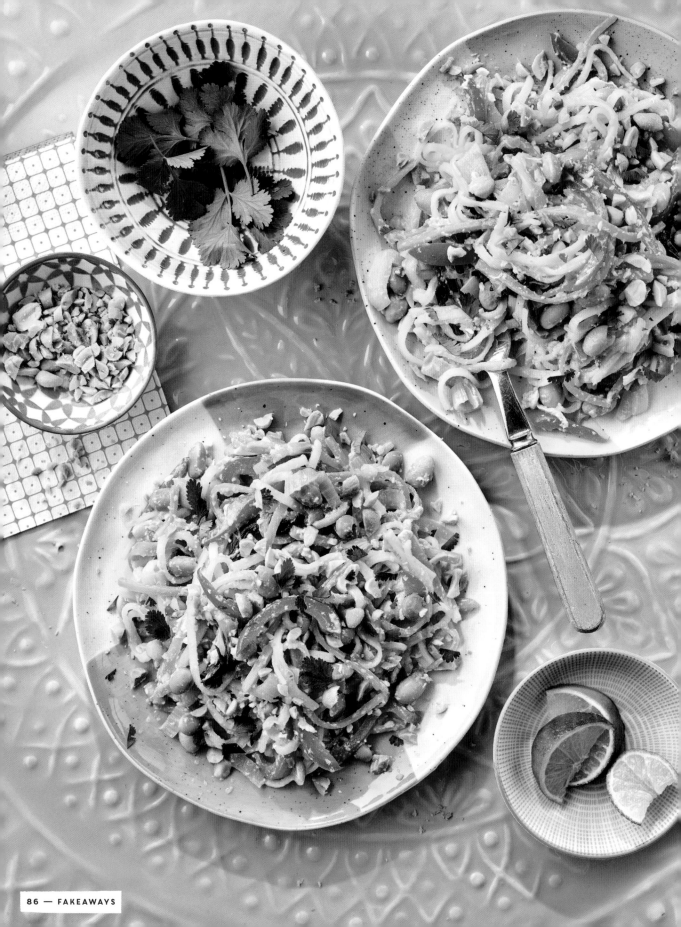

COCONUT PAD THAI NOODLES

🕐 **20 MINS** 🍲 **10 MINS** ✕ **SERVES 2**

Use GF soy sauce ↗

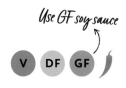

PER SERVING:
308 KCAL / 35G CARBS

75g frozen edamame beans
100g flat rice noodles
  (sometimes known
  as rice sticks)
2 tsp tamarind paste
100ml coconut dairy-free
  milk alternative
juice of ½ lime
1 tbsp vegetarian fish sauce
2 tsp low-sodium light
  soy sauce
1 tsp granulated sweetener
low-calorie cooking spray
3 spring onions, trimmed
  and sliced
½ red pepper, deseeded
  and thinly sliced
1 carrot, peeled and cut into
  matchsticks (julienne)
1 garlic clove, peeled
  and crushed
½ chilli, deseeded and
  finely chopped
1 pak choi, shredded
1 medium egg, beaten
small handful of fresh
  coriander leaves, chopped
15g salted peanuts,
  roughly chopped
lime wedges, to serve

Pad Thai is one of the most well-known Thai street-food dishes. The sweetness of coconut milk, tang of tamarind and lime, and the salty, umami fish sauce combine to make a really flavourful noodle dish. We've kept ours veggie, using edamame beans for some extra protein.

Everyday Light

Cook the edamame beans and rice noodles according to the packet instructions.

Combine the tamarind paste, coconut milk alternative, lime juice, fish sauce, soy sauce and sweetener in a small bowl.

Spray a wok or large frying pan with some low-calorie cooking spray and place over a medium-high heat. Add the spring onions, pepper and carrot and stir-fry for 2 minutes, then add the garlic, chilli, pak choi and cooked edamame beans and cook for a further minute. Pour in the sauce and cook for 2 minutes, then add the drained noodles and toss to mix well.

Push the veg mixture to the side of the wok or pan and add the beaten egg to the clear space in the pan. Stir the egg for 30 seconds, then mix in with the noodles.

Divide the Pad Thai between two plates then top with the chopped coriander leaves and peanuts. Garnish with lime wedges and serve.

SWAP THIS: If you can't find vegetarian fish sauce, replace it with 1 tablespoon of light soy sauce. Swap the rice noodles for egg noodles (adjusting the calories as necessary), and you can swap the coconut dairy-free milk alternative for coconut milk, but bear in mind it will increase the kcal.

BOLOGNESE CHEESE FRIES

🕐 **15 MINS** 🍲 **VARIABLE** (SEE BELOW) ✗ **SERVES 4**

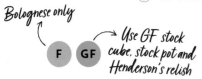

Bolognese only

F GF → *Use GF stock cube, stock pot and Henderson's relish*

PER SERVING:
379 KCAL / 49G CARBS

low-calorie cooking spray
250g 5%-fat minced beef
1 onion, peeled and diced
1 pepper (any colour),
   deseeded and diced
1 medium carrot, peeled
   and diced
3 garlic cloves, peeled
   and crushed
1 tbsp tomato puree
1 x 400g tin chopped tomatoes
200g passata
1 tbsp balsamic vinegar
1 low-salt beef stock pot
1 tsp mixed dried herbs
1 tbsp Henderson's relish or
   Worcestershire sauce
1 very low-salt beef stock cube

FOR THE FRIES
3 medium potatoes (about 700g)
50g reduced-fat mature
   Cheddar, finely grated

TO ACCOMPANY *(optional)*
75g mixed salad (+ 15 kcal
   per serving) and a drizzle
   of sriracha

> **SWAP THIS:** Swap the beef mince for pork mince. To make the dish dairy free, swap Cheddar for a dairy-free alternative.

Spaghetti bolognese is one of our go-to comfort food dishes and these fries are our tasty twist on a classic. We've swapped out the pasta for golden fries and added a rich beef bolognese and melted cheese. We've packed the sauce full of vegetables to help you get your five-a-day and using a reduced-fat cheese means that you can still enjoy some cheesy goodness without worrying about the extra calories.

Everyday Light ———————————————

HOB-TOP METHOD
🍲 **46 MINUTES**

Preheat the oven to 210°C (fan 190°C/gas mark 6).

Spray a frying pan with low-calorie cooking spray and set over a medium heat. Add the beef mince and brown the meat for 2 minutes. Add the onion, pepper, carrot and garlic and cook for a further 4 minutes. Pour in the tomato puree, chopped tomatoes and passata and stir, then add the balsamic vinegar, stock pot, mixed herbs and Henderson's relish or Worcestershire sauce, and crumble in the stock cube. Give everything a good stir and simmer over a low heat for 30 minutes, stirring occasionally, until the sauce has thickened and reduced.

While the bolognese is cooking, peel the potatoes and cut them into fries. Place the potatoes on a baking tray and spray with plenty of low-calorie cooking spray. Place in the oven and bake for 25 minutes, turning the fries halfway through, until they are golden brown.

Spoon a little of the bolognese into the bottom of an ovenproof dish and top with the fries. Spoon over the rest of the bolognese and sprinkle the grated cheese on top. Cook in the oven for 10 minutes, until the cheese is melted, and serve with your choice of accompaniment.

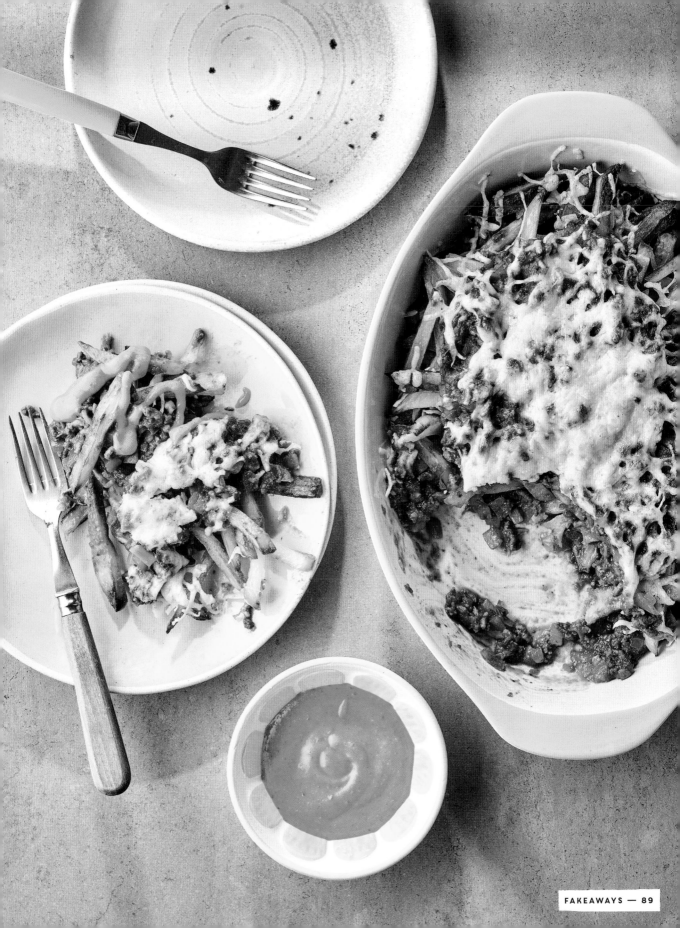

ELECTRIC PRESSURE-COOKER METHOD
🍲 35 MINS

SPECIAL EQUIPMENT
Electric pressure cooker

Preheat the oven to 210°C (fan 190°C/gas mark 6). Spray the pressure-cooker pot with low-calorie cooking spray and set to 'sauté'. Add the beef mince and brown for 2 minutes, then add the onion, pepper, carrot and garlic and cook for a further 4 minutes. If your pressure cooker doesn't have a sauté function, do this step in a saucepan on the hob, then transfer to the pressure cooker when done.

Pour in the puree, chopped tomatoes and passata and stir, then add the vinegar, stock pot, mixed herbs and Henderson's relish or Worcestershire sauce, and crumble in the stock cube. Stir well. Turn off the 'sauté' mode, cover with the lid and set the valve to 'sealing'. Pressure-cook on high for 10 minutes, then use the 'manual release' function to release pressure from the pot. Set the pressure cooker to 'sauté' and cook, stirring occasionally, until the sauce has thickened and reduced.

While the bolognese is cooking, peel the potatoes and cut them into fries. Put the fries on a baking tray and spray with plenty of low-calorie cooking spray. Bake in the oven for 25 minutes, turning them halfway through, until golden brown.

Spoon a little bolognese into the bottom of an ovenproof dish and top with fries. Spoon over the remaining bolognese and sprinkle the grated cheese on top. Cook in the oven for 10 minutes, until the cheese is melted, and serve with salad or your choice of accompaniment.

SLOW-COOKER METHOD
🍲 HIGH: 4 HOURS 10 MINS

SPECIAL EQUIPMENT
Slow cooker

Spray a frying pan with low-calorie cooking spray and set over a medium heat. Add the beef mince and brown the meat for 2 minutes, then add the onion, pepper, carrot and garlic and cook for a further 4 minutes.

Transfer to the slow-cooker pot and pour in the puree, chopped tomatoes and passata and stir, then add the vinegar, stock pot, mixed herbs and Henderson's relish or Worcestershire sauce, and crumble in the stock cube. Give everything a good stir.

Add the lid and cook on high for 4 hours. Thirty minutes before the end of cooking, preheat the oven to 210°C (fan 190°C/gas mark 6).

Peel the potatoes and cut them into fries. Place the potatoes on a baking tray and spray with plenty of low-calorie cooking spray. Place in the oven and bake for 25 minutes, turning halfway through, until they are golden brown.

Spoon a little of the bolognese into the bottom of an ovenproof dish and top with the fries. Spoon over the rest of the bolognese and sprinkle the grated cheese on top.

Cook in the oven for 10 minutes, until the cheese is melted, and serve with salad or your choice of accompaniment.

TIP: To cook the fries in an air fryer, preheat the air fryer to 190°C, spray the fries with plenty of low-calorie cooking spray and add them to the fryer. Set the timer for 25 minutes and cook until golden brown, shaking halfway through for an even colour.

CHILLI CHEESY 'NACHOS'

⏱ **5 MINS** 🍲 **40 MINS** ✕ **SERVES 4**

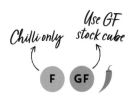

Chilli only
Use GF stock cube

F **GF**

PER SERVING:
522 KCAL / 64G CARBS

SPECIAL EQUIPMENT
30cm (12in) ovenproof dish

FOR THE POTATO WEDGES
2 baking potatoes (about
 740g in total), cut into
 wedges (unpeeled)
low-calorie cooking spray
seasoning of your choice, such
 as chip seasoning, paprika or
 salt and pepper, etc.

FOR THE CHILLI
1 large onion, peeled and
 finely diced
250g carrots, peeled and diced
250g swede, peeled and diced
3 celery sticks, diced
400g extra-lean minced beef
1 garlic clove, peeled and
 crushed
½ red chilli, deseeded
 and chopped
1 tsp chilli powder
1 x 400g tin red kidney beans
 in chilli sauce
1 x 400g tin chopped tomatoes
150ml beef stock (1 beef stock
 cube dissolved in 150ml
 boiling water)

TO FINISH
75g light spreadable cheese
20g reduced-fat Cheddar,
 finely grated
fresh coriander leaves

Dig into a delicious dinner full of different flavours and textures with melty cheese, crispy potato wedges and rich, beefy chilli! It's such a treat for any night of the week and fully customisable: try experimenting with the seasoning for the wedges to find your favourite. Prefer more of a kick? Simply add more spice for a hotter chilli! Serve with a green salad or fresh spinach leaves.

Special Occasion

FOR THE WEDGES

Preheat the oven to 220°C (fan 200°C/gas mark 7).

Microwave the potato wedges in a microwaveable bowl on high for 3 minutes. Remove, shake and return to the microwave for another 2–3 minutes. Spray a baking tray with low-calorie cooking spray, then tip the microwaved wedges onto it. Spray the wedges with more low-calorie cooking spray and sprinkle over the seasoning of your choice. Bake in the oven for about 25 minutes until golden brown, shaking the tray several times during cooking so that the wedges cook evenly.

While the wedges are in the oven, make the chilli.

CHILLI – HOB-TOP METHOD

Spray a large frying pan (that has a lid) with low-calorie cooking spray and place over a high heat, then add the onion, carrot, swede and celery and sauté for about 5 minutes until they start to soften. Add the mince, garlic, chilli and chilli powder and fry for 5 minutes until the mince is browned. Stir in the kidney beans, chopped tomatoes and stock, cover, then bring to the boil. Reduce the heat and simmer for 20–30 minutes.

Remove the lid and simmer for a few more minutes until it thickens, if necessary.

CHILLI – ELECTRIC PRESSURE-COOKER METHOD

SPECIAL EQUIPMENT
Electric pressure cooker

Set the pressure cooker to 'sauté' and spray it with a little low-calorie cooking spray. Add the onion and cook for 5 minutes until translucent, then add the minced beef and chilli powder and sauté for 5 minutes until browned. If your pressure cooker doesn't have a sauté function, do this step in a saucepan on the hob, then transfer to the pressure cooker when done.

Add the garlic, chilli powder and stock, stir, then add the tinned tomatoes and red kidney beans. Finally, tip in the diced veg. Turn off the 'saute' mode, cover with the lid and set the valve to 'sealing'. Pressure-cook on high for 15 minutes, then use the 'manual release' function to release pressure from the pot. The chilli should have thickened – if you want it thicker, cook it for a further 5–10 minutes at 'sauté' setting to reduce the liquid.

TO FINISH

Pour the chilli into the ovenproof dish and arrange the wedges around the dish. Spread the light spreadable cheese over the top of the chilli and sprinkle with the Cheddar. Bake in the preheated oven for 5–10 minutes until the cheese is melted and golden brown. Serve, scattered with coriander leaves.

"
" I just wanted to thank you so much for creating such deliciousness and sharing it with us."

—— **ABBY**

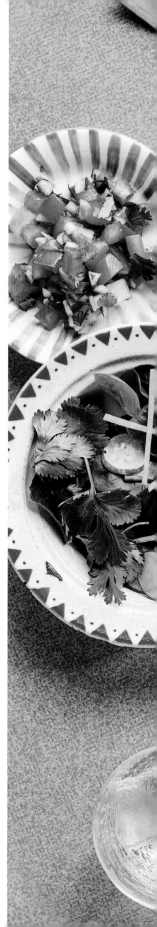

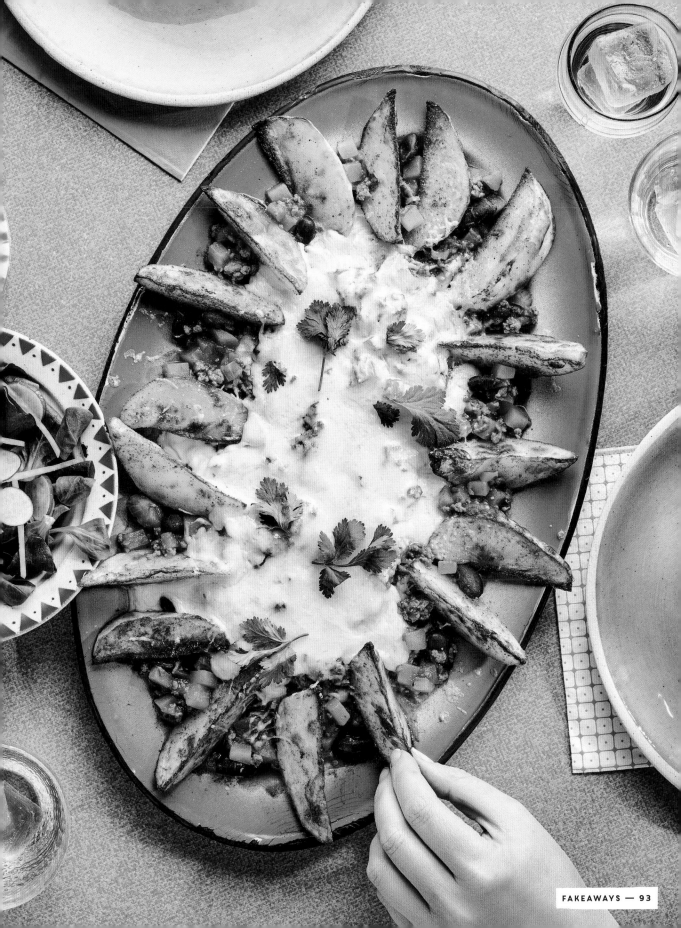

TACHOS

🕐 **20 MINS**　🗑 **15 MINS**　✕ **SERVES 4**

Beef mix only

F ❜

PER SERVING:
326 KCAL /35G CARBS

FOR THE TACO MIX
low-calorie cooking spray
1 onion, peeled and diced
1 red pepper, deseeded
　and diced
250g 5%-fat minced beef
2 garlic cloves, peeled
　and crushed
½ tsp onion granules
½tsp dried oregano
½ tsp ground cumin
½ tsp sweet smoked paprika
1 very low-salt beef stock cube
150ml boiling water
juice of ½ lime
50g lightly salted tortilla chips
10g reduced-fat Cheddar,
　finely grated

FOR THE SALSA
1 tomato, diced
1 spring onion, trimmed and
　thinly sliced
juice of ½ lime
4g fresh coriander, chopped

TO SERVE
4 low-calorie soft tortilla wraps
40g reduced-fat mature
　Cheddar, grated
30g crisp lettuce, shredded

We've combined rich beef taco mince with a layer of cheesy nachos, all wrapped up in a soft taco, and there you have it – a Tacho is born! With fresh, crisp shredded lettuce, tangy salsa and even more cheese (and a dash of hot sauce wouldn't hurt), this dish is perfect for a midweek family feast.

Everyday Light

Spray a frying pan with low-calorie cooking spray and place over a medium heat. Add the onion and pepper and fry for 2 minutes until softened, then add the minced beef and fry for 3 minutes until browned all over. Add the garlic, onion granules, dried oregano, ground cumin and paprika and cook for a further 2 minutes.

Crumble in the stock cube and pour in the boiling water, reduce the heat and let the mixture bubble for 5 minutes until the meat is coated in a rich beefy sauce. Stir in the lime juice.

While the beef is cooking, spread the tortilla chips out on a baking tray and cover with the finely grated Cheddar. Pop under a hot grill for a few minutes until the cheese has melted, then set to one side.

Combine the salsa ingredients in a small bowl and stir until everything is coated in the lime juice.

Now you are ready to assemble. Fold a tortilla wrap into a cone shape and spoon some of the beef mixture into it, then add a layer of cheesy nachos down one side of the wrap. Sprinkle some of the grated Cheddar on top of the beef and add some lettuce. Repeat with the other three tortillas.

Finish the Tachos with some of the salsa and serve.

TIPS: If you like things spicier, stir a little hot sauce through the salsa or drizzle some over the assembled tachos, for a little fiery heat! Warm the tortillas in a hot pan if you like, before shaping and filling.

SWAP THIS: Swap the beef for pork or turkey. For a dairy-free dish, swap the Cheddar for a dairy-free alternative.

MAKE IT VEGGIE: Swap the beef mince and beef stock cube for vegetarian alternatives.

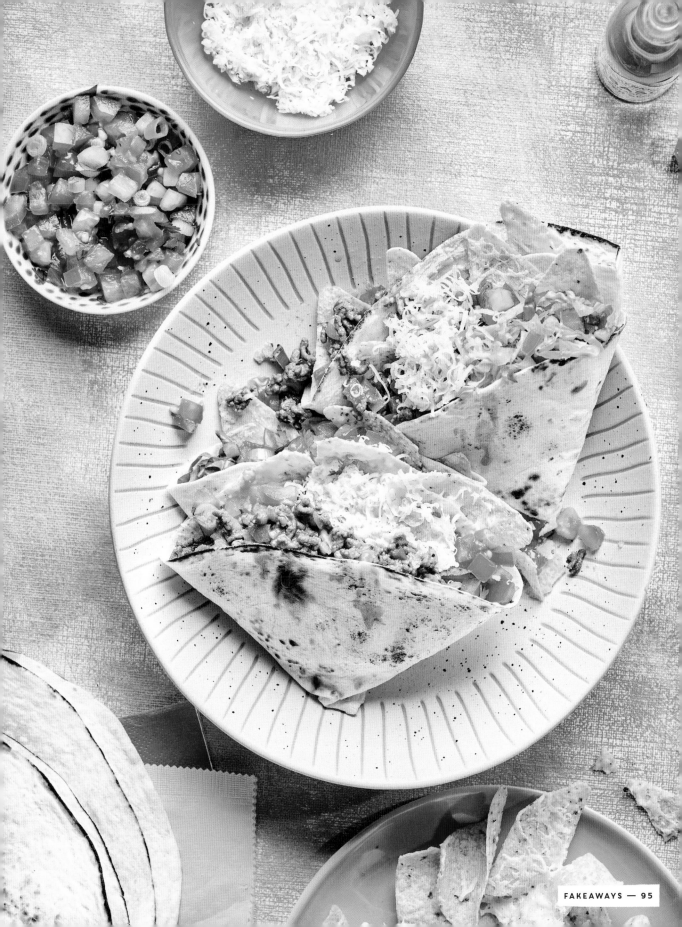

I CAN'T BELIEVE IT'S NOT BUTTER CHICKEN

🕐 **15 MINS**   🫕 **VARIABLE** (SEE BELOW)   ✕ **SERVES 4**

Use GF stock cube ↘

(F)(BF)(GF) ❯

PER SERVING:
320 KCAL /18G CARBS

FOR THE CHICKEN
low-calorie cooking spray
1 onion, peeled and thinly sliced
400g skinless, boneless
  chicken thighs (visible fat
  removed), cut into chunks
2 garlic cloves, peeled and
  finely chopped or grated
3cm (1¼in) piece of root
  ginger, peeled and finely
  chopped or grated
1 tbsp garam masala
¼ tsp ground turmeric
pinch of ground cinnamon
1 medium courgette,
  finely chopped
150g white mushrooms,
  finely chopped
1 tbsp tomato puree
1 x 400g tin chopped tomatoes
juice of ½ lemon
2 tbsp ground almonds
1 chicken stock cube
100g low-fat cream cheese
2 peppers (any colour),
  deseeded and sliced

TO ACCOMPANY
50g uncooked basmati rice
  per portion, cooked
  according to packet
  instructions (+ 173 kcal per
  125g cooked serving)

Imagine a delicious, fragrant butter chicken without the butter! This tasty chicken dish proves you don't need lashings of butter or cream to make the perfect curry. It's so simple, and you can vary the spice if you'd prefer an extra kick. Try pairing it with our raita on page 72.

Weekly Indulgence —————————————————

HOB-TOP METHOD
🫕 **35 MINS**

Spray a large frying pan with low-calorie cooking spray and place over a medium heat. Add the onion and chicken and fry for about 10 minutes until they start to colour.

After 10 minutes, stir in the garlic, ginger and ground spices. Stir for a minute, then add the courgette and mushrooms and fry for about 10 minutes until the mushrooms start to release their moisture.

Add the tomato puree, tinned tomatoes, lemon juice and ground almonds, crumble in the stock cube, and give everything a good stir. Bring to a simmer and cook for 10 minutes, then stir in the cream cheese until it has completely melted. Add the sliced peppers and simmer for a further 5 minutes. Serve!

SLOW COOKER METHOD
🫕 **HIGH: 4½ HOURS LOW: 6 HOURS**

SPECIAL EQUIPMENT
Slow cooker

Put all of the ingredients, apart from the cream cheese and sliced peppers, in the slow cooker and cook on high for 4 hours or low for 5½ hours.

Stir in the cream cheese and the sliced peppers and cook on high for a further 30 minutes. Serve!

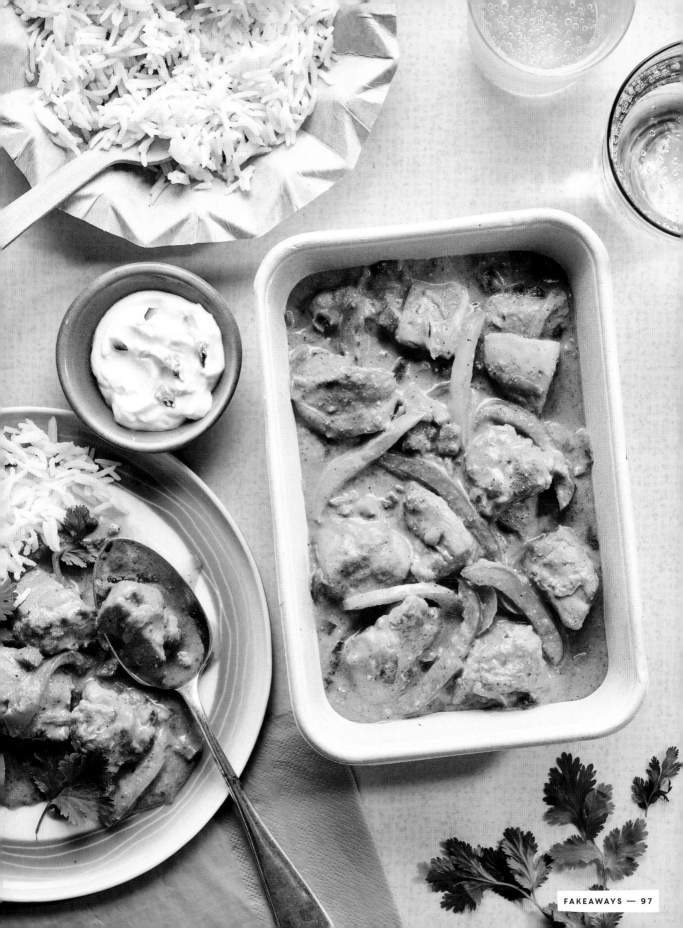

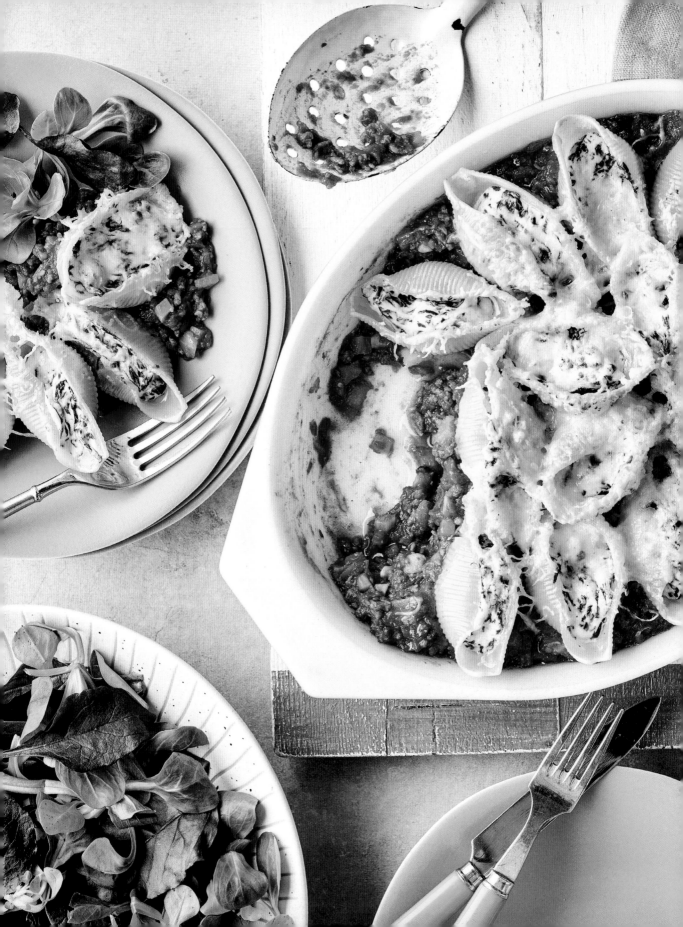

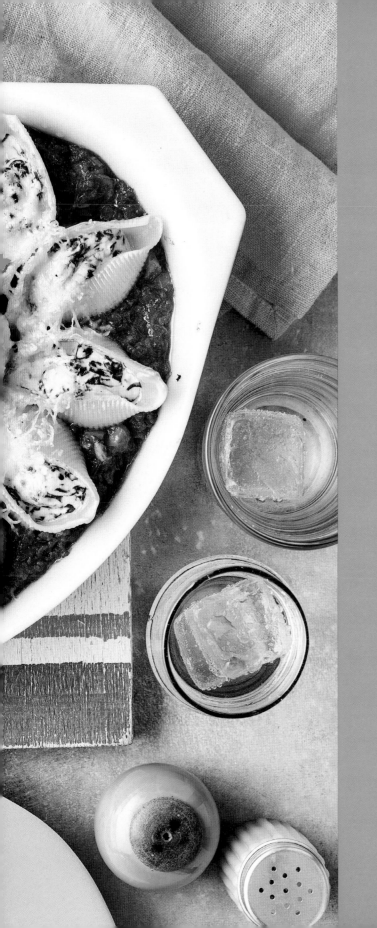

BATCH COOK

CREAMY ROASTED RED PEPPER *and* CHICKEN PASTA

Sauce only

Use GF pasta, stock pot and Henderson's relish

F **GF**

🕐 **5 MINS**   🍲 **22 MINS**   ✕ **SERVES 6**

PER SERVING:
297 KCAL / 38G CARBS

200g dried pasta, such as spaghetti, linguine, fusilli lunghi or vermicelli
3 skinless chicken breasts (visible fat removed), about 150g each, cut into 2cm (¾in) cubes
300g mushrooms, thinly sliced
sea salt and freshly ground black pepper

FOR THE SAUCE
low-calorie cooking spray
1 large red onion, peeled and sliced
4 garlic cloves, peeled and crushed
300g roasted red peppers in vinegar (drained weight), roughly chopped
500g passata
90g low-fat cream cheese
3 tbsp balsamic vinegar
1 tsp Henderson's relish or Worcestershire sauce
1 vegetable stock pot
½ tsp sweet smoked paprika
½ tsp dried basil

This tasty pasta dish uses ready-to-eat peppers for ultimate convenience, saving you time and effort. It's perfect for the fussy eaters among us, as the majority of the veg is hidden in the sauce! We love reducing food waste, and this dish works wonderfully with so many leftover veggies. Feel free to throw in whatever's waiting to be used up in the fridge and it will still taste amazing!

Everyday Light

Spray a saucepan with low-calorie cooking spray and place over a medium heat. Add the onion, garlic and red peppers and fry gently for 10 minutes, or until the onion has softened and cooked through. Add the remaining sauce ingredients (there's no need to add water with the stock pot), stir and blend with a stick blender or in a food processor until smooth. Season with salt and pepper.

Bring a large saucepan of salted water to the boil and cook the pasta according to the packet instructions.

While the pasta is cooking, spray a frying pan with low-calorie cooking spray and place over a medium heat. Add the chicken and cook gently for 5 minutes until the outside of the chicken has turned white. Add the sliced mushrooms and cook for 2 minutes until softened slightly, then add the blended sauce to the frying pan and simmer for a further 5 minutes, until the chicken is cooked through.

When the pasta is cooked, drain and mix it with the chicken and sauce. Season to taste with salt and pepper and serve.

TIP: Using jarred roasted peppers makes this dish super quick and easy. Use the ones in vinegar (not oil), otherwise you'll be adding a load of unnecessary calories!

HOW TO BATCH: The sauce can be made in bulk and frozen in portions ready for a quick dinner – it's a great alternative to supermarket pasta sauce. Cool within 2 hours of cooking, then divide the cooked recipe into portions and freeze immediately. Find detailed guidelines on reheating on page 12.

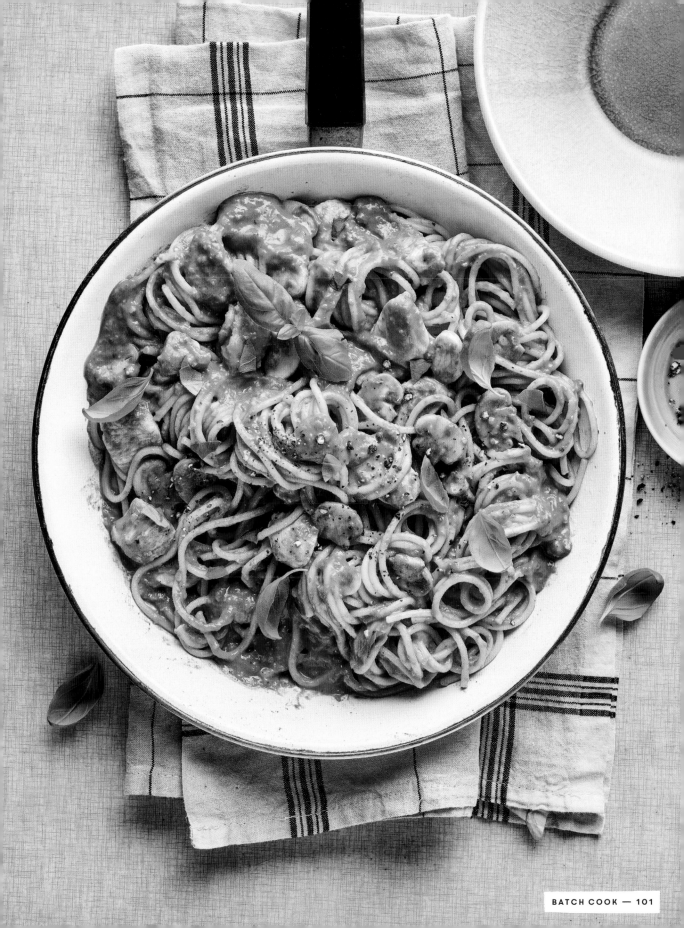

CURRIED SAUSAGES

🕐 **15 MINS** 🍲 **VARIABLE** (SEE BELOW) ✕ **SERVES 4**

Use GF sausages and stock cube ↘

F **DF** **GF** 🌶

PER SERVING:
394 KCAL / 61G CARBS

low-calorie cooking spray

1 onion, peeled and chopped

2 garlic cloves, peeled
and crushed

3 carrots, peeled and cut
into 3cm (1¼in) chunks

1 tbsp curry powder

1 tbsp madras curry powder

500ml chicken stock (1 very
low-salt chicken stock cube
dissolved in 500ml boiling
water) (300ml stock for
the slow-cooker method)

2 sweet potatoes, about 475g
in total, peeled and cut into
3cm (1¼in) chunks

1 white potato, about 210g,
peeled and cut into 3cm
(1¼in) chunks

500g butternut squash,
peeled and cut into
3cm (1¼in) chunks

6 low-fat sausages, about
360g in total, cut into chunks

2 courgettes, diced

2 red peppers,
deseeded and sliced
into strips

fresh coriander, to garnish

TO ACCOMPANY *(optional)*

50g uncooked basmati rice
per portion, cooked
according to packet
instructions (+ 173 kcal per
125g cooked serving)

This recipe came about after having a hankering for a chippy dinner one night. Sadly, a visit to the chippy and trying to lose weight don't usually work well together, so we thought we'd make our own instead! We've crammed as much veg as we can into our version of this popular Aussie dish: even the sauce is made from fresh veggies, which means it's a great way to make sure you're getting your five-a-day and is ideal for picky eaters. Serve with rice, chips, or even both!

Special Occasion

HOB-TOP METHOD
🍲 **45 MINS**

Spray a frying pan or wok with low-calorie cooking spray and place over a medium heat. Add the onion, garlic and carrots and cook for 5 minutes, stirring frequently, until the onion is browned. Add the curry powders and fry for a further minute, then add the 500ml chicken stock, both types of potatoes and butternut squash and reduce the heat to medium-low. Simmer for 20–25 minutes until the vegetables are cooked through.

Blitz the curry sauce in a blender or transfer to a bowl or Pyrex jug and blitz with a stick blender until smooth. Wipe out the frying pan, spray it with low-calorie cooking spray and place over a medium heat. Add the chopped sausages and fry for 5 minutes until lightly browned.

Return the smooth sauce to the pan. Add the diced courgettes and sliced peppers to the curry sauce and cook over a high heat for 10 minutes until the sausages are cooked.

If the sauce is too thick for your liking, simply add some more water or chicken stock. Serve garnished with coriander, with your choice of accompaniment.

> **HOW TO BATCH:** Cool the curried sausages within 2 hours of cooking, then divide into individual portions and freeze immediately. Find detailed guidelines on reheating on page 12.

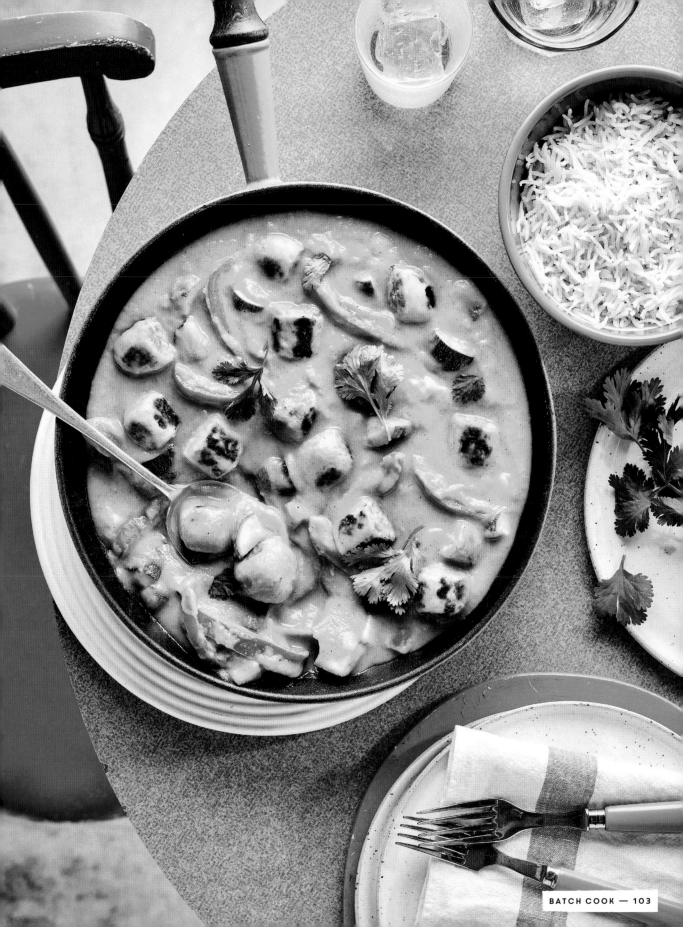

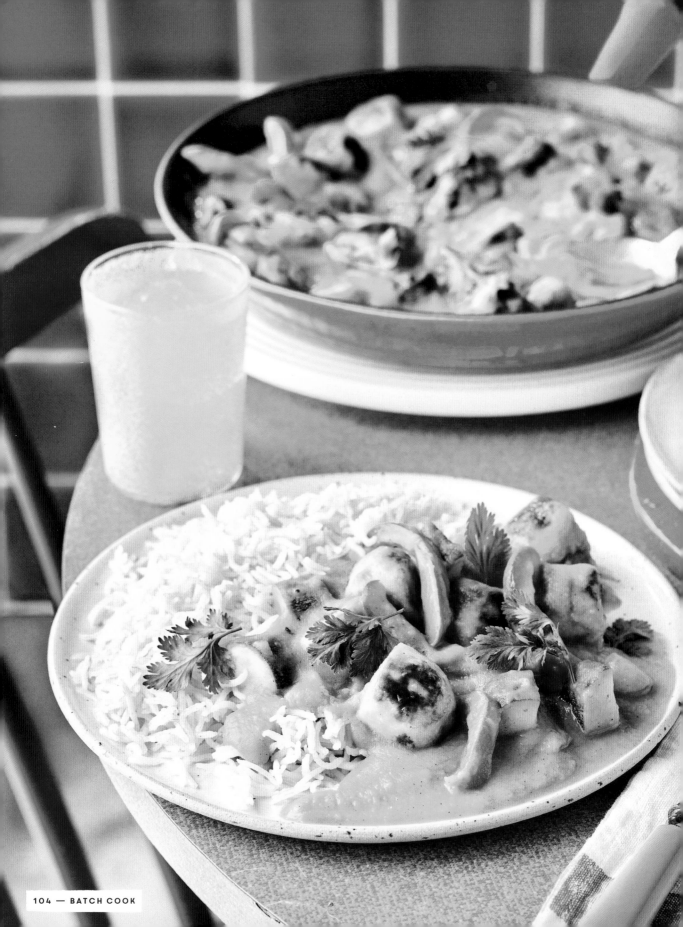

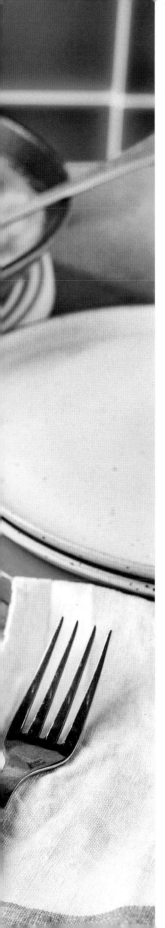

SLOW-COOKER METHOD
🏠 MEDIUM: 4 HOURS 10 MINS

SPECIAL EQUIPMENT
Slow cooker

Spray a frying pan or wok with low-calorie cooking spray and place over a medium heat. Add the onion, garlic and carrots and cook for 5 minutes, stirring frequently, until the onion is browned. Add the curry powders and fry for a further minute, then add the 300ml chicken stock, both types of potatoes and butternut squash. Transfer the contents of the frying pan or wok to the slow cooker and cook on medium for 2 hours until the vegetables are soft.

Blitz the curry sauce with a stick blender until it has a smooth consistency.

Spray a frying pan with low-calorie cooking spray and place over a medium heat. Add the chopped sausages and fry for 5 minutes until lightly browned.

Add the sausages, courgettes and peppers to the slow cooker with the curry sauce and cook on medium for a further 1–2 hours until the sausages are fully cooked and the sauce reduced. Serve garnished with coriander.

" Pinch of Nom has played a huge part in my journey."

RACHEL ———

BANGERS *and* MASH PIE

🕐 **10 MINS**   🍲 **35 MINS**   ✕ **SERVES 4**

Bangers and mash is one of our go-to weeknight dinners when we're craving something quick and comforting. We've revamped this family favourite into a pie, full of the flavours you love with a crisped-up, golden-brown top!

Weekly Indulgence

PER SERVING:
392 KCAL / 54G CARBS

FOR THE MASH
750g potatoes, peeled
  and quartered
1 medium egg, beaten
½ tsp English mustard powder
salt and black pepper

FOR THE FILLING
8 chicken chipolata sausages
  (272g in total), each sliced
  into 4 or 5 pieces
2 onions, thinly sliced
1 celery stick, finely chopped
low-calorie cooking spray
250–350ml beef stock (1 very
  low-salt beef stock cube
  dissolved in 250–350ml
  boiling water)
2 tbsp balsamic vinegar
1 tbsp Henderson's relish
1 tsp garlic granules
½ tsp dried thyme
½ tsp English mustard powder
3 tbsp tomato puree
200g frozen peas

TO ACCOMPANY
80g steamed green vegetables
  (+ 35 kcal per serving)

Preheat the oven to 220°C (fan 200°C/gas mark 7). Put the potatoes in a saucepan and cover with water, add a pinch of salt and bring to the boil. Cook for 15–20 minutes until soft.

While the potatoes are cooking, put the sausage pieces, onion and celery in a frying pan and spray with low-calorie cooking spray. Cook over a medium heat for 5 minutes, until the sausage has started to brown and the onion starts to soften. Add the stock, vinegar, Henderson's relish, garlic granules, thyme and mustard powder, then reduce the heat and simmer for 5–10 minutes until the onions are soft and glossy. Remove from the heat and stir in the tomato puree. The mix should be coated in a thick gravy but add a splash of water to loosen it if you need to. Stir through the peas and set aside while you prepare the mash.

When the potatoes are done, drain the water and mash the potatoes until creamy. Add the egg and mustard powder and mix through. Season with salt and pepper.

Spread the sausage mix in a roasting dish or pie dish. Spoon the mash on top and use the back of the spoon to smooth it out. Place in the preheated oven and bake for 15 minutes, or until the top is golden and the pie is piping hot throughout.

SWAP THIS: We used chicken chipolata sausages in this dish, but you can swap them for your preferred low-fat sausage, or even chunks of chicken breast!

MAKE IT VEGGIE: Switch to vegetarian sausages and vegetable stock.

HOW TO BATCH: Cool the pie within 2 hours of cooking, then divide the cooked recipe into individual portions and freeze immediately. Find detailed guidelines on reheating on page 12.

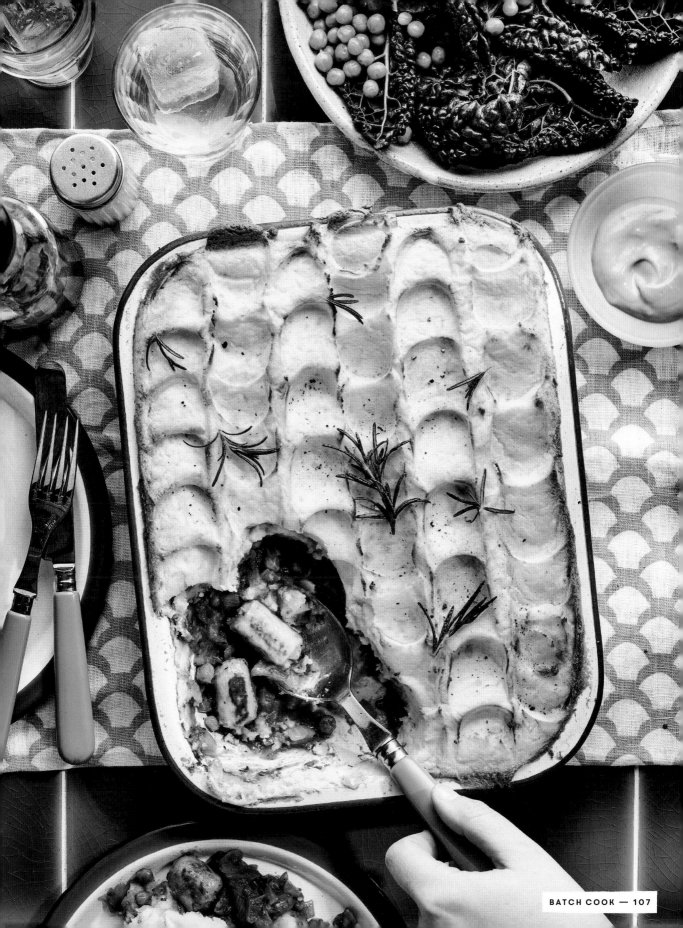

SWEET POTATO CHILLI

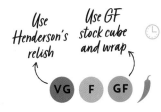

Use Henderson's relish *Use GF stock cube and wrap*

VG **F** **GF**

🕐 **10 MINS** 🍲 **VARIABLE** (SEE BELOW) ✕ **SERVES 4**

This Sweet Potato Chilli has all of the delicious flavours you'd expect from a classic chilli, but without the meat. We think it has a really subtle kick, but you can easily modify how spicy it is by adjusting the chilli powder.

PER SERVING:
346 KCAL / 57G CARBS

low-calorie cooking spray
2 onions, peeled and diced
1 pepper (any colour), deseeded and diced
4 garlic cloves, minced
450g sweet potato, peeled and cut into 1cm (½in) chunks
300ml vegetable stock (1 vegetable stock cube dissolved in 300ml boiling water) (200ml stock for the slow-cooker method)
3 tbsp balsamic vinegar
2 tsp Henderson's relish or Worcestershire sauce
2 tsp smoked paprika
2 tsp chilli powder, or to taste
2 tsp ground coriander
2 x 400g tins chopped tomatoes
1 x 400g tin kidney beans, drained and rinsed
1 x 400g tin green lentils, drained and rinsed
sea salt and freshly ground black pepper
fresh coriander and red onion, to serve

TO ACCOMPANY *(optional)*
50g uncooked basmati rice per portion, cooked according to packet instructions (+ 173 kcal per 125g cooked serving) or 4 low-calorie tortilla wraps (+ 104 kcal per wrap)

Special Occasion ─────────────────

HOB-TOP METHOD
🍲 **40 MINS**

Spray a saucepan with low-calorie cooking spray and place over a medium heat. Add the onions, pepper and garlic and fry for 5 minutes until the onions start to soften, then add the sweet potato, 300ml stock, vinegar, relish, paprika, chilli powder and ground coriander. Stir and cook for a further 5 minutes. Add the tomatoes, beans and lentils and stir well. Once it's bubbling, reduce the heat and cover. Cook for 30 minutes, stirring occasionally, until the sweet potato is tender and the sauce is rich and thick. Loosen it with a splash of water if it seems too thick. Season and serve with rice or wraps, coriander and red onion.

SLOW-COOKER METHOD
🍲 **HIGH: 3–4 HOURS LOW: 6–8 HOURS**

Spray a frying pan with low-calorie cooking spray and place over a medium heat. Add the onions, pepper and garlic and fry for 5 minutes until the onions start to soften, then add the sweet potato, 200ml stock, balsamic vinegar, relish, paprika, chilli powder and ground coriander. Stir and cook for a further 5 minutes. Transfer everything to the slow cooker, add the tomatoes, beans and lentils and stir well. Cover and cook for 3–4 hours on high or 6–8 hours on low. When it's ready the sweet potato will be tender and the sauce rich and thick. Loosen with a splash of water if it seems too thick. Season and serve with your choice of accompaniment, coriander and red onion.

> **HOW TO BATCH:** Cool within 2 hours of cooking, then divide the cooked recipe into individual portions and freeze immediately. Find detailed guidelines on reheating on page 12.

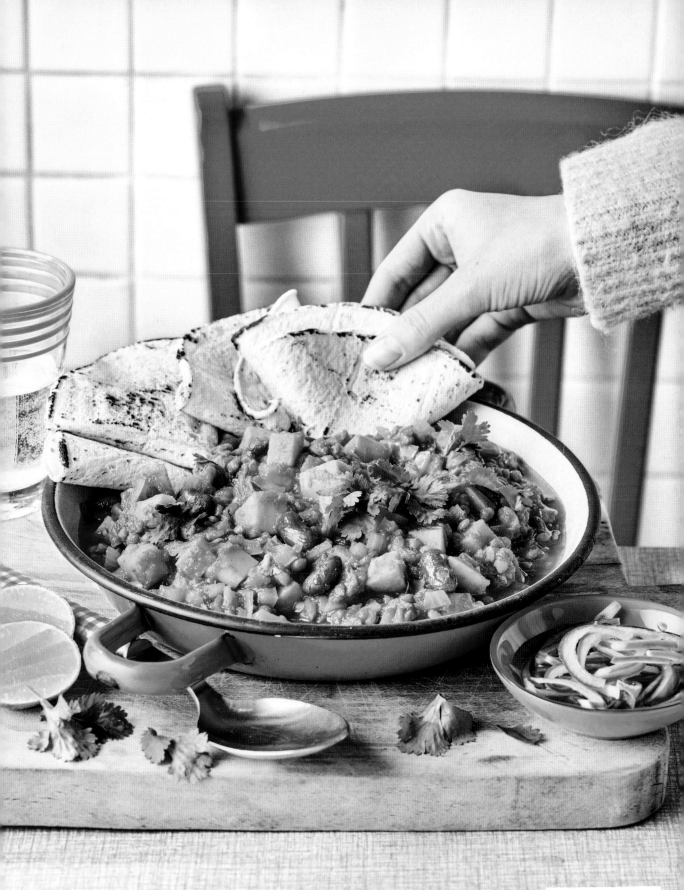

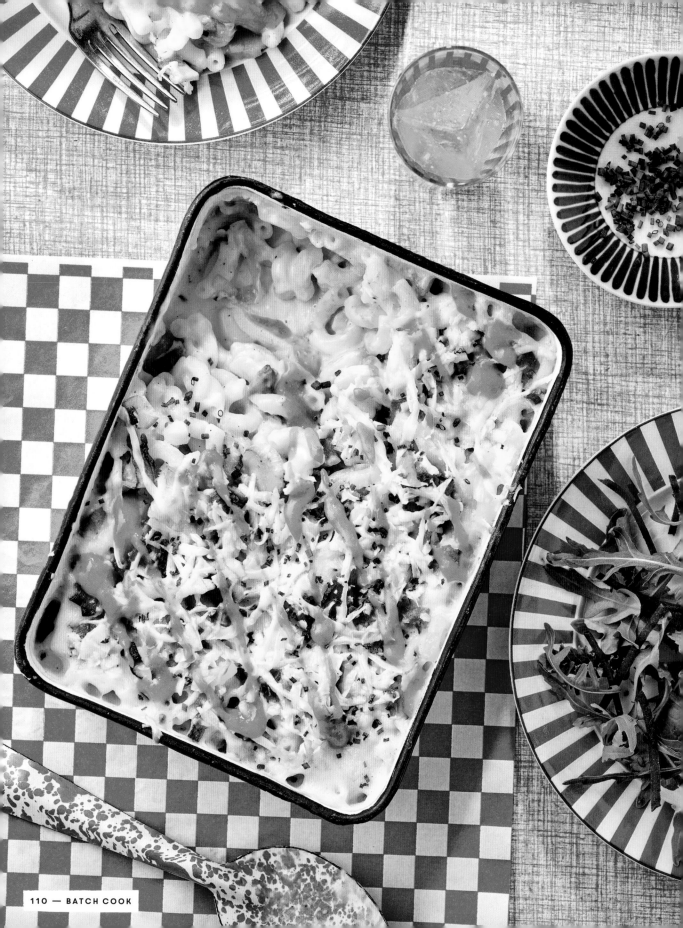

BACON *and* LEEK MAC 'N' CHEESE

⏰ **10 MINS**　🍲 **35 MINS**　✕ **SERVES 4**

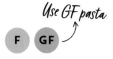

Use GF pasta ↘

F　**GF**

PER SERVING:
459 KCAL / 50G CARBS

SPECIAL EQUIPMENT
18 x 27cm (7 x 10½in)
ovenproof dish

200g dried macaroni
low-calorie cooking spray
1 leek, washed and chopped
6 smoked bacon medallions
　(about 180g), diced

FOR THE CHEESE SAUCE
500ml skimmed milk
25g reduced-fat spread
2 tbsp cornflour
100g reduced-fat mature
　Cheddar, finely grated
¼ tsp English mustard powder
sea salt and freshly ground
　black pepper

FOR THE TOP
20g reduced-fat mature
　Cheddar, finely grated

TO ACCOMPANY *(optional)*
75g mixed salad (+ 15 kcal per
　serving), a drizzle of hot sauce

We've added bacon and leeks to this comfort-food favourite to give it an extra twist. Using skimmed milk, reduced-fat spread and reduced-fat cheese means that we keep the calories down without compromising on that classic, cheesy flavour. Using strong mature reduced-fat Cheddar really boosts the cheesiness!

Weekly Indulgence

Put the macaroni in a large saucepan of boiling water, then lower the heat and partially cover with a lid. Simmer for about 10 minutes or until al dente. Drain and return to the pan, covering to keep it warm. Set aside off the heat.

Now make the cheese sauce. Pour the milk into a small saucepan, add the reduced-fat spread, and heat gently until steaming hot and the reduced-fat spread has melted. Take care not to let the milk boil over.

Mix the cornflour with 2 tablespoons of water in a bowl until smooth, then pour the cornflour mixture into the hot milk, stirring constantly with a balloon whisk or wooden spoon. Simmer for 3–5 minutes, stirring, until the sauce is smooth and has thickened slightly. Stir in the grated cheese and mustard. Season if needed and remove from the heat.

Spray a frying pan with low-calorie cooking spray and place over a medium heat. Add the leek and cook for 10 minutes or until softened, then add the bacon and cook for a further 5 minutes. Mix the leek and bacon with the macaroni in the saucepan, then stir in the cheese sauce. Tip into the ovenproof dish, sprinkle with the remaining cheese and place under a hot grill for a few minutes to brown the top. Serve with your choice of accompaniment.

SWAP THIS: Swap the bacon for cooked ham, and try using different small pasta shapes, such as penne.

HOW TO BATCH: Cool within 2 hours of cooking, then divide the cooked recipe into individual servings and freeze immediately. Find detailed guidelines on reheating on page 12.

SLOW-COOKER STROGANOFF

🕐 **10 MINS**   🍲 **VARIABLE** (SEE BELOW)   ✕ **SERVES 4**

Use GF stock pot or cube and Henderson's relish ↘

PER SERVING:
261 KCAL / 8.5G CARBS

low-calorie cooking spray
500g diced, lean stewing
 steak, trimmed of any
 visible fat
1 onion, peeled and
 finely diced
4 garlic cloves, peeled
 and crushed
200ml beef stock (1 very
 low-salt beef stock
 cube dissolved in
 200ml boiling water)
2 tsp Henderson's relish or
 Worcestershire sauce
300g mushrooms, cut into
 chunky slices
180g low-fat cream cheese
2–3 tbsp Dijon mustard
fresh parsley, to garnish

Stroganoff is traditionally a dish cooked quickly in a frying pan, using prime steak. We've had so many requests for a slow-cooker version of our beef stroganoff, so we had to try it! Slow cooking isn't only extra-convenient for busy days, but it allows you to use cheaper cuts of meat too, which is always a bonus! Slow cooking this dish also gives it a deeper, richer flavour and the steak becomes fall-apart tender. It's great served with rice, pasta or potatoes.

Everyday Light ————————————————

SLOW-COOKER METHOD
🍲 **LOW: 6–7 HOURS**

SPECIAL EQUIPMENT
Slow cooker

Spray a frying pan with low-calorie cooking spray and place over a medium-high heat. Add the steak and onion and fry for 3 minutes until the meat is sealed and the onion has softened, then add the garlic, stir well and transfer everything to the slow-cooker bowl.

Add the stock and Henderson's relish or Worcestershire sauce and cook on low for 6–7 hours.

Half an hour before serving, spray the frying pan with low-calorie cooking spray and sauté the mushrooms over a medium heat for 3 minutes.

Add the mushrooms to the slow cooker (still on the low setting), stir in the cream cheese and the Dijon mustard, close the lid and allow 20 minutes for the cream cheese to heat through.

Serve sprinkled with parsley and with your choice of accompaniment.

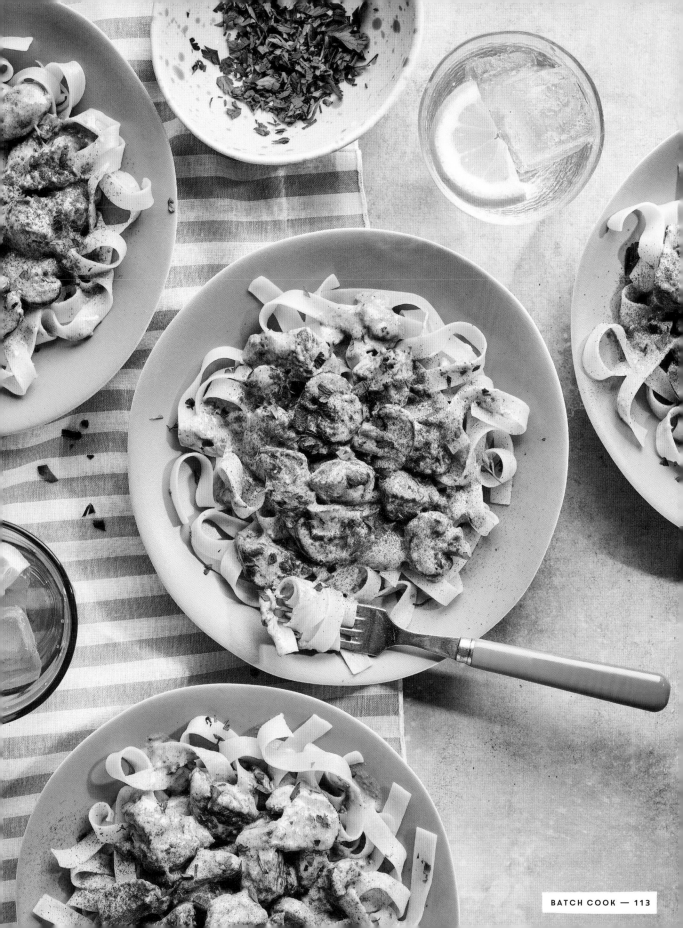

ELECTRIC PRESSURE-COOKER METHOD
🍲 40 MINS

SPECIAL EQUIPMENT
Electric pressure cooker

Spray the pressure cooker with low-calorie cooking spray and set to 'sauté'. Add the steak and onion and fry for 5 minutes to seal the meat and soften the onion, then add the garlic and cook for 30 seconds. If your pressure cooker doesn't have a sauté function, do this in a pan on the hob then transfer to the pressure cooker. Turn off the 'sauté' mode, add the stock and relish, cover with the lid and set the valve to 'sealing'. Pressure-cook on high for 20 minutes, then release pressure naturally for 10 minutes. Release the remaining pressure using the 'quick release' function. Towards the end of cooking, spray a frying pan with low-calorie cooking spray and sauté the mushrooms over a medium heat for 3 minutes. Add the cream cheese, mustard and mushrooms to the pressure cooker. The cheese can cool the stroganoff a little so set the pressure cooker to 'sauté' for a couple of minutes to reheat it if needed. Serve sprinkled with parsley and your choice of accompaniment.

HOW TO BATCH:
Cool the stroganoff within 2 hours of cooking, then divide it into individual portions and freeze immediately. Find detailed guidelines on reheating on page 12.

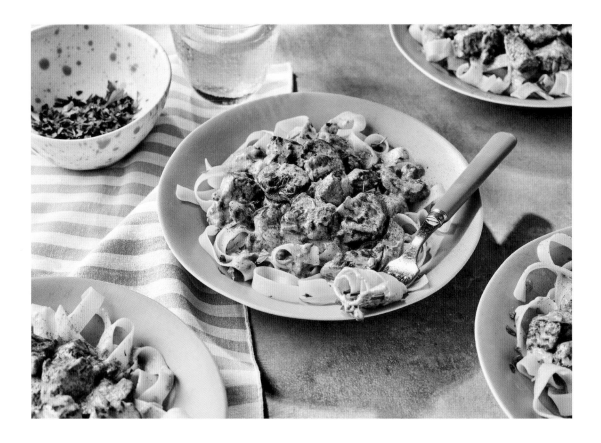

ONE-POT SUNDAY BEEF

 Use GF stock cube and Henderson's relish

🕐 **15 MINS**   🍲 **VARIABLE** (SEE BELOW)   ✕ **SERVES 4**

(F) (DF) (GF)

PER SERVING:
462 KCAL / 29G CARBS

low-calorie cooking spray

1kg silverside or topside beef joint, all visible fat removed and meat tied with string

1 large onion, peeled and sliced

2 garlic cloves, peeled and crushed

400g new potatoes, left whole if small, or halved if larger

1 large parsnip, peeled and quartered lengthways

200g small carrots, peeled and left whole

800ml beef stock (1 very low-salt beef stock cube dissolved in 800ml boiling water) (300ml for the slow cooker, 350ml for the pressure cooker)

2 dried bay leaves

1 tsp dried thyme

1 tsp dried oregano

1 tbsp Dijon mustard

1 tbsp tomato puree

1 tbsp Worcestershire sauce or Henderson's relish

1 tsp balsamic vinegar

sea salt and freshly ground black pepper

TO ACCOMPANY
80g steamed green vegetables (+ 35 kcal per serving)

Our One-pot Sunday Beef is a tasty alternative to a traditional Sunday lunch and means that you won't have to spend hours in the kitchen. The beef is deliciously tender and, as it produces its own gravy as it cooks, the potatoes, parsnips and carrots are super-full of flavour too. This is a real 'meat and two veg' (or three veg in this case!) kind of meal and is perfect served with some steamed green vegetables or our Loaded Cauliflower Cheese (page 224) and Marmite Roasties (page 229).

Weekly Indulgence

OVEN METHOD
🍲 **3 HOURS 45 MINS**

Preheat the oven to 180°C (fan 160°C/gas mark 4).

Spray a large frying pan with low-calorie cooking spray and place over a high heat. Add the beef joint (string on) and sear for about a minute on each side until lightly browned. Transfer to a large casserole dish.

Reduce the heat and spray the frying pan again with low-calorie cooking spray. Add the onion and cook for about 10 minutes, until the onions are softening and are lightly golden, scraping any meaty bits off the bottom of the frying pan and stirring them into the onion. Add the garlic for the last 2 minutes of cooking.

Add the onion, garlic, potatoes, parsnip and carrots to the beef in the casserole dish.

Mix the 800ml hot stock with the bay leaves, thyme, oregano, mustard, tomato puree, Worcestershire sauce or Henderson's relish and balsamic vinegar. Stir, then add to the beef and veg in the casserole dish and cover tightly with a lid. Cook in the preheated oven for 3½ hours, or until the beef is tender. Check occasionally that there is enough stock and add a little boiling water if needed.

Remove the beef from the casserole dish, wrap it in foil and leave it to stand for 5 minutes.

Using a slotted spoon, remove the potatoes, parsnip and carrots from the casserole dish and place them on a large warmed serving plate, leaving the onions in the cooking liquid.

Remove the bay leaves from the cooking liquid and discard. Using a stick blender, blitz the cooking liquid, onions and any other small pieces of cooked vegetables that may still be in the casserole dish until smooth. Taste the gravy and season with salt and pepper if needed.

Unwrap the beef, remove the string and cut it into slices using a large serrated knife. Arrange the beef slices on the serving plate with the vegetables and pour some gravy over the meat if desired, or serve the gravy separately.

Serve with accompaniments of your choice.

SLOW-COOKER METHOD
🍲 HIGH: 4–5 HOURS

SPECIAL EQUIPMENT
Slow cooker

Spray a large frying pan with low-calorie cooking spray and place over a high heat. Add the beef joint and sear for about a minute on each side until lightly browned. Transfer to the slow-cooker pot.

Lower the heat and spray the frying pan again with low-calorie cooking spray. Add the onion and cook for about 10 minutes, until the onions are softening and are lightly golden, scraping any meaty bits off the bottom of the frying pan and stirring them into the onion. Add the garlic for the last 2 minutes of cooking.

Add the onion, garlic, potatoes, parsnip and carrots to the beef in the slow cooker. Mix the 300ml hot beef stock with the bay leaves, thyme, oregano, Dijon mustard, tomato puree, Worcestershire sauce or Henderson's relish and balsamic vinegar.

Stir, then add to the beef and vegetables in the slow cooker and cover with the lid. Turn the slow cooker onto high setting and cook for 4–5 hours until the beef is tender.

Remove the beef joint from the slow cooker using a large slotted spoon, wrap it in foil and leave it to stand for 5 minutes.

Use the slotted spoon to remove the potatoes, parsnip and carrots from the slow cooker and place them on a large warmed serving plate, leaving the onions in the cooking liquid.

Remove the bay leaves from the cooking liquid and discard. Using a stick blender, blitz the cooking liquid, onions and any other small pieces of cooked vegetables that may still be in the slow cooker until smooth. Taste the gravy and season with salt and pepper if needed.

Unwrap the beef, remove the string and cut it into slices using a large serrated knife. Arrange the beef slices on the serving plate with the vegetables and pour some gravy over the meat if desired, or serve the gravy separately.

Serve with accompaniments of your choice.

> **TIP:** Use new potatoes or waxy potatoes as they will hold together during cooking. Don't use floury potatoes as they will fall apart during cooking.

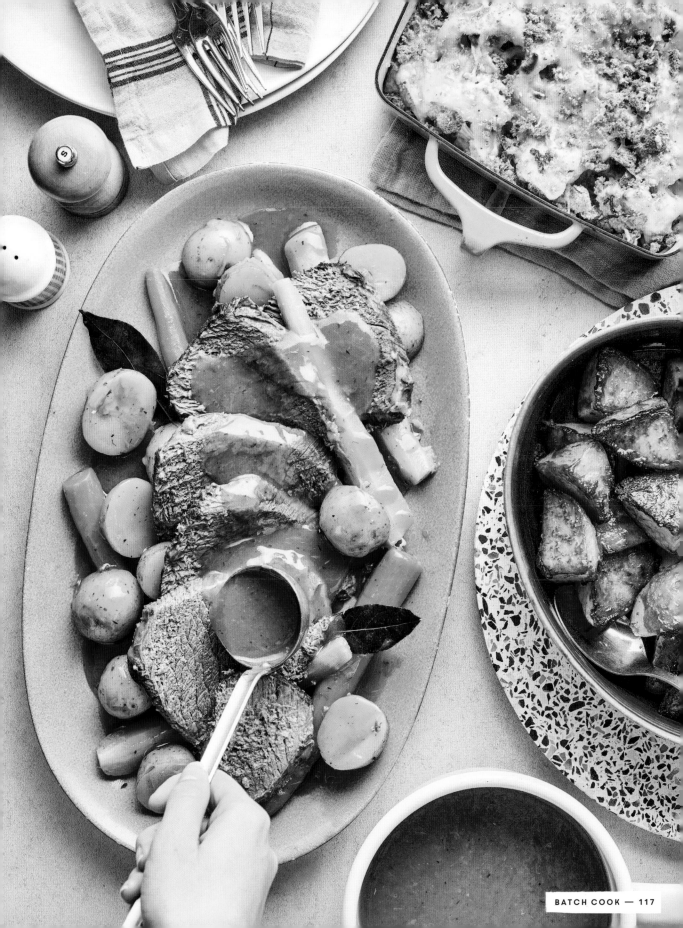

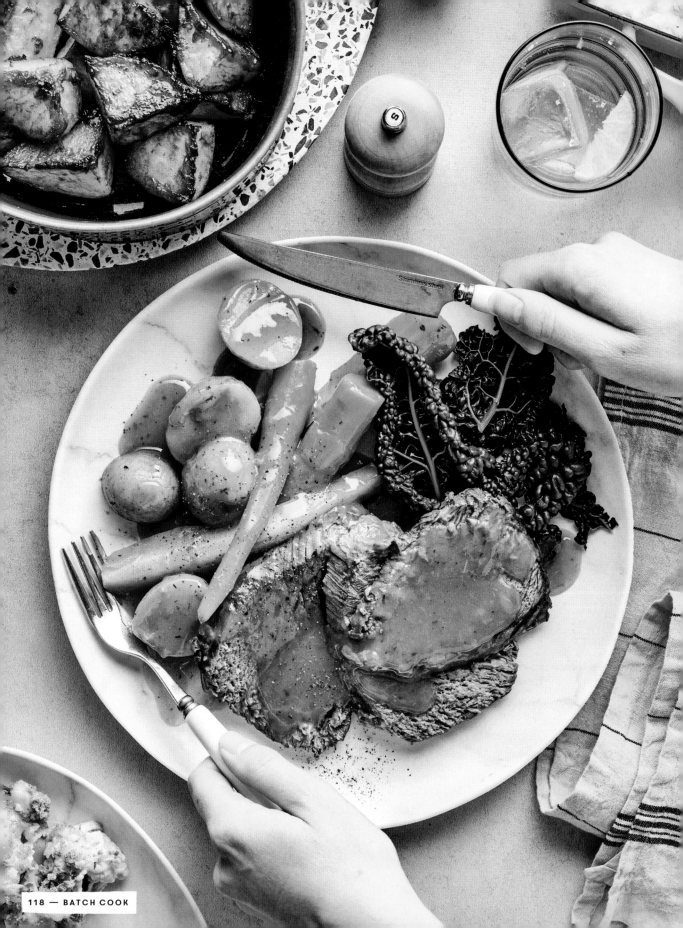

ELECTRIC PRESSURE-COOKER METHOD
🍲 1 HOUR 5 MINS

SPECIAL EQUIPMENT
Electric pressure cooker

Spray the pressure-cooker pot with low-calorie cooking spray and set the pressure cooker to 'sauté'. Add the beef joint and sear for about a minute on each side to seal and lightly brown. Remove from the pressure cooker and transfer to a plate. If your pressure cooker doesn't have a sauté function, do this step in a frying pan on the hob, then transfer to the pressure cooker when done.

Add the onion to the pressure cooker and sauté for about 10 minutes or until softened and golden, scraping any meaty bits off the bottom and stirring them into the onion. Add the garlic for the last 2 minutes of cooking. Return the beef to the pressure cooker, placing it on top of the onions.

Mix the 350ml hot beef stock with the bay leaves, thyme, oregano, Dijon mustard, tomato puree, Worcestershire sauce or Henderson's relish and balsamic vinegar. Stir, then add to the beef and onions.

Cover with the lid and set the valve to 'sealing'. Pressure-cook on high for 55 minutes, then use the 'quick pressure release' function to release pressure from the pot, taking great care not to place yourself anywhere near the escaping steam. When the float valve has gone down, open the lid.

Add the potatoes, parsnip and carrots to the beef. Cover with the lid and set the valve to 'sealing' again. Pressure-cook on high for 10 minutes. Use the 'quick pressure release' function to release pressure from the pot, again taking care near the escaping steam. When the float valve has gone down, open the lid.

Remove the beef joint from the pressure cooker using a large slotted spoon and wrap it in foil. Leave it to stand for 5 minutes. Use the slotted spoon to remove the potatoes, parsnip and carrots from the pressure cooker and place them on a large warmed serving plate, leaving the onions in the cooking liquid.

Remove the bay leaves from the cooking liquid and discard. Using a stick blender, blitz the cooking liquid, onions and any other small pieces of cooked vegetables that may still be in the pressure cooker until smooth. Taste the gravy and season with salt and pepper if needed.

Unwrap the beef, remove the string and cut it into slices using a large serrated knife. Arrange the beef slices on the serving plate with the vegetables and pour some gravy over the meat if desired, or serve the gravy separately.

Serve with accompaniments of your choice.

TIP: If you find the gravy is too thick for your taste, thin it down with a small amount of boiling water, adding a little at a time. If you find the gravy is too thin for your taste, place it in a small saucepan and simmer, uncovered, until reduced down to the desired thickness.

HOW TO BATCH: Cool the beef within 2 hours of cooking, then divide into individual portions and freeze immediately. Find detailed guidelines on reheating on page 12.

SPANISH RICE

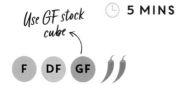

Use GF stock cube ↗

F **DF** **GF** 〃

🕐 **5 MINS**　　🍲 **VARIABLE** (SEE BELOW)　　✕ **SERVES 4**

PER SERVING:
383 KCAL / 65G CARBS

low-calorie cooking spray
1 onion, peeled and finely diced
2 garlic cloves, peeled
　and crushed
1 red pepper, deseeded
　and finely diced
½ red chilli, deseeded
　and finely diced
65g sweet (dulce) cooking
　chorizo, diced
2 tsp ground cumin
2 tsp smoked paprika
2 tsp sriracha sauce
2 tsp tomato puree
300g basmati rice, rinsed
1 litre vegetable stock
　(1 vegetable stock cube
　dissolved in 1 litre boiling
　water) (700ml stock for the
　pressure-cooker method)
2 tbsp fresh lime juice
30g pitted green olives,
　quartered

MAKE IT VEGGIE:
Swap chorizo for a
plant-based sausage
alternative.

HOW TO BATCH:
Cool the dish within 1 hour
of cooking, then divide the
dish into individual portions
and freeze immediately.
Find detailed guidelines on
reheating rice on page 12.

This one-pot recipe is absolutely packed full of delicious Spanish-inspired flavours, including smoked paprika and sweet chorizo. Perfect for the family if you're looking for a fuss-free midweek meal that won't leave you with tons of washing up at the end!

Everyday Light

HOB-TOP METHOD
🍲 **20 MINS**

Spray a large saucepan with low-calorie cooking spray and place over a medium heat. Add the onion and garlic and fry for 3 minutes until just softening, then add the red pepper and red chilli and fry for a further 2 minutes. Once the vegetables are soft, add the chorizo, cumin, paprika, sriracha and tomato puree and fry for a minute.

Add the rice to the pan, pour in the litre of stock and give everything a good stir. Bring to the boil and cover with a lid, lowering to a simmer. Cook for 6 minutes, stir, re-cover with the lid and cook for a further 6 minutes.

Turn off the heat, stir through the lime juice and olives and serve.

ELECTRIC PRESSURE-COOKER METHOD
🍲 **10 MINS**

SPECIAL EQUIPMENT
Electric pressure cooker

Spray the pressure cooker pot with low-calorie cooking spray and set to 'sauté'. Add the onion and garlic and fry for 2 minutes until just softening, then add the red pepper and red chilli and fry for a further 2 minutes. Once the vegetables are soft, add the chorizo, cumin, paprika, sriracha and tomato puree and fry for a minute. If your pressure cooker doesn't have a sauté function, do this step in a pan on the hob then transfer to the pressure cooker when done.

Add the rice to the pan, pour in the 700ml of stock and stir well. Turn off the 'sauté' mode, cover with the lid and set the valve to 'sealing'. Pressure-cook on high for 3 minutes, then use the 'manual release' function to release pressure from the pot for 3 minutes. Set the valve to 'venting', remove the lid, stir through the lime juice and green olives and serve.

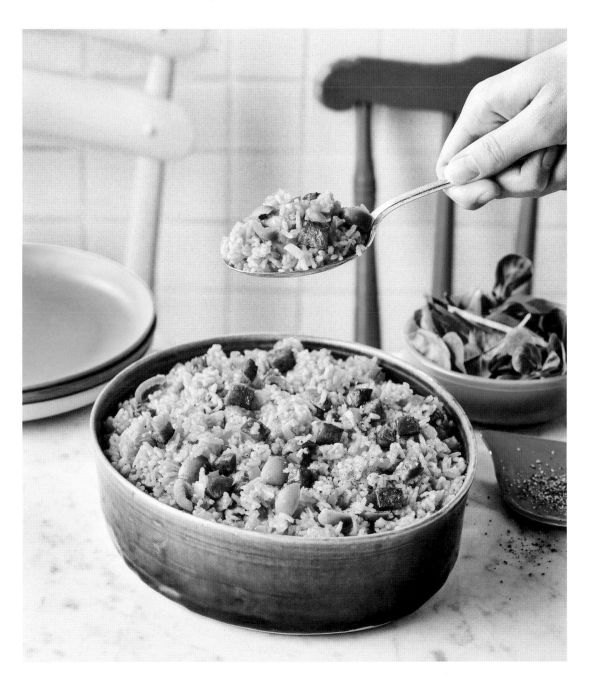

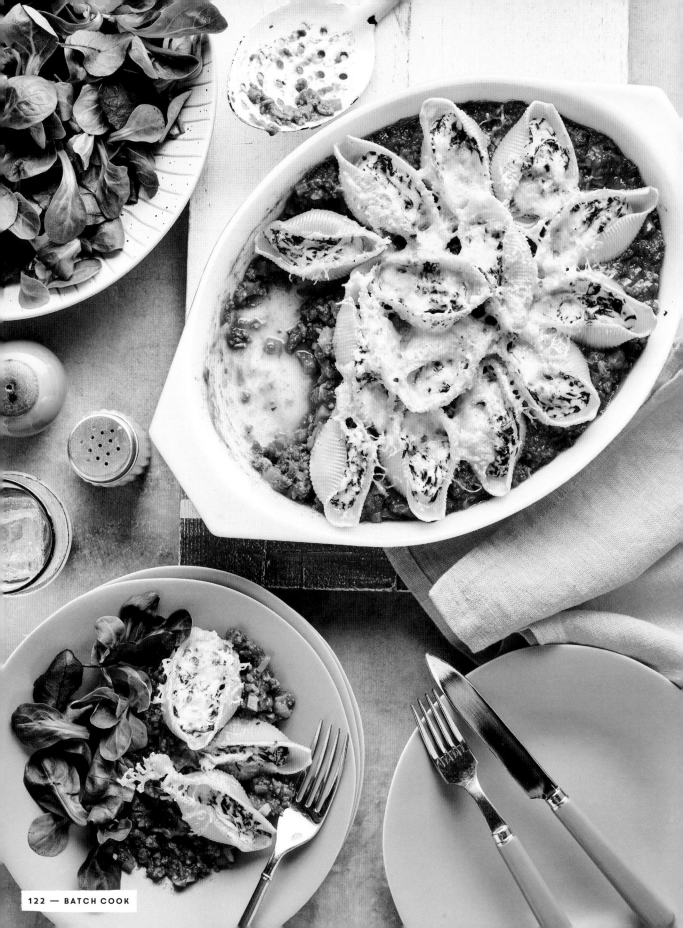

STUFFED PASTA BOLOGNESE

Use GF pasta, stock cube, and Henderson's relish

🕐 **10 MINS** 🍲 **VARIABLE** (SEE BELOW) ✕ **SERVES 6**

F **GF**

PER SERVING:
417 KCAL / 34G CARBS

FOR THE BOLOGNESE
low-calorie cooking spray
1 onion, peeled and diced
1 pepper (any colour),
    deseeded and diced
4 garlic cloves, peeled
    and crushed
400g 5%-fat minced beef
1 carrot, peeled and diced
1 celery stick, diced
80g mushrooms, diced
2 x 400g tins chopped
    tomatoes
1 tbsp Henderson's relish or
    Worcestershire sauce
1 tbsp tomato puree
1 tbsp Italian mixed herbs
1 very low-salt beef stock cube
sea salt and freshly ground
    black pepper

FOR THE STUFFED SHELLS
175g extra-large pasta shells
    (about 20 shells)
70g fresh baby spinach leaves
150g low-fat cream cheese
150g ricotta
1 tsp Italian mixed herbs
½ tsp garlic granules or powder
40g reduced-fat Cheddar,
    finely grated

TO ACCOMPANY
75g mixed salad
    (+ 15 kcal per serving)

This stuffed pasta dish is a real showstopper! It takes some time to prepare, but we promise it's worth it. With rich, meaty stuffing inside tender pasta shells and topped with plenty of melty cheese, what's not to love?

Weekly Indulgence

OVEN METHOD
🍲 **1 HOUR 20 MINS**

Preheat the oven to 200°C (fan 180°C/gas mark 6).

Spray a frying pan or casserole dish with low-calorie cooking spray and place over a medium heat. Add the onion and fry for about 4 minutes until softened, then add the pepper and garlic and cook for 2 minutes. Add the mince and fry for 5 minutes until browned, breaking it up with a wooden spoon. Add the remaining ingredients for the bolognese, crumbling in the stock cube. Let it bubble for 2 minutes, then remove from the heat and season. If you've used a frying pan, pour the bolognese into an ovenproof dish and cover with a lid or foil. Cook in the oven for 45 minutes until the sauce is rich and thick.

Meanwhile, cook the pasta for a minute less than the packet instructions, then drain in a colander. Rinse under cold water to stop it from cooking further and drain well.

Wilt the spinach in a saucepan over a medium heat for 3 minutes, stirring, then remove from the heat and add the cream cheese, ricotta, mixed herbs, garlic granules and a pinch of salt. Stir well – the mixture should be a smooth paste. Spoon the spinach mixture into the par-cooked pasta shells or use a food bag with the end cut off to pipe the mixture into the shells. Place the shells on a plate, cover with a clean cloth and chill until the bolognese sauce is ready.

When the bolognese is cooked, season it and increase the oven temperature to 220°C (fan 200°C/gas mark 7). Place the shells on top of the bolognese, making sure they're nestled in well so they continue cooking in the sauce. Top with the cheese and bake in the oven for 20 minutes.

SLOW-COOKER METHOD
🍲 HIGH: 5 HOURS 20 MINS LOW: 9 HOURS 20 MINS

SPECIAL EQUIPMENT
Slow cooker

Put all of the ingredients for the bolognese into the slow cooker and cook on high for 5 hours or low for 9 hours. While the bolognese is cooking, cook the pasta for one minute less than the cooking time shown on the packet instructions, then drain in a colander. Run the pasta under cold water to prevent the pasta from cooking further and drain well.

Place a saucepan over a medium heat and add the spinach. Stir for about 3 minutes until it wilts. Remove the pan from the heat and add the cream cheese, ricotta, Italian herbs, garlic powder and a pinch of salt. Stir well until combined – the mixture should have the consistency of a smooth paste.

Spoon the spinach mixture into the par-cooked pasta shells or use a food bag with the end cut off to pipe the mixture into the shells. Place the shells on a plate, cover with a clean cloth and refrigerate until the bolognese sauce is ready.

Preheat the oven to 220°C (fan 200°C/gas mark 7).

Place the shells on top of the bolognese sauce, making sure they're nestled in well so they continue cooking in the sauce. Top with the grated cheese and bake in the oven for 20 minutes.

TIPS: You can make the bolognese sauce in advance and keep it in the freezer. Please make sure it is fully defrosted before reheating. You can also serve the stuffed pasta shells as a dish on their own – just cook the pasta a little longer and according to the time stated on the packet instructions.

HOW TO BATCH: Cool within 2 hours of cooking, then divide the cooked recipe into individual portions and freeze immediately. Find detailed guidelines on reheating on page 12.

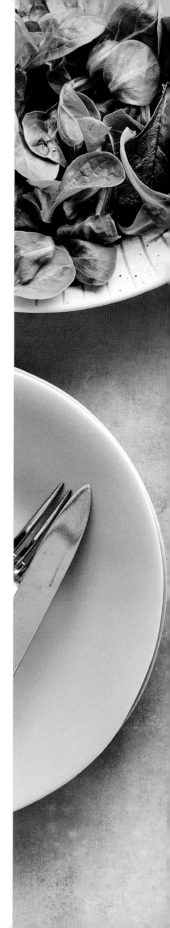

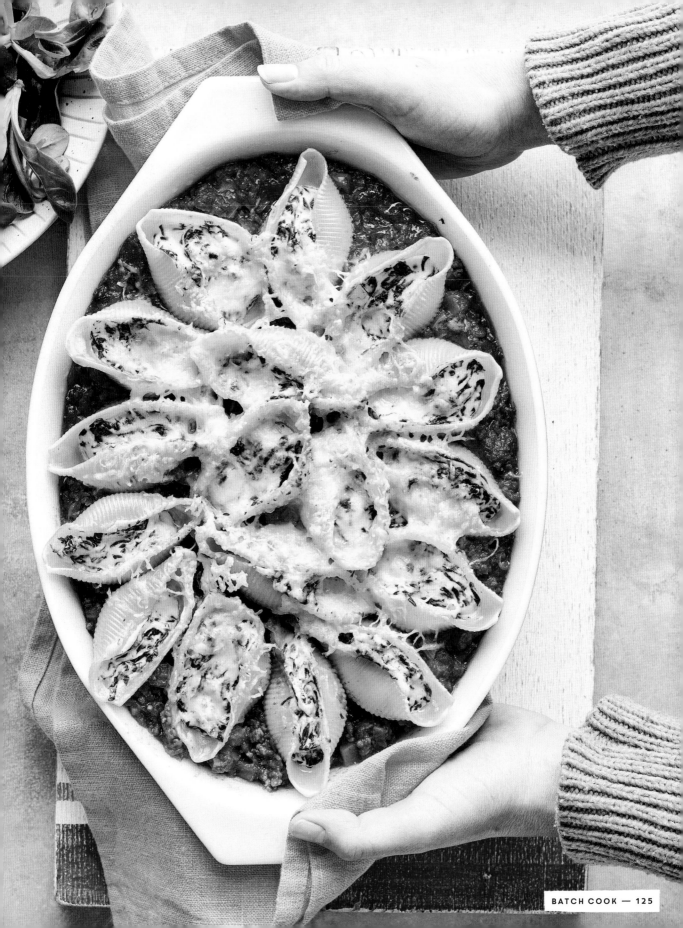

PULLED HAM *in a* MUSTARD SAUCE

🕐 **5 MINS**   🍲 **VARIABLE** (SEE BELOW)   ✕ **SERVES 10**

Use GF stock cube ↘

PER SERVING:
191 KCAL / 1.9G CARBS

FOR THE HAM
1.4kg unsmoked
  gammon joint
600ml chicken stock
  (1 very low-salt chicken stock
  cube dissolved in 600ml
  boiling water)

FOR THE MUSTARD SAUCE
150ml semi-skimmed milk
180g low-fat cream cheese
2 tsp Dijon mustard
2 tbsp finely chopped chives
freshly ground black pepper

TO ACCOMPANY
80g steamed green
  vegetables (+ 35 kcal
  per serving)

> **TIPS:** Some gammon joints need to be soaked in water for a few hours then drained before cooking or they will be too salty. To test if yours needs soaking, cut a small piece off the joint and fry it in a pan. If it's too salty once cooked, soak it first. This recipe coats the shredded meat in sauce. If you want it saucier, double the sauce ingredients. This will add an extra 54 kcal to each portion.

This simple recipe is a great main to pair with any of your favourite sides, and it's perfect for batch cooking so you always have a delicious dinner ready in the freezer!

Everyday Light ——————————————

OVEN METHOD
🍲 **2 HOURS**

FOR THE HAM

Preheat the oven to 190°C (fan 170°C/gas mark 5).

Remove any visible fat from the outside of the gammon joint and discard. Cut the joint into eight chunks, removing any large veins of fat you find while cutting it.

Put the gammon chunks in an ovenproof dish, pour over the stock and cover with a lid. If you don't have a suitable pan with a lid you can use some folded foil and scrunch it well around the top. Put the dish in the preheated oven and cook for 2 hours, or until the ham can be shredded with a fork.

Remove from the oven, carefully take out the meat and transfer it to a bowl. Pour the stock into a jug and set aside. Use two forks to shred the meat and cover with foil to keep warm while you prepare the sauce.

FOR THE SAUCE

Separate any fat from the stock by running the juices through a fat separator. If you don't have a fat separator you can tilt the jug and spoon off the fat that has floated to the top. Discard the fat.

Place the dish you cooked the ham in on the hob over a medium heat. If it's not suitable for the hob, use another saucepan for this step. Add the milk, cream cheese, mustard and 2 tablespoons of the stock, mix well and

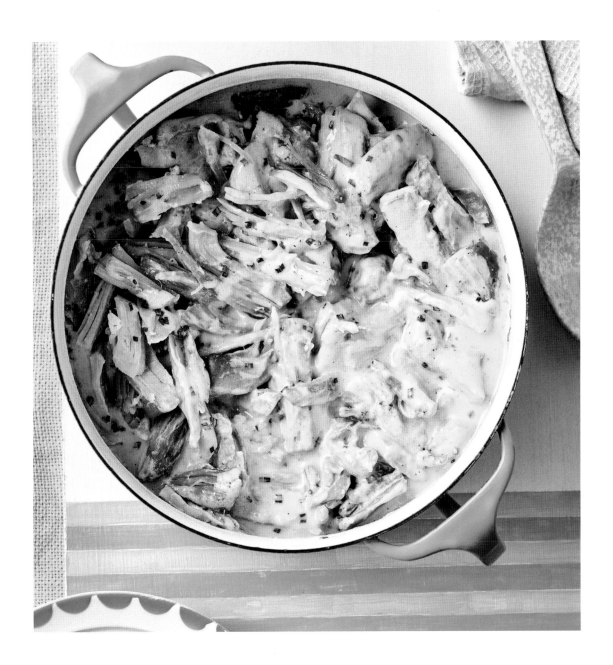

TIPS: Confused between ham and gammon? It's gammon when it's raw and ham when it's cooked! You don't need all the stock for this dish, so once it's cool, you can freeze it in an ice-cube tray ready to use in your stews and soups.

warm over the heat until smooth, then stir in the chives. Season to taste with pepper.

You don't need any more of the stock for this dish but once it's cool freeze it in an ice-cube tray ready to use in your stews and soups.

Tip your ham back into the pan and turn off the heat. Mix to coat the meat with the sauce and serve.

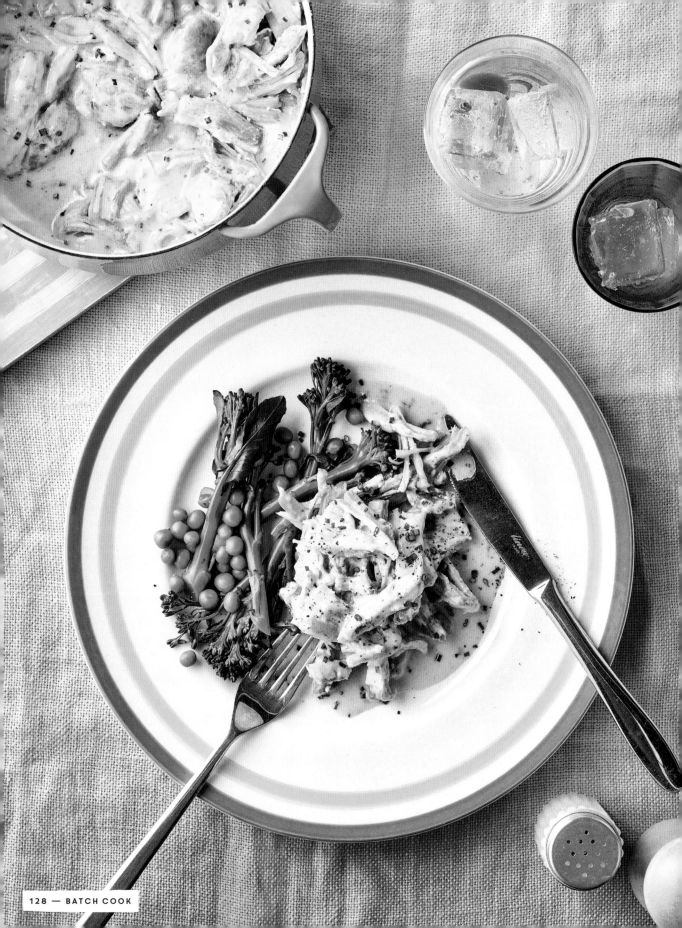

ELECTRIC PRESSURE-COOKER METHOD
🍲 40 MINS

SPECIAL EQUIPMENT
Electric pressure cooker

FOR THE HAM

Remove any visible fat from the outside of the gammon joint and discard. Cut the joint into eight chunks, removing any large veins of fat you find while cutting it.

Put the gammon chunks in the pressure cooker, pour in the stock, cover with the lid and set the valve to 'sealing'. Pressure-cook on high for 40 minutes, then leave the valve shut so the pressure releases naturally. Once the pressure has released, remove the lid, carefully take out the meat and transfer it to a bowl. Pour the stock into a jug and set aside. Use two forks to shred the meat and cover with foil to keep warm while you prepare the sauce.

FOR THE SAUCE

Separate any fat from the stock by running the juices through a fat separator. If you don't have a fat separator you can tilt the jug and spoon off the fat that has floated to the top. Discard the fat.

Set the pressure cooker to 'sauté'. Add the milk, cream cheese, mustard and 2 tablespoons of the stock. Mix well over the heat until smooth, then stir in the chives. Season to taste with pepper. If your pressure cooker doesn't have a sauté function, do this in a pan on the hob then transfer to the pressure cooker when done.

Tip your ham back into the pressure cooker and turn it off. Mix to coat the meat with the sauce and serve.

SLOW-COOKER METHOD
🍲 HIGH: 4–5 HOURS LOW: 7–8 HOURS

SPECIAL EQUIPMENT
Slow cooker

FOR THE HAM

Remove any visible fat from the outside of your gammon joint and discard. Cut the joint into eight chunks, removing any large veins of fat you find while cutting it.

Put the gammon chunks in the slow cooker, pour over the stock and place on the lid. Cook on high for 4–5 hours or low for 7–8 hours.

Once cooked, remove the lid from your slow cooker, carefully take out the meat and transfer it to a bowl. Pour the stock into a jug and set aside. Use two forks to shred the meat and cover with foil to keep warm while you prepare the sauce.

FOR THE SAUCE

Separate any fat from the stock by running the remaining juices through a fat separator. If you don't have a fat separator you can tilt the jug and spoon off the fat that has floated to the top. Discard the fat.

Turn your slow cooker to high and add the milk, cream cheese, mustard and 2 tablespoons of the stock. Mix well over the heat until smooth and then stir in the chives. Season to taste with pepper.

Tip your ham back into the slow cooker and turn it off. Mix to coat the meat with the sauce and serve.

HOW TO BATCH: Cool the ham and sauce within 2 hours of cooking, then divide into individual portions and freeze immediately. Find detailed guidelines on reheating on page 12.

CHEESY AUBERGINE BAKE

🕐 **15 MINS** 🍲 **1 HOUR** ✗ **SERVES 4**

PER SERVING:
188 KCAL /19G CARBS

3 aubergines (750–800g), cut
  into 1cm (½in)-thick chunks
2 red onions, peeled and
  thickly sliced
3 garlic cloves, peeled
  and crushed
low-calorie cooking spray
2 x 400g tins chopped
  tomatoes
2 tbsp balsamic vinegar
½ tsp dried basil
½ tsp dried oregano
½ tsp sweet smoked paprika
pinch of granulated sweetener
sea salt and freshly ground
  black pepper
45g feta cheese, crumbled
40g reduced-fat mature
  Cheddar, finely grated
basil leaves, to garnish

TO ACCOMPANY *(optional)*
80g steamed green vegetables
  (+ 35 kcal per serving)

This comforting veggie main meal is made all in one dish, so it's not only super easy and delicious, but requires minimum effort and fuss too.

Everyday Light ────────────────────

Preheat the oven to 210°C (fan 190°C/gas mark 6).

Put the aubergine, onions and garlic in a large roasting dish, spray well with low-calorie cooking spray and toss to make sure everything's well coated. Place the dish in the oven and roast the vegetables for 25 minutes.

Remove the dish from the oven, add the tinned tomatoes, balsamic vinegar, basil, oregano, paprika, sweetener and some salt and pepper, and mix well. Sprinkle the crumbled feta and the grated Cheddar over the top and place the dish back in the oven for 25–30 minutes, or until the aubergines are soft and tender and the top is melted.

Remove from the oven, garnish with basil and serve with your choice of accompaniment.

TIP: Better-quality tinned tomatoes will really make the difference in this dish. If the ones you are using are a little watery, add a tablespoon of tomato puree.

SWAP THIS: The recipe is so versatile. If you're not an aubergine fan, use courgette instead. If you don't like feta, add extra Cheddar or another cheese of your choice!

HOW TO BATCH: Cool within 2 hours, then divide the recipe into portions and freeze immediately. Find detailed reheating guidelines on page 12.

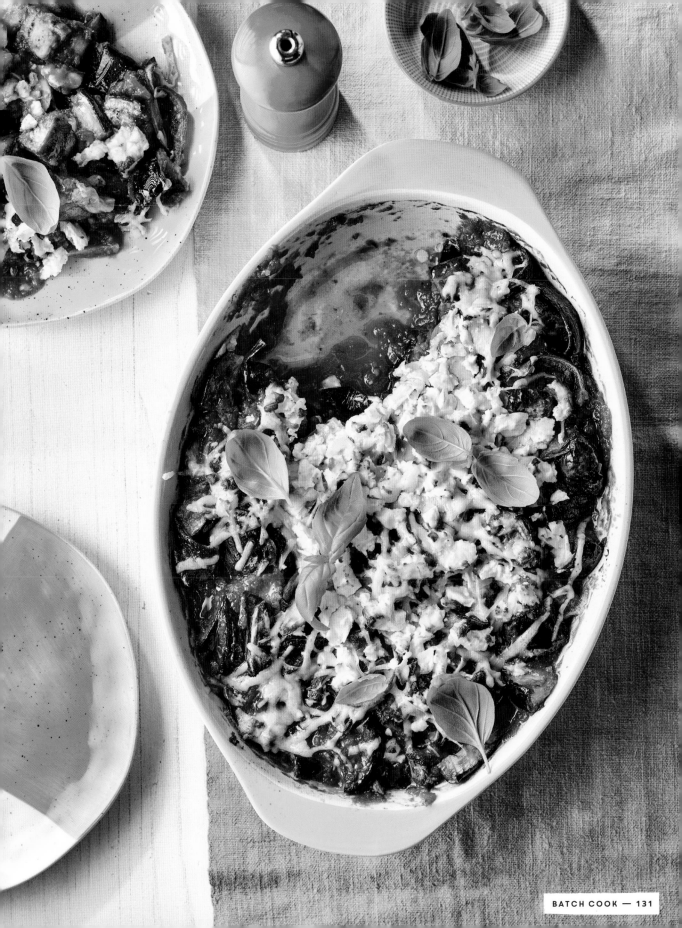

PAPRIKA CHICKEN

🕐 **10 MINS**   🍲 **VARIABLE** (SEE BELOW)   ✕ **SERVES 4**

Use GF stock cube and stock pot

F **GF** 🌶

PER SERVING:
273 KCAL / 13G CARBS

low-calorie cooking spray
1 onion, peeled and diced
2 garlic cloves, peeled and
    crushed
1 red pepper,
    deseeded and sliced
1 yellow pepper,
    deseeded and sliced
600g diced chicken breast
1 tbsp sweet smoked paprika
1 tbsp regular paprika
¼ tsp freshly ground
    black pepper
1 tsp dried oregano
2 tbsp tomato puree
400ml chicken stock
    (1 very low-salt chicken
    stock cube and 1 reduced-
    salt chicken stock pot
    dissolved in 400ml boiling
    water) (200ml stock for the
    pressure-cooker method)
75g reduced-fat cream cheese

TO ACCOMPANY
50g uncooked basmati rice
    per portion, cooked
    according to packet
    instructions (+ 173 kcal
    per 125g cooked serving)

> **SWAP THIS:** For a
> dairy-free dish, swap
> the cream cheese for
> a dairy-free alternative.

This super-easy Paprika Chicken can be cooked in just one pot, which means there's very little faffing around and hardly any washing up either. We've combined sweet and smoked paprika in this dish to give it a slightly smoky flavour, but if you only have one kind then you could also use 2 tablespoons of the same paprika instead. Serve with rice or mashed potatoes for a super hearty, comforting dinner.

Weekly Indulgence

HOB-TOP METHOD
🍲 **40 MINS**

Spray a frying pan with low-calorie cooking spray and place over a medium heat. Add the onion and fry for 5 minutes until lightly golden, then add the garlic and peppers and cook for a further 2 minutes. Add the diced chicken to the pan and brown on all sides for 4 minutes.

Add the smoked paprika, paprika, black pepper, oregano and tomato puree and give everything a stir. Add the 400ml stock to the pan, reduce the heat so that the mixture is just bubbling and simmer for 25 minutes until the sauce has reduced.

Remove from the heat and stir through the cream cheese until dissolved and combined. Serve with your choice of accompaniment.

ELECTRIC PRESSURE-COOKER METHOD
🍲 **25 MINS**

SPECIAL EQUIPMENT
Electric pressure cooker

Spray the pressure-cooker pot with low-calorie cooking spray and set the pressure cooker to 'sauté'. Add the onion and fry for 2 minutes, then add the garlic, peppers and chicken and cook for a further 2 minutes until the chicken is browned on all sides. If your pressure cooker doesn't have a sauté function, do this in a pan on the hob then transfer to the pressure cooker when done. Add the smoked paprika, paprika, black pepper, oregano and tomato puree and stir. Pour in the 200ml stock, turn off the 'sauté' mode, cover with the lid and set the valve to 'sealing'. Pressure-cook on high for 5 minutes, then use the 'manual release' function to release pressure from the pot for 10 minutes.

Set the valve to 'venting', taking care with the hot steam. Set the pot to 'sauté' and simmer for 5 minutes until the sauce is reduced and thickened. Add the cream cheese and stir until dissolved and combined. Serve with your choice of accompaniment.

HOW TO BATCH: Cool the chicken within 2 hours of cooking, then divide the cooked recipe into individual portions and freeze immediately. Find detailed guidelines on reheating on page 12.

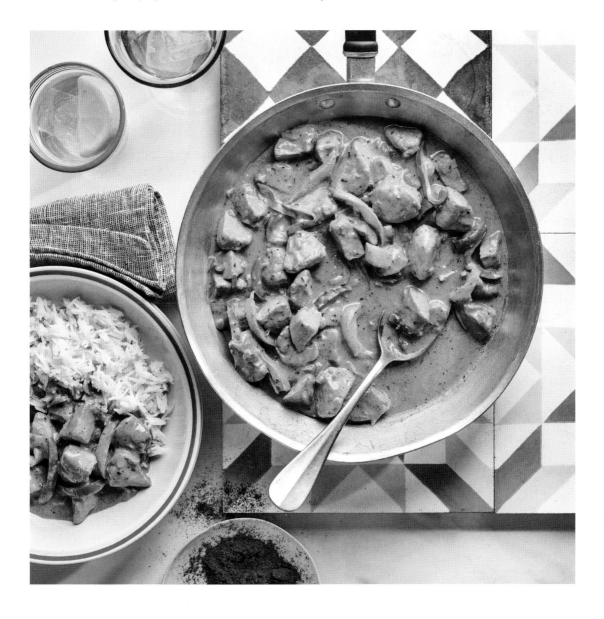

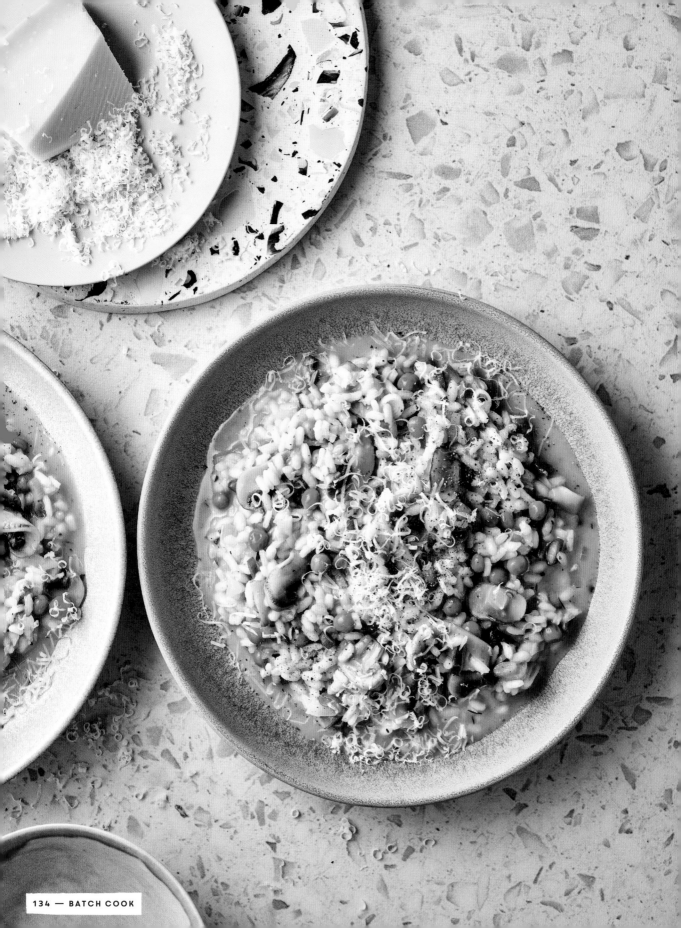

CREAMY, CHEESY GARLIC MUSHROOM RISOTTO

🕐 **15 MINS**　🍲 **40 MINS**　✕ **SERVES 4**

Use vegetarian Italian-style hard cheese and Henderson's relish

Use GF stock cubes

V　F　GF

PER SERVING:
406 KCAL / 69G CARBS

low-calorie cooking spray
1 onion, peeled and diced
400g white mushrooms,
   sliced, leave any smaller
   mushrooms whole
4 garlic cloves, peeled and
   crushed or finely chopped
1 tsp dried Italian herbs
2 tsp white wine vinegar
1 tbsp Henderson's relish
   or Worcestershire sauce
300g Arborio rice
1 litre vegetable stock
   (2 vegetable stock
   cubes dissolved in
   1 litre boiling water)
juice of 1 lemon
1 bunch of spring onions,
   trimmed and thinly sliced
150g frozen peas
60g Parmesan, finely grated
sea salt and freshly ground
   black pepper

Risotto is one of our favourite Italian dishes that can be enjoyed all year round. This satisfying oven-baked version takes away the need to constantly stir, so you can still enjoy a creamy, cheesy risotto but with even less effort!

Weekly Indulgence

Preheat the oven to 200°C (fan 180°C/gas mark 6).

Spray an ovenproof pan (that has a lid) with low-calorie cooking spray and place over a medium heat. Add the diced onion and cook for 2 minutes until softened slightly, then add the mushrooms and fry for about 5 minutes until the mushrooms start to release water. Add the garlic, dried Italian herbs, white wine vinegar and Henderson's relish, stir well and cook for a further 2 minutes, then add the rice and stir. Pour in the stock and bring the mixture to the boil.

Remove the pan from the heat and place the lid tightly on the pan. Place in the preheated oven and cook for 25 minutes.

Remove from the oven and stir in the lemon juice, spring onions and peas. Cover with the lid and return to the oven for a final 5 minutes.

Remove the lid and sprinkle with the grated cheese, and season with salt and pepper.

Serve!

TIP: If you don't have an ovenproof pan, use a large frying pan up to step 3, then transfer to an ovenproof dish with a lid to cook in the oven.

HOW TO BATCH: Cool within 1 hour of cooking, then divide the cooked recipe into individual portions and freeze immediately. Find detailed guidelines on reheating rice on page 12.

HOMITY PIE

 20 MINS **1 HOUR 10 MINS** ✕ **SERVES 6**

PER SERVING:
288 KCAL / 40G CARBS

SPECIAL EQUIPMENT
23cm (9in) round, loose-
bottomed, shallow cake tin,
or oval/round baking dish

reduced-fat spread, for greasing
low-calorie cooking spray
1 large onion, peeled and
  finely chopped
2 large leeks, trimmed,
  washed and thinly sliced
2 garlic cloves, peeled
  and crushed
3 medium potatoes
  (about 450g), peeled
  and cut into chunks
100ml semi-skimmed milk
1 tbsp fresh thyme leaves,
  finely chopped
2 medium eggs, beaten
  with a fork
80g reduced-fat mature
  Cheddar, grated
sea salt and freshly ground
  black pepper
8 sheets (160g) of filo pastry
  (24cm/9½in squares)
1 small egg, beaten, for glazing

HOW TO BATCH:
Cool the pie within 2 hours
of cooking, then divide
the cooked recipe into
individual portions and
freeze immediately. Find
detailed guidelines on
reheating on page 12.

Homity Pie is believed to date back to the Second World War, when it was created to give basic food rations a new lease of life. Budget friendly and really filling, this dish is packed full of potatoes, onions, cheese and leeks, which means it's a great way to help you get plenty of vegetables. It's also delicious cold for lunch the next day!

Everyday Light

Preheat the oven to 180°C (fan 160°C/gas mark 4) and grease the tin or baking dish with some reduced-fat spread.

Spray a large frying pan with low-calorie cooking spray and place over a medium heat. Add the onion and leeks and fry for 15–20 minutes, adding the garlic for the last 5 minutes. The onions and leeks should be softened and golden brown.

Meanwhile, cook the potatoes in a pan of boiling water for 15–20 minutes or until tender. Drain well, return to the pan and mash with the milk. Add the onion, leeks and garlic, then the thyme, beaten eggs and 60g of the cheese. Stir well and season to taste.

Place a single sheet of filo in the bottom of the greased tin or dish and allow the excess pastry to overhang the edge. Brush the pastry all over with some of the small beaten egg. Place another single sheet of filo on top of the first sheet, at an angle. Again, allow the excess pastry to overhang the edge of the tin and brush with egg for glazing. Repeat until all the filo has been used to line the tin. The base of the tin should be completely covered with overlapping sheets of filo. Brush egg all over the final layer.

Spoon your potato mixture into the prepared pastry case and spread it out evenly. Sprinkle the remaining cheese on the top and place on a baking tray. Bake in the oven for 30–35 minutes until hot through and golden brown.

Remove from the oven and cool slightly in the tin or dish, then carefully remove from the tin and place on a plate or leave in the dish. Serve warm.

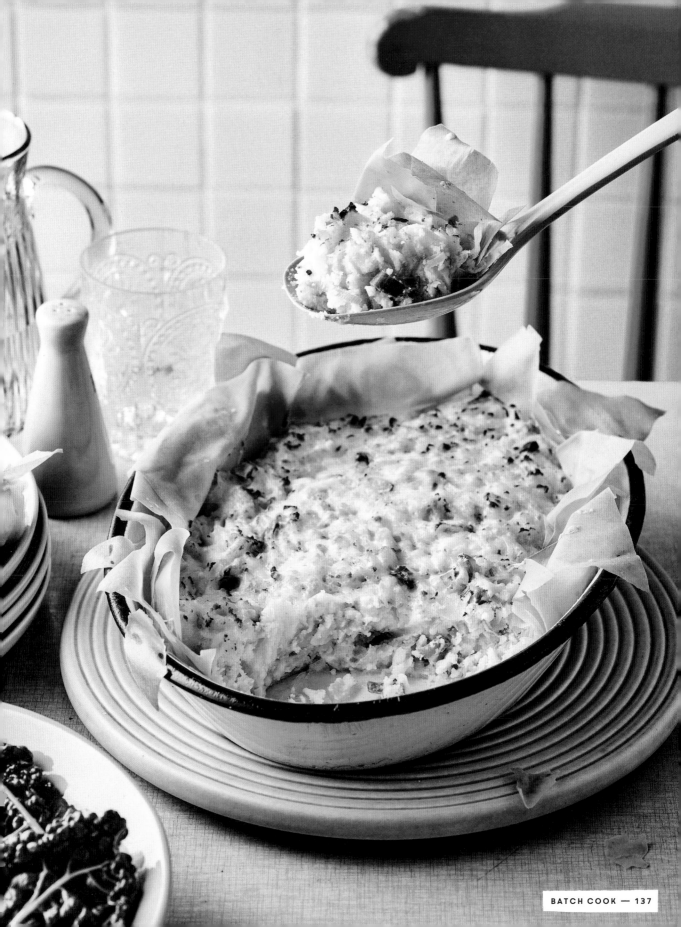

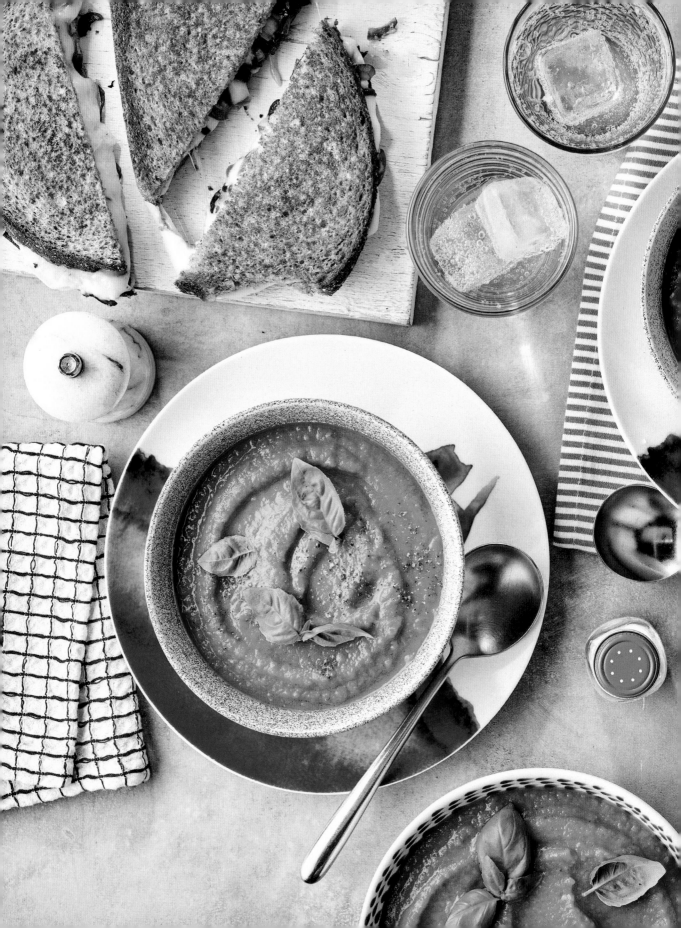

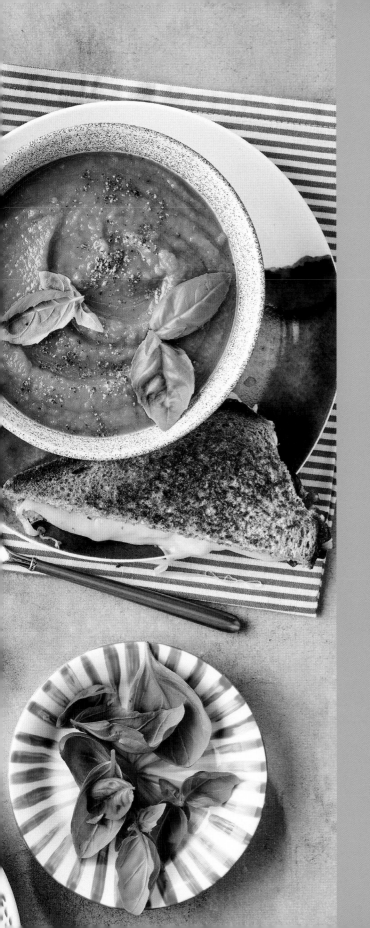

STEWS
· and ·
SOUPS

MATZO BALL SOUP

🕐 **15 MINS** 🍲 **45 MINS** ✕ **SERVES 6**

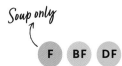

Soup only

F **BF** **DF**

PER SERVING:
171 KCAL / 17G CARBS

FOR THE MATZO BALLS
2 medium eggs, beaten
100ml sparkling water
60g matzo meal
¼ tsp sea salt
¼ tsp freshly ground
  black pepper
¼ tsp garlic granules
¼ tsp onion granules
4g fresh parsley, chopped

FOR THE SOUP
low-calorie cooking spray
1 onion, peeled and diced
2 garlic cloves, peeled
  and crushed
3 carrots, peeled and sliced
1 parsnip, peeled and sliced
2 celery sticks, sliced
2 very low-salt chicken
  stock cubes
1 chicken stock pot
½ tsp freshly ground pepper
1.5 litres boiling water
2 skinless chicken breasts
  (visible fat removed),
  about 150g each
a few sprigs of fresh dill

> **TIP:** If you wanted to make the kcal count even lower, then you could use panko breadcrumbs instead of matzo meal to achieve the same fluffy results for only 168 calories per serving.

Our take on a traditional Jewish dish, this soup uses chicken broth as its base and cooks the vegetables and chicken all together to create a really great depth of flavour. Matzo balls are a dumpling often eaten during Jewish Passover, and we've used the traditional matzo meal for this recipe to give the dish that authentic taste.

Everyday Light

Combine the matzo ball ingredients in a mixing bowl and bring everything together with a fork. Cover and refrigerate for 30 minutes.

While the matzo ball mixture is in the fridge, spray a large saucepan with low-calorie cooking spray and place over a medium heat. Add the onion and fry for 2 minutes until softened, then add the garlic, carrots, parsnip and celery and fry for a further 3 minutes.

Combine the stock cubes, stock pot and pepper in the boiling water in a heatproof jug and stir. Add the chicken breasts to the saucepan and pour over the stock. Bring the soup to the boil, cover, reduce the heat to a simmer and cook for 20 minutes – the liquid should be just bubbling, not boiling.

Remove the pan from the heat, transfer the chicken to a plate or board and shred it with two forks, then return it to the pan.

Spray your hands with plenty of low-calorie cooking spray (to stop the mixture sticking to your hands and make sure the matzo balls are smooth), take small walnut-sized amounts of the chilled matzo mixture and roll them in your hands to make 12 smooth balls.

Add the matzo balls to the pan of soup, cover, place over a low heat so that the pan is just bubbling, and cook for 20 minutes.

Remove from the heat, sprinkle with dill sprigs and serve.

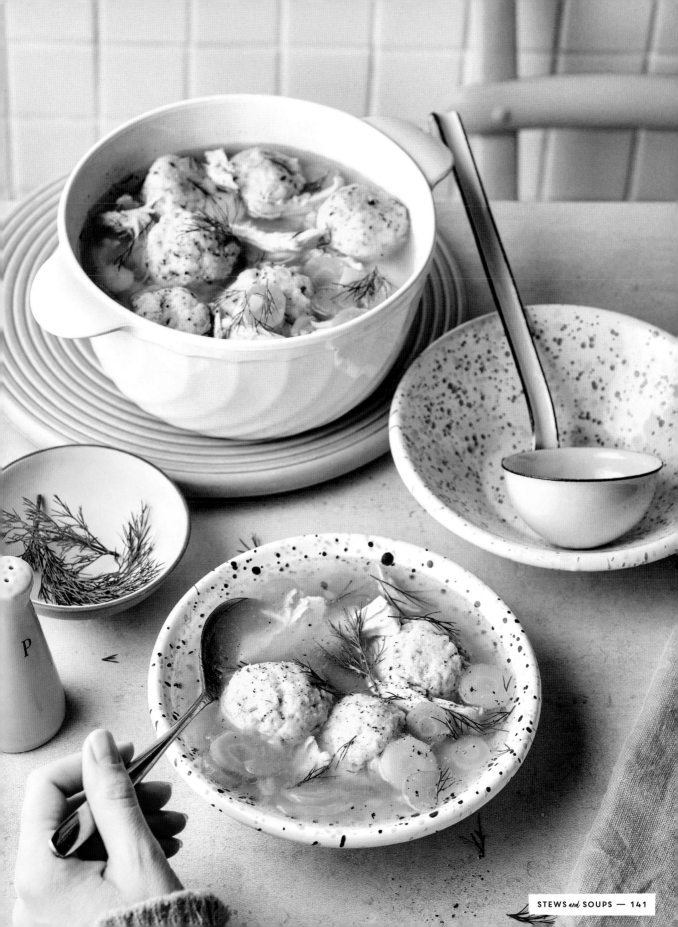

BEEF *and* BAKED BEAN STEW

Use GF stock cube and Henderson's relish ←

🕐 **10 MINS**   🍲 **VARIABLE** (SEE BELOW)   ✕ **SERVES 6**

PER SERVING:
313 KCAL / 35G CARBS

low-calorie cooking spray
500g diced stewing beef,
  all visible fat removed
½ tsp ground black pepper
1 large carrot, peeled and sliced
1 onion, peeled and chopped
400g potatoes, peeled
  and quartered
700ml beef stock (1 very
  low-salt beef stock cube
  dissolved in 700ml boiling
  water) (use 600ml stock for
  slow-cooker method)
1 beef stock pot
2 tbsp Henderson's relish or
  Worcestershire sauce
2 x 410g tins baked beans
sea salt and freshly ground
  black pepper

Baked beans may seem like an unusual addition to a stew but when you combine them with tender, fall-apart beef and fresh veggies, they add a unique richness as well as packing in some extra protein. This filling, hearty beef stew is cooked over several hours for all of the flavours to combine beautifully. Just add a crusty wholemeal roll to mop up the juices!

Everyday Light ─────────────────────

OVEN METHOD
🍲 **3 HOURS 30 MINS**

Preheat the oven to 190°C (fan 170°C/gas mark 5).

Spray a lidded frying pan (ovenproof if possible, but a regular frying pan is fine) with low-calorie cooking spray, add the beef and brown over a medium heat for 2–3 minutes, turning the pieces halfway through so they colour evenly. If your frying pan isn't ovenproof, transfer the beef to an ovenproof casserole dish. Add the pepper, carrot, onion, potatoes, 700ml beef stock, stock pot and Henderson's relish to the casserole dish or pan. Add the baked beans, stir, cover and put in the oven for 3 hours. Remove the lid and cook for a further 30 minutes. Season with salt and pepper and serve.

SLOW-COOKER METHOD
🍲 **HIGH: 6–7 HOURS**

SPECIAL EQUIPMENT
Slow cooker

Spray a frying pan with low-calorie cooking spray, add the beef and brown over a medium heat for 2–3 minutes, turning the pieces halfway through so they colour evenly. Transfer the browned beef to the slow cooker and add the pepper, carrot, onion, potatoes, 600ml beef stock, stock pot and Henderson's relish. Add the baked beans, stir, cover with the lid and cook on high for 4½ hours. Remove the lid and cook for a further 1½–2 hours. Season and serve.

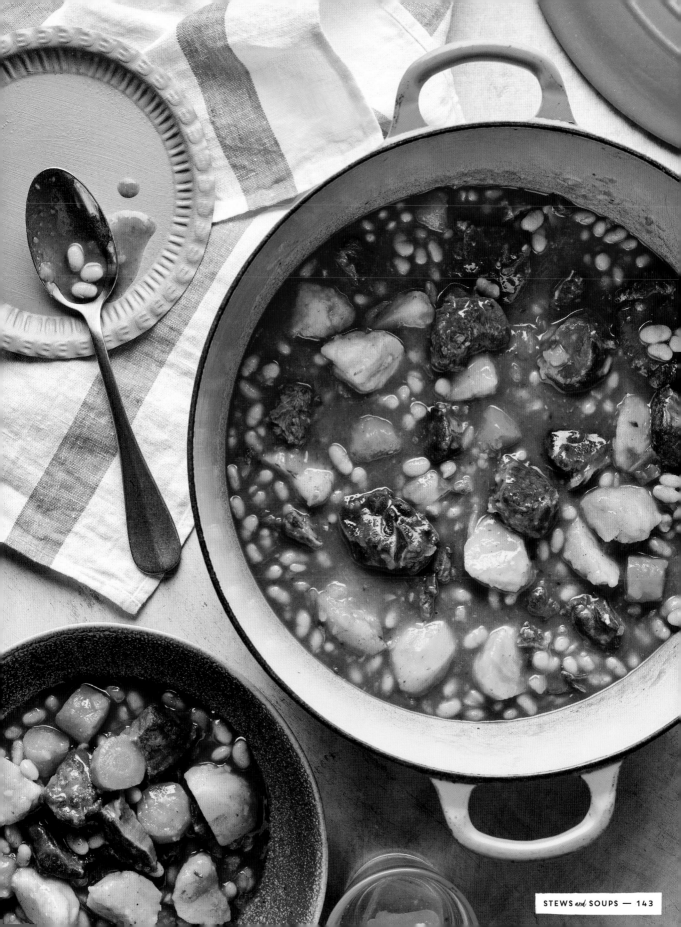

GERMAN POTATO SOUP

🕐 **20 MINS** 🍲 **55 MINS** ✕ **SERVES 6**

Use non-dairy cream cheese

Use GF stock cube and rolls

(F) (BF) (DF) (GF)

PER SERVING:
161 KCAL / 25G CARBS

low-calorie cooking spray
1 large onion, peeled
  and chopped
1 garlic clove, peeled
  and crushed
3 smoked bacon medallions,
  diced
3 medium potatoes (about
  600g in total), peeled and
  cut into 2cm (¾in) dice
3 medium carrots, peeled and
  cut into 2cm (¾in) dice
1 celery stick, chopped
1 large leek, trimmed,
  washed and chopped
1 litre chicken stock
  (1 chicken stock cube
  dissolved in 1 litre
  boiling water)
1 bay leaf
2 tsp fresh thyme leaves,
  chopped
1 tsp fresh rosemary
  leaves, chopped
50g low-fat cream cheese
5g fresh parsley, chopped
sea salt and freshly ground
  black pepper

TO ACCOMPANY *(optional)*
60g wholemeal bread rolls
  (+ 152 kcal per roll)

You simply cannot beat a bowl of steaming hot soup on a chilly autumn or winter's day! This is our version of a popular German soup known as 'Kartoffelsuppe': a creamy and comforting soup packed with vegetables and bacon. Using lighter cream cheese keeps it thick and indulgent without a pot of full-fat cream in sight!

Everyday Light

Spray a large saucepan (with a lid) with low-calorie cooking spray and place over a medium heat. Add the onion and cook for 10 minutes, until golden and softening, then add the garlic and bacon and cook for 5 minutes. Add the potatoes, carrots, celery and leek and stir, then pour in the chicken stock and add the bay leaf, thyme and rosemary. Cover and simmer over a medium heat for 35–40 minutes, stirring occasionally, until the vegetables have softened and the soup is slightly thickened.

Remove the bay leaf and discard. Stir in the cream cheese until completely blended in, then stir in the chopped parsley and season to taste with salt and pepper.

Serve alone, or with your choice of accompaniment.

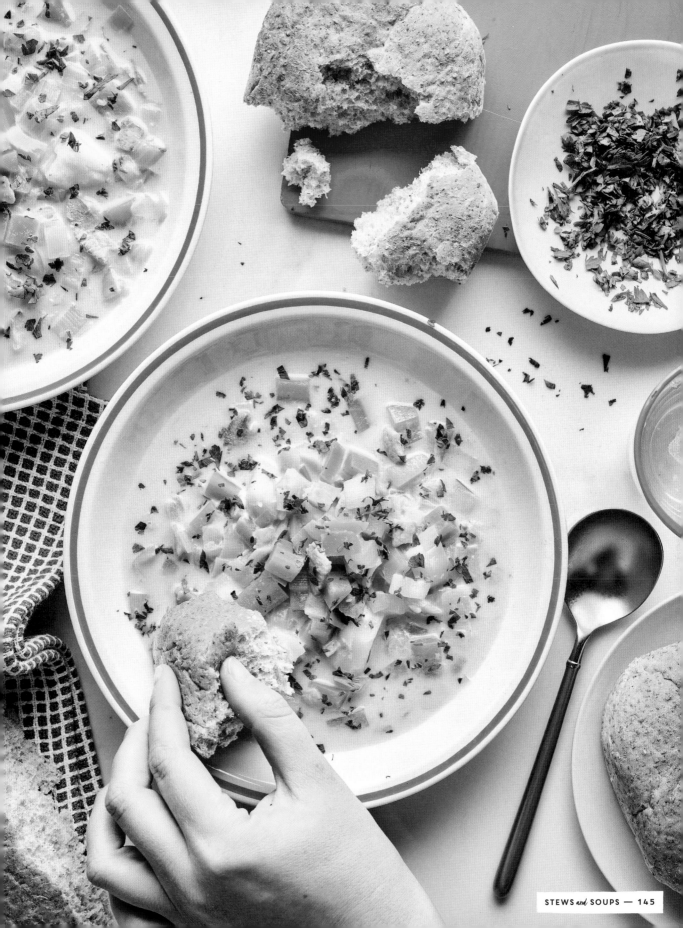

CURRIED CHICKEN
and RICE SOUP

🕐 **15 MINS**   🍲 **VARIABLE** (SEE BELOW)   ✕ **SERVES 4**

Use GF stock cubes

(**F**) (**GF**) 🌶

PER SERVING:
274 KCAL / 35G CARBS

2 skinless chicken breasts
(visible fat removed),
about 150g each
low-calorie cooking spray
2 large carrots, peeled and
cut into 1cm (½in) dice
1 onion, peeled and diced
1 pepper (any colour),
deseeded and cut into
1cm (½in) dice
3 garlic cloves, peeled
and crushed
2cm (¾in) piece of root ginger,
peeled and grated
4 tsp curry powder
1 tbsp tomato puree
2 very low-salt chicken
stock cubes
100g basmati rice
juice of ½ lemon
1 tbsp mango chutney
50g reduced-fat cream cheese
handful of fresh coriander
leaves, roughly chopped

SWAP THIS: Swap the
chicken breast for the same
weight of turkey breast.

MAKE IT VEGGIE:
Leave out the meat, change
to a vegetable stock cube
and add extra veggies.

Super-thick and deliciously filling, this creamy Curried
Chicken and Rice Soup is a twist on a mulligatawny.
Warming Indian spices help to make this chunky soup
ideal for colder months, and light cream cheese gives
it that indulgent, creamy taste without tons of extra
calories. It's a great way to use up any chicken that
you might have left over from your Sunday lunch!

Everyday Light ───────────────────

HOB-TOP METHOD
🍲 **35 MINS**

Place the whole chicken breasts in a pan of water, so they
are just covered, and bring to a gentle simmer. Cook for
10–12 minutes, until no pink remains. You may need to cook
them a little longer if the breasts are particularly thick.
While cooking, skim off any white bits that rise to the top,
as you will use the cooking liquor later.

While the chicken breasts are poaching, spray a large
saucepan with low-calorie cooking spray and place over
a medium-low heat. Add the carrots, onion and pepper
and sauté for 8 minutes until softened, then add the garlic,
ginger and curry powder and cook for a further minute to
release the flavours. Add the tomato puree and remove
from the heat.

Remove the chicken from the pan, reserving the poaching
liquor, and shred the meat with two forks. Dissolve the
two stock cubes in the cooking liquor and make it up to
1.4 litres, adding more boiling water as necessary. Put the pan
back over the heat, add the stock along with the shredded
chicken and bring to a simmer. Cook for 10 minutes.

Add the rice and cook for a further 15 minutes. The soup
should be broth-like and the rice cooked. When the rice is
cooked, stir in the lemon juice, chutney and cream cheese.
Ladle into warm bowls, sprinkle with coriander and serve.

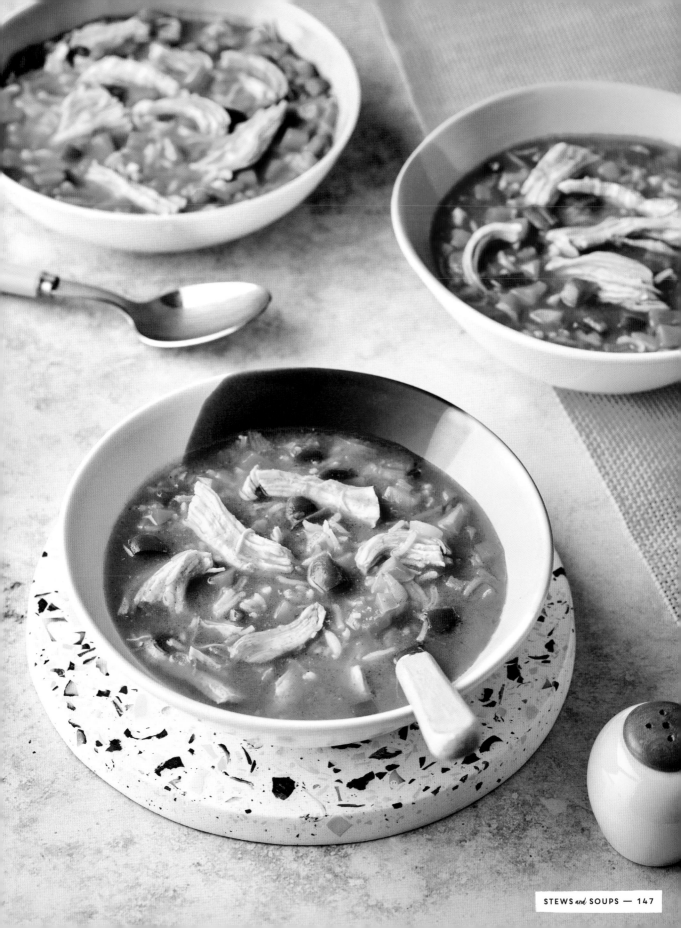

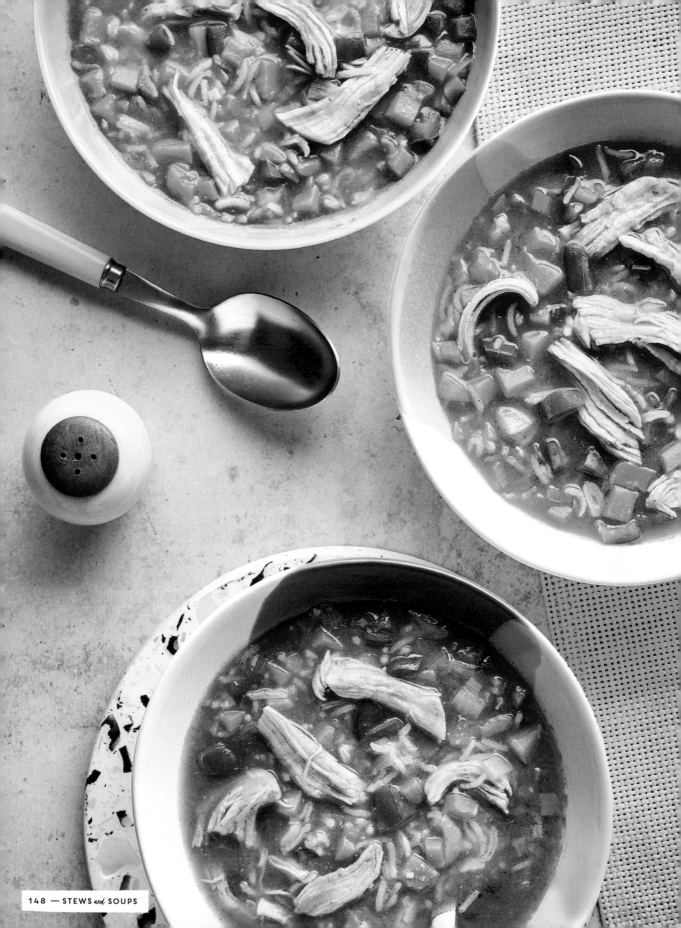

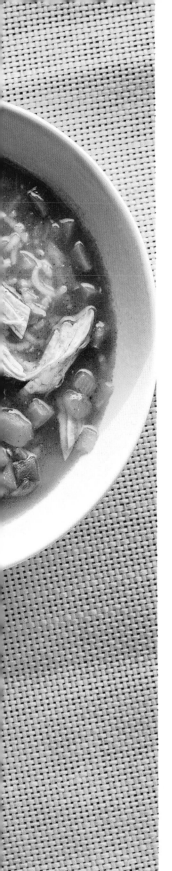

SLOW-COOKER METHOD
🍲 6 HOURS

SPECIAL EQUIPMENT
Slow cooker

Dissolve the two stock cubes in 1.2 litres of boiling water.

Place the onion, carrots, pepper, garlic, ginger, curry powder, tomato puree and stock in the slow cooker and stir well. Add the whole chicken breasts and cook on low for 5 hours.

Remove the chicken breasts and shred with two forks.

Put the shredded chicken back in the slow-cooker bowl and stir in the rice, mango chutney and lemon juice. Continue cooking for 45 minutes–1 hour, until the rice is cooked. The soup should be broth-like when it's ready. Stir in the cream cheese until it is melted and serve in warmed bowls, sprinkled with chopped coriander.

> **TIP:** You can use leftover chicken for this, but do remember any leftover soup must be discarded as chicken should not be reheated more than once.

"Quick, delicious and healthy meals for all of us to enjoy without having to think too much or spend hours in the kitchen."

KATE ——

GREEK POTATO STEW

🕐 **15 MINS** 🍲 **45 MINS** ✕ **SERVES 4**

V **F** **GF**

PER SERVING:
215 KCAL / 34G CARBS

low-calorie cooking spray
2 onions, peeled and sliced
1 red pepper,
   deseeded and sliced
4 garlic cloves, peeled
   and crushed
1 tsp dried oregano
1 x 400g tin chopped tomatoes
300ml vegetable stock
   (1 vegetable stock cube
   dissolved in 300ml
   boiling water)
600g new potatoes, cut into
   2.5cm (1in) chunks
8 stoned olives, sliced
juice of ½ lemon
freshly ground black pepper
65g reduced-fat
   Greek-style salad cheese
   or reduced-fat feta

TO ACCOMPANY *(optional)*
75g mixed salad (+ 15 kcal
   per serving) and a 60g
   wholemeal bread roll
   (+ 152 kcal per roll)

Sometimes simple fresh flavours are the best! This Greek Potato Stew might be really quick and simple to make, but it's full of delicious flavours and is super versatile too. This recipe works best with waxy potatoes that hold their shape, like Charlotte, Maris Peer or Jersey Royals – just make sure that you keep an eye on them so that they don't disintegrate into the sauce while they cook.

Weekly Indulgence

Spray a saucepan with low-calorie cooking spray and place over a medium heat. Add the sliced onions and pepper and sauté for 8 minutes, until soft, then add the garlic and oregano and cook for a further minute or two.

Add the tomatoes and stock and stir in the potatoes. Bring to the boil, then reduce the heat to medium-low, cover and simmer for 25 minutes, until the potatoes are almost cooked.

Stir in the olives and lemon juice and continue cooking, uncovered, for another 10 minutes, or until a knife slides easily into the potatoes.

Season with a little black pepper, then crumble the Greek-style salad cheese or feta on top.

Serve with your choice of accompaniment.

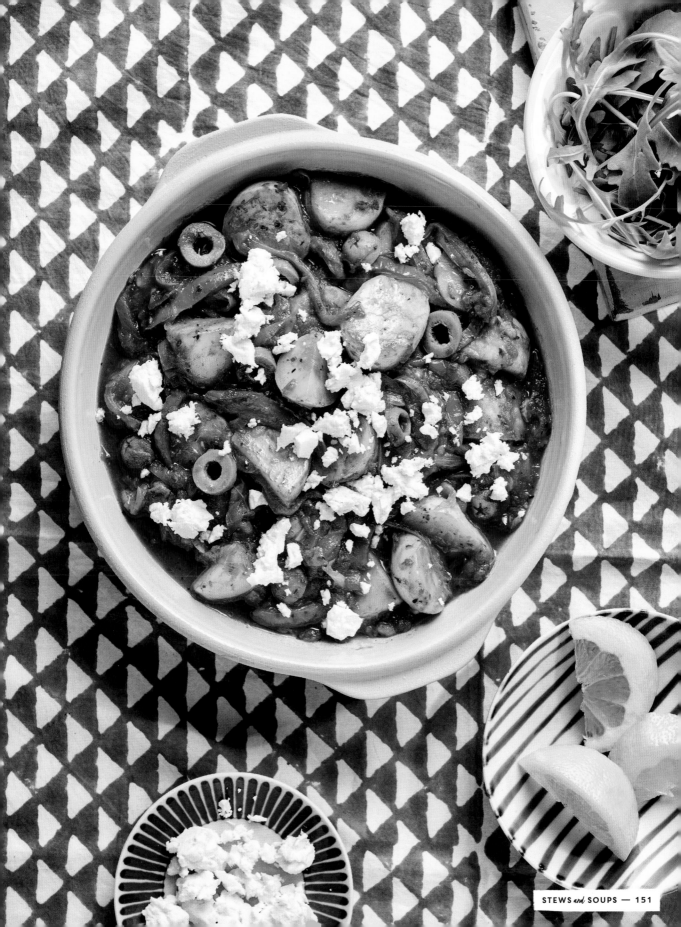

CREAMY CHICKEN SOUP

⏱ **10 MINS**　🍲 **VARIABLE** (SEE BELOW)　✕ **SERVES 4**

 Use GF stock cubes

(F) (DF) (GF)

PER SERVING:
172KCAL /26G CARBS

low-calorie cooking spray
2 onions, peeled and
　roughly sliced
3 garlic cloves, peeled
　and crushed
1 celery stick, roughly chopped
2 skinless, boneless chicken
　thighs (visible fat removed),
　about 150g in total
1 large potato (about 400g),
　peeled and cut into 2cm
　(¾in) chunks
1.2 litres chicken stock
　(2 very low-salt chicken
　stock cubes dissolved in
　1.2 litres boiling water)
　(use 1 litre stock for the
　pressure-cooker method)
1 tbsp white wine vinegar
2 bay leaves
½ tsp dried thyme
½ tsp dried tarragon
1 small head of cauliflower,
　florets only
sea salt and freshly ground
　black pepper

This Creamy Chicken Soup is like a big warm hug from the inside and is perfect for when you're feeling a bit under the weather or need warming up on a cold winter's day. This simple dairy-free recipe has all of the flavours you'd expect, but without any of the extra calories, so you can enjoy it guilt free.

Everyday Light —————————————————————

HOB-TOP METHOD
🍲 **45 MINS**

Spray a large saucepan with low-calorie cooking spray and place over a medium heat. Add the onions, garlic and celery and cook gently for 5 minutes, until the onions begin to soften, then add the rest of the ingredients to the saucepan and give it a stir. Bring to the boil, turn down the heat to a simmer and place the lid on the pan. Cook for 35–40 minutes, until the potatoes are tender and the chicken is cooked through.

Take the pan off the heat, remove the bay leaves and discard. Transfer the chicken thighs to a bowl and shred the meat with two forks.

Using a stick blender in the pan, or a food processor, blend the rest of the ingredients until the soup is smooth. Stir in the shredded chicken, season to taste with salt and pepper and serve.

SWAP THIS: We recommend using chicken thighs in this soup as we think the flavour is better, but you could use a large chicken breast instead if you prefer – it'll be totally delicious either way!

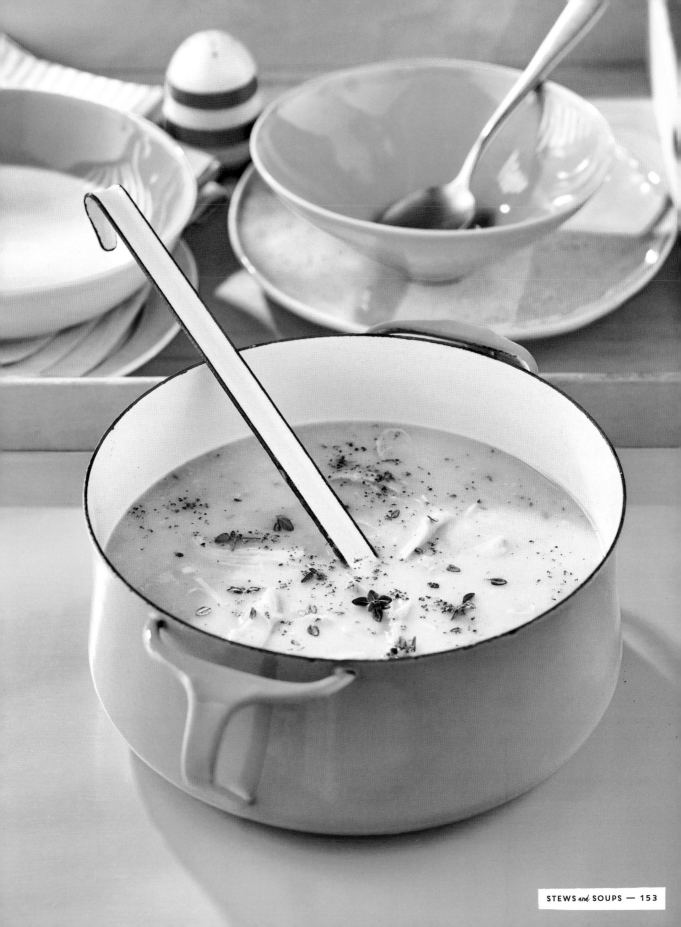

SLOW-COOKER METHOD
🍲 HIGH: 3–4 HOURS LOW: 6–7 HOURS

SPECIAL EQUIPMENT
Slow cooker

Spray a frying pan with low-calorie cooking spray and place over a medium heat. Add the onions, celery and garlic and cook gently for 5 minutes, until the onions begin to soften.

Transfer the contents of the frying pan to the slow cooker. Add the rest of the ingredients and give it a stir. Place the lid on the slow cooker and cook for 3–4 hours on high or 6–7 hours on low, until the potatoes are tender and the chicken is cooked through.

Turn off the slow cooker, remove the bay leaves and discard. Transfer the chicken thighs to a bowl and shred the meat with two forks.

Using a stick blender in the slow cooker, or a food processor, blend the rest of the ingredients until the soup is smooth. Stir in the shredded chicken, season to taste with salt and pepper and serve.

ELECTRIC PRESSURE-COOKER METHOD
🍲 17 MINS

SPECIAL EQUIPMENT
Electric pressure cooker

Spray the pressure-cooker pot with low-calorie cooking spray and set the pressure cooker to 'sauté'. Add the onions, celery and garlic and cook gently for 5 minutes, until the onions begin to soften. If your pressure cooker doesn't have a sauté function, you can do this step in a saucepan on the hob and transfer it to the pressure cooker once done.

Turn off the 'sauté' mode. Add the rest of the ingredients to the pressure cooker (remember to use 1 litre of chicken stock, not 1.2 litres) and give it a stir, making sure nothing is stuck to the bottom of the bowl. Cover with the lid and set the valve to 'sealing'. Pressure-cook on high for 12 minutes. After 12 minutes, use the 'manual release' function to release pressure from the pot.

Once the pressure has released, remove the lid. Remove the bay leaves and discard. Transfer the chicken thighs to a bowl and shred the meat with two forks.

Using a stick blender in the pressure cooker, or a food processor, blend the rest of the ingredients until the soup is smooth. Stir in the shredded chicken, season to taste with salt and pepper and serve.

TIPS: You could use meat with bones for added flavour – just make sure the skin is removed before cooking and all the bones are removed after it's cooked! If you want a thicker soup, use 1 litre of stock in the slow-cooker and hob-top methods, or reduce the soup over the heat at the end of cooking (removing the slow-cooker lid for the last hour of cooking). If you want it thinner, just add a little splash of water at a time and stir until it's to your liking.

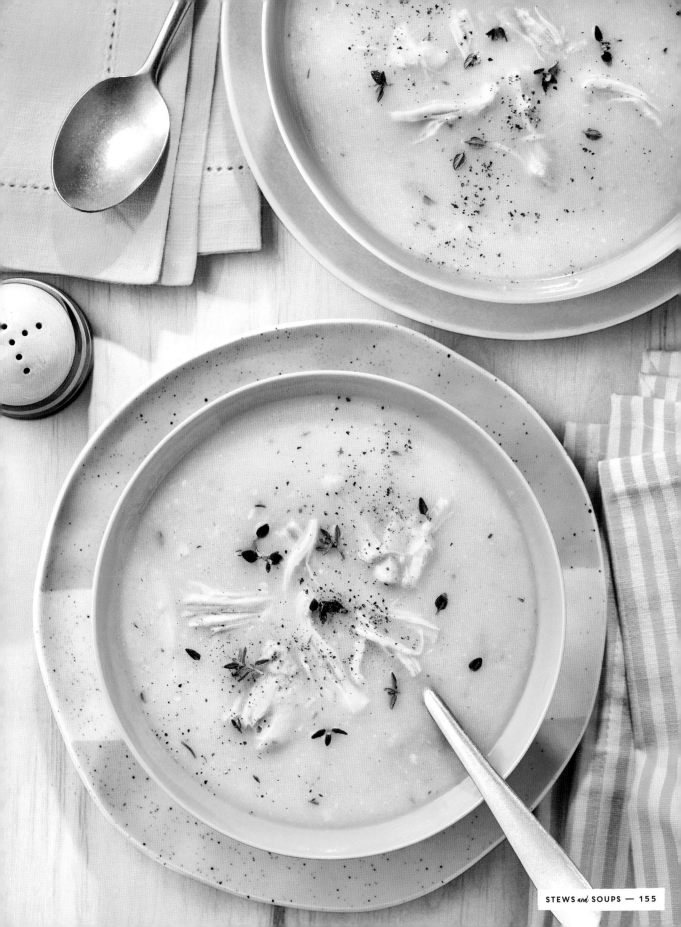

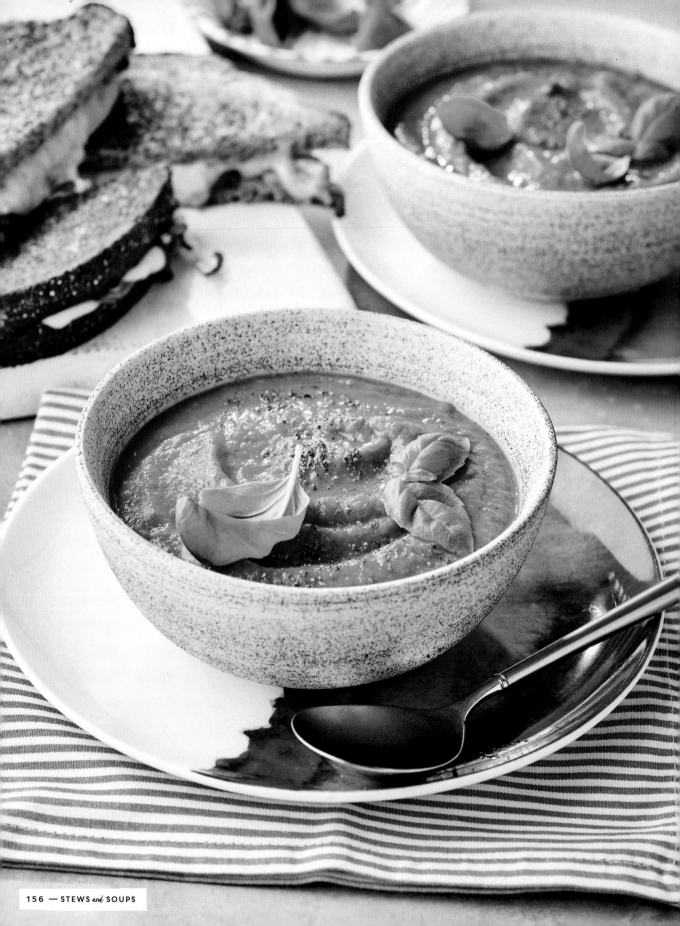

CREAMY TOMATO SOUP

🕐 **10 MINS**　🍲 **40 MINS**　✕ **SERVES 4**

Use Henderson's relish

Use GF stock cubes and Henderson's relish

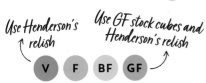

V F BF **GF**

PER SERVING:
166 KCAL / 26G CARBS

low-calorie cooking spray
2 small onions, peeled
　and diced
2 medium carrots, peeled
　and diced
1 celery stick, sliced
1 garlic clove, peeled
　and crushed
2 fresh bay leaves or
　a pinch of dried basil
2 tbsp tomato puree
1 potato (about 200g),
　peeled and diced
400ml vegetable stock
　(2 very low-salt vegetable
　stock cubes dissolved in
　400ml boiling water)
2 x 400g tins chopped
　tomatoes
1 tbsp white wine vinegar
2 tbsp Henderson's relish or
　Worcestershire sauce
1 tbsp low-fat cream cheese
sea salt and freshly ground
　black pepper
fresh basil leaves, to garnish

We think this creamy, warming soup is better than what you'd find in a tin, and it's full of extra goodness from hidden veggies. You can even make up a large batch and freeze it for later! Fancy a larger lunch? Pair it with The Ultimate Grilled Cheese (page 232) – this will increase the calories per serving to 700 kcal.

Everyday Light

Spray a large saucepan with low-calorie cooking spray and place over a medium heat. Add the onions, carrots, celery, garlic and bay leaves or dried basil and fry for 6–8 minutes until they soften and the onions start to brown. Add the tomato puree and fry for a further 2 minutes, then add the potato, stock, chopped tomatoes, white wine vinegar and Henderson's relish or Worcestershire sauce. Reduce the heat and simmer for 30 minutes.

After 30 minutes, stir in the cream cheese.

Remove the pan from the heat, discard the bay leaves and blitz with a stick blender or in a food processor until smooth. If the soup is a little too thick for your liking, loosen it with an extra splash of water.

Season to taste with salt and pepper, garnish with basil leaves and serve.

FISH CHOWDER

🕐 **15 MINS**   🍲 **45 MINS**   ✕ **SERVES 6**

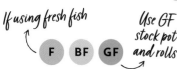

If using fresh fish ↘   *Use GF stock pot and rolls* ↙

(**F**) (**BF**) (**GF**)

PER SERVING:
270 KCAL / 30G CARBS

low-calorie cooking spray

1 onion, peeled and chopped

2 smoked bacon medallions,
   cut into 2cm (¾in) squares

2 garlic cloves, peeled
   and crushed

700g floury potatoes, peeled
   and cut into 2.5cm
   (1in) chunks

700ml fish stock (1 fish
   stock pot dissolved in
   700ml boiling water)

1 dried bay leaf

2 sprigs of fresh thyme

180g skinless, boneless smoked
   haddock, cut into 2.5cm
   (1in) pieces

380g skinless, boneless cod,
   cut into 2.5cm (1in) pieces

175g cooked peeled
   prawns, drained

1 x 160g tin sweetcorn, drained

300ml skimmed milk

45g low-fat cream cheese

2 tsp lemon juice

sea salt and freshly ground
   black pepper (optional)

a few chives, chopped,
   to garnish

TO ACCOMPANY *(optional)*
60g wholemeal bread rolls
   (+ 152 kcal per roll)

Inspired by the fish chowder that's popular in New England, USA, our version skips the cream to save on calories! This is a comforting, chunky fish soup that's bursting with seafood flavours. Substantial enough to serve alone, or with a crusty wholemeal roll, this dish makes the perfect hearty, filling and slimming-friendly lunch!

Weekly Indulgence

Spray a large saucepan (that has a lid) with low-calorie cooking spray and place over a medium heat. Add the onion and cook for 5 minutes until it starts to soften, then add the bacon and garlic and cook for a further 5 minutes.

Add the potato, fish stock, bay leaf and thyme, bring to the boil, then reduce the heat, cover and simmer for 20 minutes, until the potato is tender.

Add the haddock, cod, prawns, sweetcorn and milk and simmer over a low heat for 10–15 minutes, until the fish is opaque and beginning to flake. Remove from the heat and stir in the cream cheese.

Add the lemon juice, remove the bay leaf and any thyme stalks, taste and season with salt and pepper if needed.

Serve sprinkled with a few chopped chives.

TIP: You could use frozen fish instead of fresh – just follow the manufacturer's instructions for cooking.

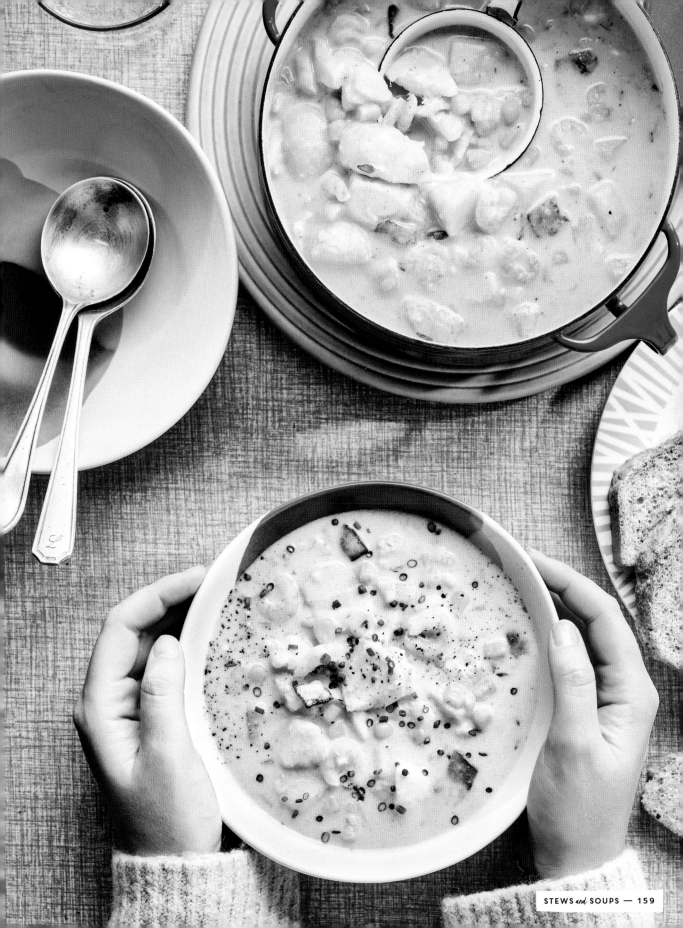

SMOKY CHICKPEA STEW

⏱ **15 MINS**   🍲 **VARIABLE** (SEE BELOW)   ✕ **SERVES 4**

Use GF stock cube and stock pot

PER SERVING:
253 KCAL / 42G CARBS

low-calorie cooking spray
2 onions, peeled and diced
2 carrots, peeled and cut into
  5mm (¼in)-thick slices
2 celery sticks, sliced
1 tbsp smoked sweet paprika
2 garlic cloves, peeled
  and crushed
1 tbsp tomato puree
1.3 litres vegetable stock
  (1 vegetable stock cube
  dissolved in 1.3 litres boiling
  water) (use 600ml water for
  slow-cooker method)
1 red wine stock pot
2 bay leaves
500g potatoes, peeled and
  cut into 2.5cm (1in) dice
1 x 400g tin chickpeas,
  drained and rinsed
1 tsp red wine vinegar
sea salt and freshly ground
  black pepper
small handful of fresh
  flat-leaf parsley, chopped

TIP: Smoked paprika and smoked sweet paprika (used here) are the same thing. Hot smoked paprika has a fiery chilli kick so only use it if you love heat.

SWAP THIS: Swap the tinned chickpeas for tinned white beans, such as haricot or cannellini.

Rustling up this warming veggie stew couldn't be simpler. Prep the chunky veg the night before and let the slow cooker do the hard work, so you can look forward to arriving home to a mouth-watering aroma filling the kitchen and a smoky stew that's ready to serve.

Everyday Light ————————————————

HOB-TOP METHOD
🍲 **1 HOUR 30 MINS**

Spray a saucepan with low-calorie cooking spray and place over a medium heat. Add the onions, carrots and celery and sauté for 8–10 minutes, then add the smoked paprika and garlic and cook for a further minute to release the aromas. Stir in the tomato puree, then add the 1.3 litres of stock, red wine stock pot and bay leaves. Bring to the boil, cover, then reduce the heat to medium-low and simmer for 20 minutes.

Add the potatoes, chickpeas and red wine vinegar and cook for a further 50 minutes–1 hour, uncovered, until the vegetables are soft and the sauce is thick.

Season to taste with salt and pepper, remove the bay leaves and serve sprinkled with chopped parsley.

SLOW-COOKER METHOD
🍲 **HIGH: ABOUT 4 HOURS LOW: 7–8 HOURS**

SPECIAL EQUIPMENT
Slow cooker

Put all the ingredients (600ml stock), except the parsley, into the slow-cooker bowl and stir well. It might look as if there is not enough liquid, but don't worry, the vegetables will release liquid as they cook, producing a rich sauce.

Cook on high for 4 hours or low for 7–8 hours. Remove the bay leaves, stir, season with salt and pepper and serve sprinkled with the chopped parsley.

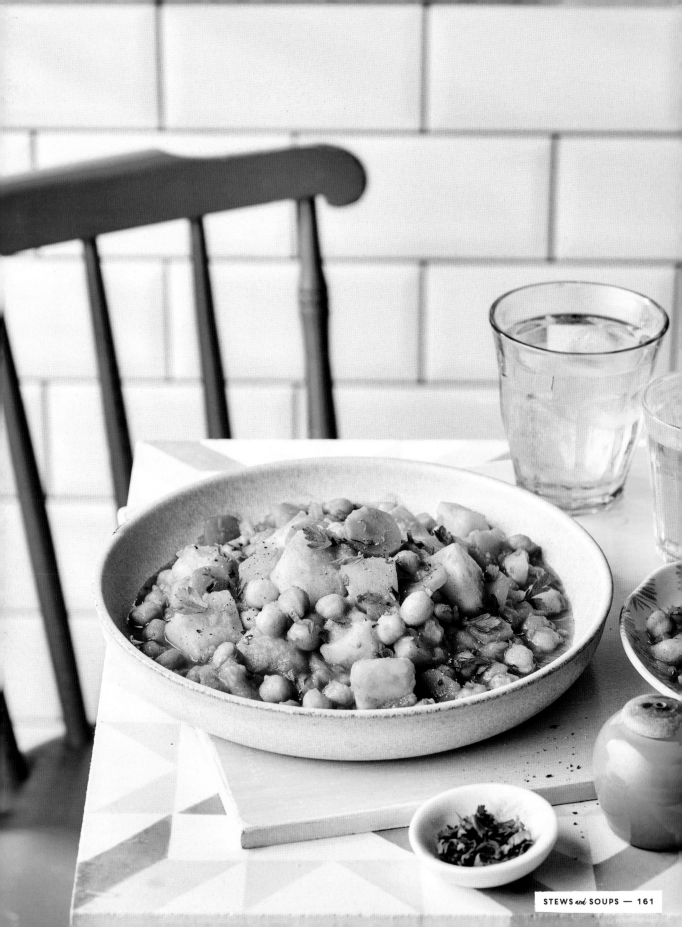

BEEF STEW *and* DUMPLINGS

🕙 **10 MINS**   🍲 **VARIABLE** (SEE BELOW)   ✕ **SERVES 4**

PER SERVING:
463 KCAL / 57G CARBS

FOR THE STEW
low-calorie cooking spray
2 onions, peeled and diced
400g diced stewing beef
  (all visible fat removed)
½ tsp garlic granules
½ tsp onion granules
½ tsp beef extract, such
  as Bovril
½ tbsp balsamic vinegar
1 tbsp Worcestershire sauce
  or Henderson's relish
2 large carrots (about 120g
  each), peeled and diced
8 shallots, peeled and
  cut in half
1 celery stick, roughly chopped
200g swede, peeled and diced
100g button mushrooms,
  left whole
300g potato, peeled and cut
  into chunks
500ml beef stock (1 very
  low-salt beef stock cube and
  1 beef stock pot dissolved
  in 500ml boiling water) (use
  400ml beef stock for the
  slow-cooker method)
15g cornflour

FOR THE DUMPLINGS
100g self-raising flour
¼ tsp baking powder
pinch of salt
2 egg yolks

Tender beef stew and dumplings is as close as you can get to a hug in a bowl! In our lower-calorie version of this classic comfort food, we've used egg yolks in the dumplings. This keeps the taste and texture of traditional dumplings but with no suet in sight.

Weekly Indulgence ──────────────

OVEN METHOD
🍲 **2 HOURS 40 MINS**

Preheat the oven to 180°C (fan 160°C/gas mark 4).

Spray a casserole dish with low-calorie cooking spray and place over a medium heat. Add the onions and cook for 5 minutes until softened, then add the beef and cook for a further 5 minutes until browned all over. Add the garlic and onion granules, beef extract, balsamic vinegar and Worcestershire sauce or Henderson's relish and stir. Add the remaining stew ingredients, except the cornflour, cover with a lid and cook in the oven for 2 hours.

While the stew is cooking, make the dumplings.

Sift the flour and baking powder into a bowl, add the salt and egg yolks and mix slightly with a fork. Using your hands, rub in the egg yolk the same way you would if using fat, until the mixture resembles breadcrumbs. Add 4 tablespoons of cold water, a little at a time, until it comes together to form a dough. You will need a firm dough that's not too wet, so the amount of water you need will depend on the size of your egg yolks. Shape the dough into four equally sized dumplings and set aside in the fridge for later.

After the stew has been cooking for 2 hours, mix the cornflour with a little water, then stir it into the stew. Add the dumplings to the stew, replace the lid and cook for another 30 minutes, until the stew has thickened and the dumplings are puffed up. Remove the lid for the last 10 minutes if you want the dumplings to be browned a little.

Remove from the oven and serve.

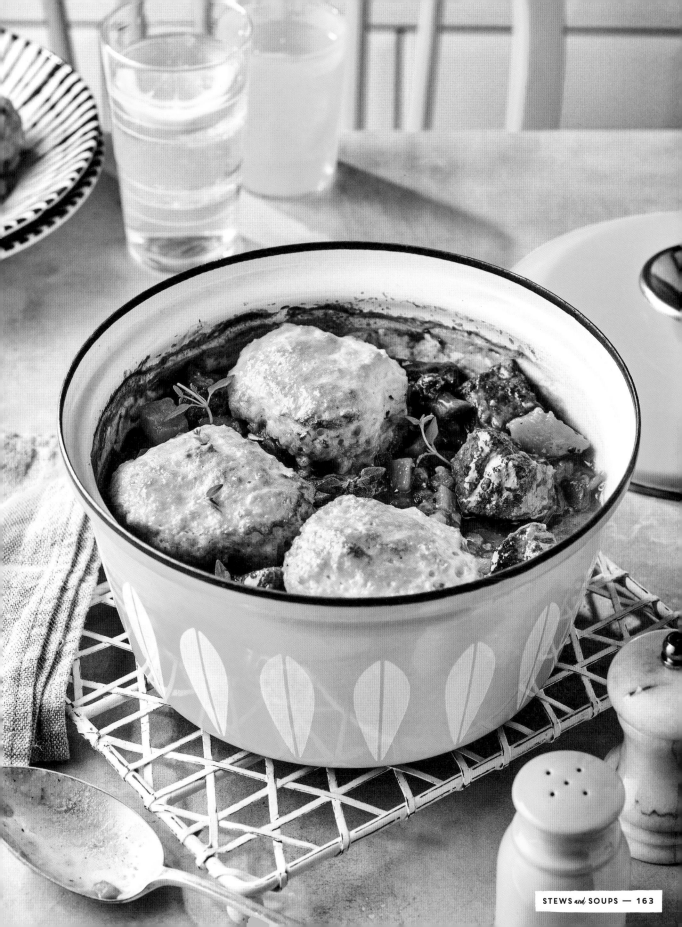

SLOW-COOKER METHOD
🍲 HIGH: 4 HOURS LOW: 6–7 HOURS

SPECIAL EQUIPMENT
Slow cooker

Put all the stew ingredients, except the cornflour and low-calorie cooking spray, into the slow-cooker pot, cover with the lid and cook on high for 4 hours, or low for 6–7 hours.

While the stew is cooking, make the dumplings.

Sift the flour and baking powder into a bowl, add the salt and egg yolks and mix slightly with a fork. Using your hands, rub in the egg yolk the same way you would if using fat, until the mixture resembles breadcrumbs. Add 4 tablespoons of water, a little at a time, until it comes together to form a dough. You will need a firm dough that's not too wet, so the amount of water you need will depend on the size of your egg yolks. Shape the dough into four equally sized dumplings and set aside in the fridge for later.

Forty minutes before the end of the cooking time, check to see if the meat is tender. If it is, mix the cornflour with a little water, then stir it into the stew. Add the dumplings, cover with the lid and cook on high for the final 40 minutes, until the stew has thickened and the dumplings are puffed up. Serve!

TIP: The dumplings can be made in advance and kept in the fridge until they are needed.

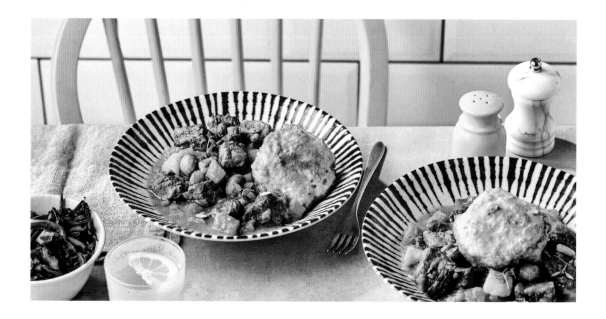

LAMB SCOUSE

🕐 **10 MINS**   🍲 **VARIABLE** (SEE BELOW)   ✕ **SERVES 8**

   F **BF** **DF** **GF**

PER SERVING:
396 KCAL / 44G CARBS

low-calorie cooking spray
800g diced lamb, all visible
  fat removed
sea salt and freshly ground
  black pepper
3 onions, peeled and
  roughly diced
6 carrots, peeled and
  thickly sliced
1.5kg potatoes, peeled, half
  of them thinly sliced
400ml beef stock (1 very
  low-salt beef stock cube
  dissolved in 400ml
  boiling water)
1 beef stock pot
2 tbsp Henderson's relish or
  Worcestershire sauce
fresh parsley, to garnish

As the name suggests, Lamb Scouse has been a staple dinner for those of us in the Merseyside area for as far back as we can remember! It's been one of our go-to comfort foods for so long and we couldn't wait to share our take on this nostalgic dish. Cheap, cheerful and a hearty one-pot dinner, it's sure to become one of your family favourites in no time. Try teaming it with our Balsamic Roasted Onions (page 222).

Everyday Light ─────────────

OVEN OR HOB-TOP METHOD
🍲 **2 HOURS 30 MINS**

Preheat the oven to 180°C (fan 160°C/gas mark 4) – or you can cook the dish on the hob.

Spray a casserole dish with low-calorie cooking spray and place over a medium heat. Season the meat well with salt and pepper, then brown it in the dish on all sides for 5–6 minutes. Transfer to a plate and set aside.

Spray some more low-calorie cooking spray in the dish, then add the onions and carrots and sauté for about 5 minutes until they start to colour slightly.

Place the sliced potatoes on top of the veg in an even layer, then place the browned meat on top. Add the beef stock to the dish, cover and cook in the oven or over a medium heat on the hob for 1 hour 20 minutes.

After 1 hour 20 minutes add the beef stock pot and Henderson's relish or Worcestershire sauce, then stir to break up the sliced potatoes (this will thicken the Scouse).

Cut the remaining potatoes into chunks, then add them and stir. You may need to add a little extra water if it looks a little too dry. Replace the lid and cook for another hour or so, or until the potatoes are cooked and the lamb is tender. Remove from the heat, check the seasoning, sprinkle with parsley and serve.

ELECTRIC PRESSURE-COOKER METHOD
🍲 45 MINS

SPECIAL EQUIPMENT
Electric pressure cooker

Spray the pressure-cooker pot with some low-calorie cooking spray and set the pressure cooker to 'sauté'. Season the meat well with salt and pepper, then sauté it for about 5 minutes until brown on all sides. Transfer to a plate and set aside.

Spray some more low-calorie cooking spray in the pot, then add the onions and carrots and sauté for 5 minutes until they start to brown. If your pressure cooker doesn't have a sauté function, sauté the meat then the onions and carrots in a frying pan on the hob, then transfer the onions and carrots to the pressure cooker when done.

Place the sliced potatoes on top of the veg, then place the browned meat on top. Add the beef stock to the pressure cooker, cover with the lid and set the valve to 'sealing'. Pressure-cook on high for 30 minutes, then let the pressure release naturally.

When the pressure is released, carefully remove the lid and add the Worcestershire sauce or Henderson's relish and stock pot. Stir well to break up the sliced potatoes (this will thicken the Scouse).

Cut the remaining potatoes into chunks, then add them and stir. Replace the lid and set the pressure-cook on high for 5 minutes, letting the pressure release naturally before serving.

Check the lamb is tender and the potato is cooked, then taste and season if needed, sprinkle with parsley and serve.

"
"So good to have healthy meals full of flavour!"

—— REBECCA

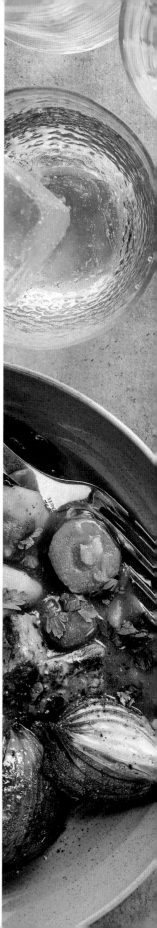

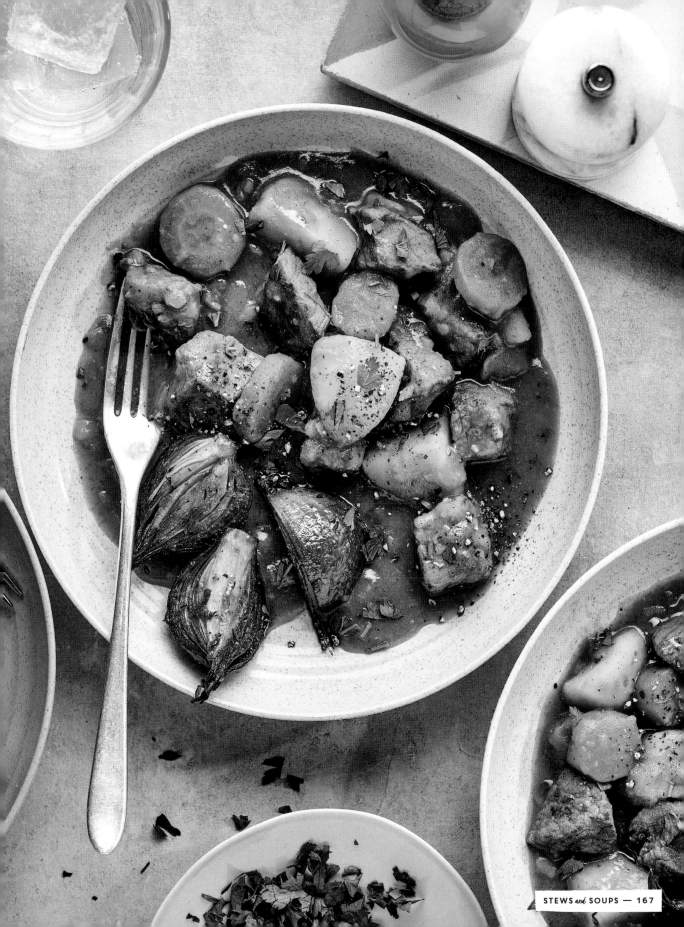

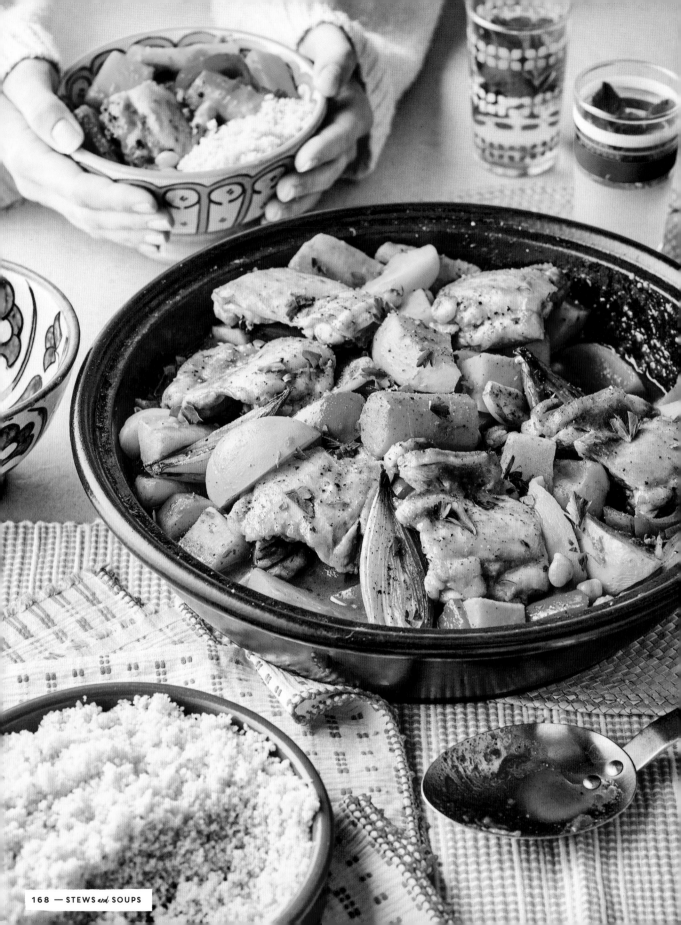

KATE'S TAGINE

🕐 **15 MINS**   🍲 **1 HOUR 30 MINS–2 HOURS**   ✗ **SERVES 4**

Use GF stock cubes ↘

 F **BF** **DF** **GF**

PER SERVING:
460 KCAL /45G CARBS

FOR THE SPICE MIX
2 tsp ground ginger
1 tsp ground cumin
2 tsp ground coriander
1 tsp ground cinnamon
1 tsp ground white pepper
½ tsp ground allspice
½ tsp ground turmeric

FOR THE TAGINE
low-calorie cooking spray
8 skinless, boneless chicken
  thighs (visible fat removed),
  about 600g in total
6 garlic cloves, peeled and
  cut in half
6 shallots, peeled and cut in half
200g carrots, peeled and
  cut into chunks
200g swede, peeled and
  cut into chunks
200g parsnips, peeled and
  cut into chunks
250ml chicken stock
  (2 very low-salt chicken
  stock cubes dissolved in
  250ml boiling water)
1 x 400g tin chopped tomatoes
200g peeled and deseeded
  butternut squash, cut into chunks
1 pepper (any colour),
  deseeded and diced
1 x 400g tin chickpeas,
  drained and rinsed
1½ tbsp tomato puree
1 x 410g tin sliced peaches in
  natural juice, drained

A tagine is a North African dish, named after the earthenware pot it is cooked in. Don't worry if you don't have a tagine, you can cook this dish in a covered pan in the oven like we have and it will taste just as good! This is our take on the traditional dish of chicken, garlic and Moroccan spices.

Weekly Indulgence

Preheat the oven to 200°C (fan 180°C/gas mark 6). Combine all the spice mix ingredients in a bowl and set aside.

Spray a large casserole dish or tagine with low-calorie cooking spray and place over a medium heat. Add the chicken thighs and cook them for 2–3 minutes on each side until browned (no need for them to be cooked through). Remove from the dish and set aside.

Add the garlic and shallots to the casserole dish or tagine and cook for about 5 minutes until slightly browned, then add the carrots, swede, parsnips and 1 tablespoon of the spice mix. Stir in the chicken, stock and chopped tomatoes, cover with a lid and place in the oven for 30 minutes.

After 30 minutes, stir in the butternut squash, diced pepper, chickpeas, tomato puree and sliced peaches. Cover and cook for a further 45 minutes. If there is still a lot of liquid after 45 minutes, leave the lid off for 30 minutes so the liquid reduces.

Serve!

TIPS: Be sure to use sliced peaches in natural juices not in syrup as this will affect the calories. The leftover Moroccan spice mix can be stored in an airtight container ready for next time!

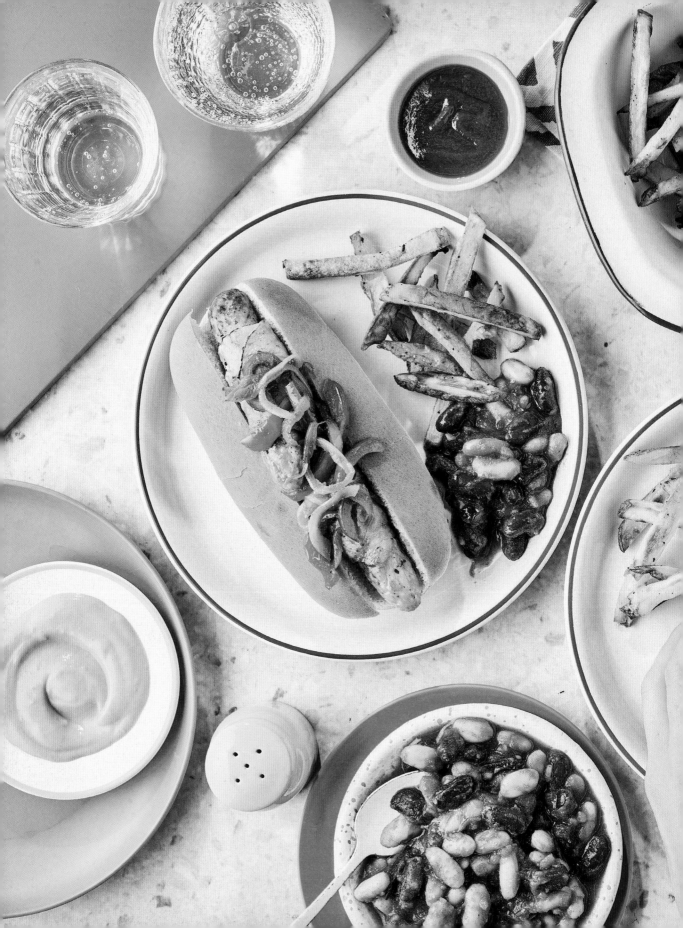

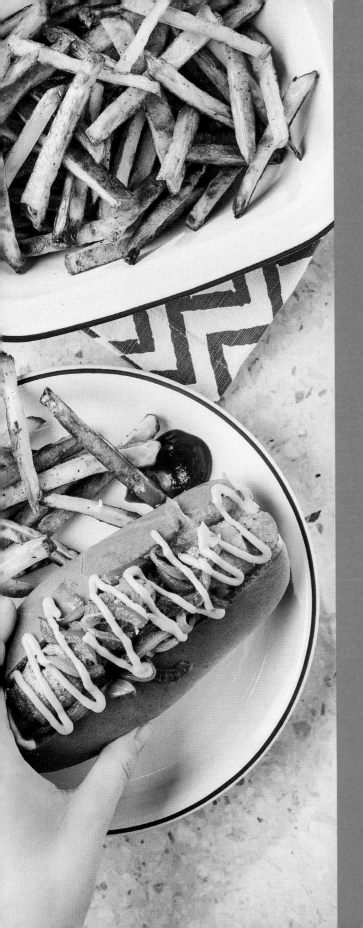

BAKES
&
ROASTS

CHICKEN, BACON *and* LEEK COTTAGE PIE

🕐 **15 MINS**   🍲 **1 HOUR**   ✕ **SERVES 4**

PER SERVING:
403 KCAL / 39G CARBS

740g potatoes, peeled and
   quartered
low-calorie cooking spray
1 large leek, trimmed, washed
   and sliced
1 onion, peeled and
   finely chopped
500g diced chicken breast
100g unsmoked bacon
   medallions, cut into strips
2 tsp English mustard powder
325ml chicken stock
   (1 very low-salt chicken
   stock cube dissolved in
   325ml boiling water)
100g low-fat cream cheese
1 sprig of fresh thyme,
   leaves chopped
10g fresh parsley
   leaves, chopped
sea salt and freshly ground
   black pepper
25g reduced-fat
   Cheddar, grated

A comforting cottage pie, but not as you know it! Adding the classic combo of chicken and bacon brings a wonderful flavour that's a little different to your typical pies. Serve with a glug of gravy and steamed veggies if you like, for an easy family dinner.

Weekly Indulgence

Preheat the oven to 220°C (fan 200°C/gas mark 7).

Put the potatoes in a saucepan with enough water to cover, add a pinch of salt and bring to the boil. Cook for 15–20 minutes until soft.

Meanwhile, spray a frying pan with low-calorie cooking spray and place over a medium heat. Add the leek and onion and fry for 2–3 minutes until soft, then add the chicken and bacon and cook for 5 minutes. Add the mustard powder, then stir 300ml of the chicken stock into the pan. Bring to a simmer and cook for 10 minutes.

Add 75g of the cream cheese and all the thyme leaves to the chicken, stir until well mixed, then transfer to a medium ovenproof dish.

When the potatoes are cooked, drain and leave for a few minutes to dry, then mash until smooth.

Add the remaining 25g of the cream cheese, the chopped parsley and the remaining chicken stock to the mashed potatoes and mix. Season to taste with salt and pepper. Spoon the potato over the chicken mix and level it out using the back of a fork. Sprinkle with the grated cheese and cook in the preheated oven for 25–30 minutes until golden brown.

Remove from the oven and serve.

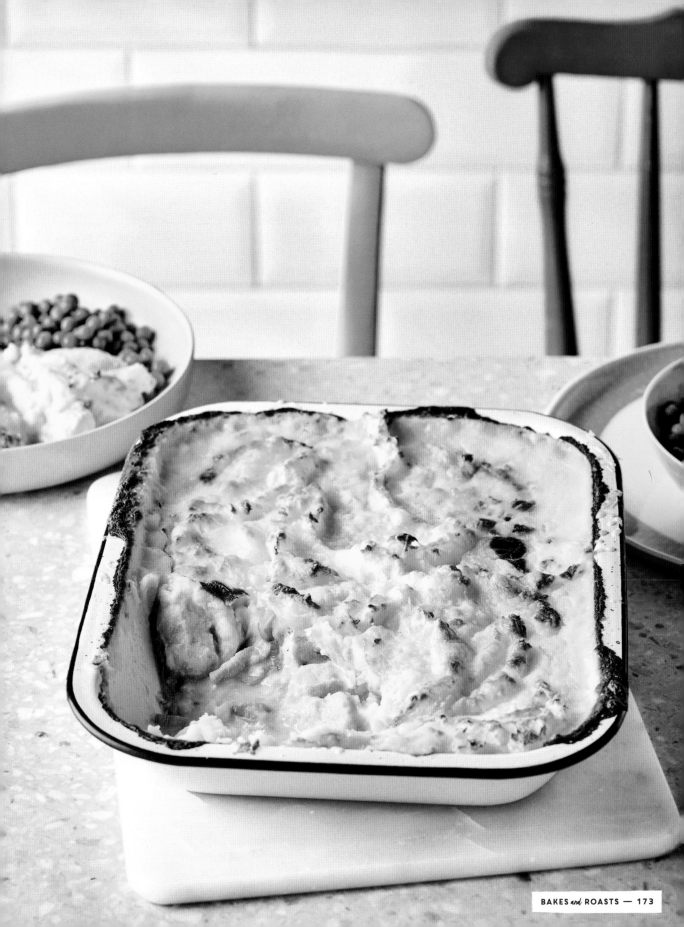

TIPSY BBQ CHICKEN

Use GF stock cube and BBQ seasoning ↱

F BF DF GF

🕐 **5 MINS**   🍲 **20 MINS**   ✕ **SERVES 4**

This is one of those dishes that can be enjoyed in so many ways! It makes a fab Texas BBQ-inspired dinner or can be eaten cold with a fresh salad for lunch. Try it cooked in the oven, the air fryer or even on the BBQ!

Weekly Indulgence

Preheat the oven to 220°C (fan 200°C/gas mark 7).

In a large bowl, whisk together the BBQ seasoning, white wine vinegar, hot pepper sauce, crumbled stock cube, Bourbon whiskey, BBQ sauce and honey. Add the onion, making sure to separate the onion into rings as you put it in the bowl, then add the chicken thighs. Mix really well, making sure that the chicken gets well coated in the mixture.

Spray a roasting tin with low-calorie cooking spray. Tip the contents of the bowl into the roasting tin and cook in the preheated oven for 15–20 minutes until the chicken is cooked through. The chicken should show no sign of pinkness and the juices should run clear.

Serve with your choice of accompaniment.

PER SERVING:
190 KCAL /15G CARBS

1 tbsp BBQ seasoning
1 tsp white wine vinegar
1 tsp hot pepper sauce
1 beef stock cube, crumbled
1 tbsp Bourbon whiskey
4 tbsp BBQ sauce
1 tbsp runny honey
1 red onion, peeled and thinly sliced
400g skinless, boneless chicken thighs (visible fat removed)
low-calorie cooking spray

TO ACCOMPANY *(optional)*
75g mixed salad (+ 15 kcal per serving) and baked potato, 225g raw weight (+ 225 kcal per serving)

TIP: You can also cook this dish in the air fryer for 15 minutes at 200°C, making sure the chicken is cooked through.

SWAP THIS: To make this dish extra decadent, take the chicken out of the oven after 10 minutes and top with grated Cheddar. Place back in the oven for the remaining 5–10 minutes. Remember to adjust the calories accordingly!

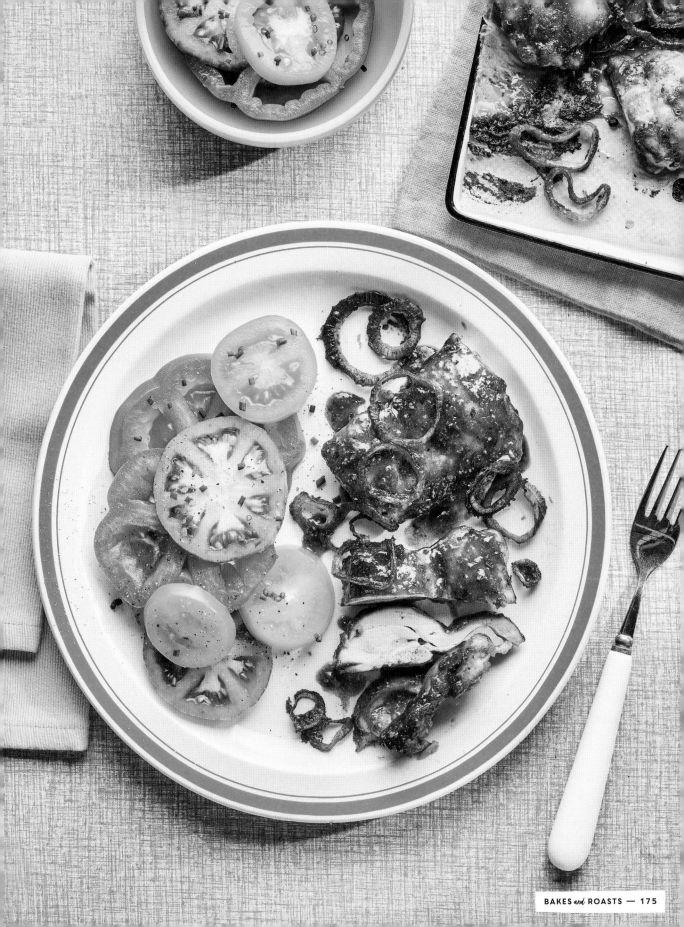

VEGETARIAN COTTAGE PIE JACKETS

🕐 **10 MINS** 🍲 **1–1¾ HOURS** ✕ **SERVES 4**

Use Henderson's relish ↑

(V) (F) (DF)

PER SERVING:
454 KCAL / 77G CARBS

4 baking potatoes (about 1.5kg total), pierced with a fork
low-calorie cooking spray
1 onion, peeled and finely diced
1 carrot, finely diced
1 celery stick, finely diced
2 garlic cloves, peeled and minced
250g Quorn mince
250ml vegetable stock (1 vegetable stock cube dissolved in 250ml boiling water)
½ tsp dried thyme
¼ tsp dried rosemary
1 tbsp Henderson's relish or Worcestershire sauce
100g frozen peas
1 medium egg, beaten
¼ tsp English mustard powder
sea salt and black pepper

TO ACCOMPANY *(optional)*
80g steamed green vegetables (+ 35 kcal per serving) and
2 tbsp tomato ketchup (+ 15 kcal per tbsp)

SWAP THIS: Use a drained, rinsed tin of green lentils instead of Quorn, or make it meaty with 250g 5%-fat minced beef and beef stock, adjusting the calories.

Why pick between a cottage pie and a crispy, golden baked potato when you don't have to? These comforting jackets are stuffed with a vegetarian cottage pie filling and topped with fluffy mash for the ultimate twist on a British classic. Try them with steamed veggies and a jug of gravy (see page 79 or use our Gravy from *Quick & Easy*) on the side for a satisfying family dinner.

Special Occasion

Preheat the oven to 220°C (fan 200°C/gas mark 7).

First, cook the potatoes. We like to cook them in the microwave for 20 minutes on high before crisping them up in the oven. (If you don't have a microwave you can cook them in the oven instead, individually wrapped in foil, for 1–1½ hours – just put them in ahead of time!) Spray the potatoes with low-calorie cooking spray and crisp up the skin in the oven or preheated air fryer for 10 minutes.

While the potatoes are crisping up, spray a lidded frying pan with low-calorie cooking spray and place over a medium heat. Add the onion, carrot, celery and garlic and cook for 5 minutes, until the onions are softening, then add the Quorn, stock, dried herbs and Henderson's relish. Stir and bring to the boil, cover, reduce the heat and simmer for 20 minutes, removing the lid for the final 5 minutes to allow any remaining stock to reduce and the mixture to thicken. Remove from the heat and stir in the peas.

Halve the cooked potatoes and scoop out the flesh – they will be very hot so do this with an oven glove or let them cool a little first! Put the flesh in a bowl with the egg and mustard powder, season and mash until creamy. Fill the hollow potato skins with the filling mixture and place on a baking tray. Add a dollop of mash to each potato half, using a fork to roughen up the top of the mash. Bake in the oven for 15 minutes, or until the mash has a golden crust. Serve with your choice of accompaniment.

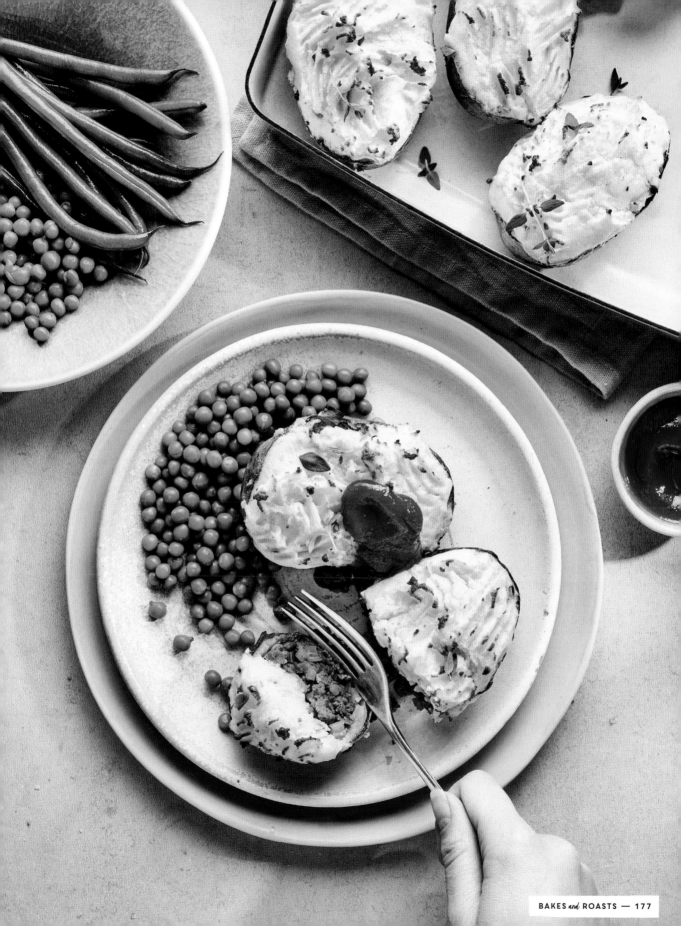

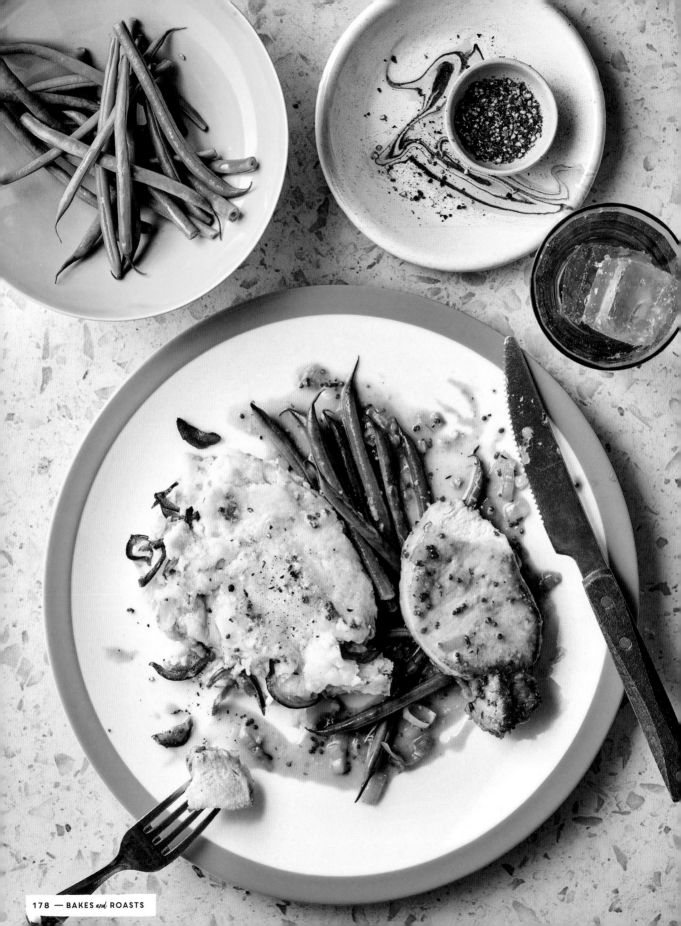

HONEY *and* MUSTARD PORK

🕐 **10 MINS**　🍲 **30 MINS**　✕ **SERVES 4**

PER SERVING:
252 KCAL / 22G CARBS

low-calorie cooking spray
1 onion, peeled and
　finely chopped
1 medium leek, trimmed,
　washed, halved lengthways
　and thinly sliced
2 garlic cloves, peeled
　and crushed
4 lean pork loin steaks,
　trimmed of all visible fat
　(about 100g each after
　removing fat)
½ tsp dried thyme
½ tsp dried sage
4 tbsp clear honey
3 tbsp wholegrain mustard
1 tbsp Henderson's relish or
　Worcestershire sauce
½ tsp balsamic vinegar
3 tbsp apple juice
sea salt and freshly ground
　black pepper (optional)

TO ACCOMPANY *(optional)*
baked potato, 225g raw
　weight (+ 225 kcal per
　serving), 80g steamed
　green vegetables
　(+ 35 kcal per serving)

These super-simple pork steaks are pan-fried with leek and onion and coated with a sweet and sticky mustard glaze. Delicious served alongside some fresh green vegetables, or even with a fluffy baked potato, they are super-hearty and comforting. They're ready in no time at all, which makes them the perfect choice for a midweek meal.

Special Occasion

Spray a large frying pan with low-calorie cooking spray and place over a medium heat. Add the onion, leek and garlic and fry for about 10 minutes until softened and golden. Move the vegetables to the edges of the frying pan and add the pork. Seal the pork for 2 minutes on each side until lightly golden.

In a small mixing bowl, mix together the thyme, sage, honey, wholegrain mustard, Henderson's relish or Worcestershire sauce, balsamic vinegar and apple juice.

Reduce the heat, add the honey and mustard mixture and cook gently for 10–15 minutes, stirring occasionally, until the pork is cooked through. When the meat is cooked, the juices will run clear and it will no longer be pink in the middle. Taste and season with salt and pepper if needed.

Serve at once, with your choice of accompaniment.

TIP: Using wholegrain mustard will ensure you get a clear, sticky glaze on the pork. Using other mustards such as Dijon or English will not produce the clear, sticky glaze.

SWAP THIS: Swap the pork steaks for the same weight of pork medallions or lean pork chops.

CREAMY GARLIC *and* PARMESAN CHICKEN

 10 MINS   **35 MINS**   **SERVES 4**

Use GF stock cube and bread

PER SERVING:
258 KCAL / 4.7G CARBS

low-calorie cooking spray
500g diced chicken breast
1 small onion, peeled and
   finely chopped
4 garlic cloves, peeled
   and crushed
475ml chicken stock
   (1 very low-salt chicken
   stock cube dissolved in
   475ml boiling water)
30g wholemeal bread
60g Parmesan, grated
3 tsp dried chives
100g reduced-fat
   cream cheese
150g broccoli, cut into
   small florets
freshly ground black
   pepper (optional)

TO ACCOMPANY
80g steamed veg (+ 35 kcal
   per serving) or Stir-fried
   Savoy Cabbage, page 221
   (+ 38 kcal per serving)

> **TIP:** If you do not have
> a pan suitable for the oven
> and hob, cook the chicken
> and sauce in a large frying
> pan and transfer to an
> ovenproof dish before
> sprinkling with breadcrumbs
> and putting in the oven.

If you're a cheese lover, then this is the dish for you! The double whammy of cheese in this recipe means that it's hard to believe that it's slimming friendly, but it's surprisingly low on calories. We've used strong-flavoured Parmesan as a little goes a long way and it helps to keep the calories down. Serve with our Stir-fried Savoy Cabbage (page 221) for a super-satisfying dinner that tastes as good as it looks.

Everyday Light

Spray a large ovenproof pan or casserole pan with low-calorie cooking spray and place over a high heat. Add the chicken and cook for 2–3 minutes until sealed. Remove from the pan, cover and put to one side. Give the pan another spray with low-calorie cooking spray and return to a medium heat. Add the onion and sauté for 5 minutes until beginning to soften, then add the garlic and cook for a further minute. Pour in the stock and bring to the boil, reduce the heat and simmer for 10 minutes.

While the stock simmers, preheat the oven to 200°C (fan 180°C/gas mark 6) and blitz the bread in a blender to make breadcrumbs. Mix the crumbs with half the Parmesan and 1 teaspoon of the chives in a small bowl. Set aside.

Add the cream cheese, the remaining Parmesan and another teaspoon of the chives to the stock and stir until well mixed. Test the consistency of the sauce – it should lightly coat the back of a spoon like thin cream. If it is too thin, simmer it for a couple more minutes until the correct consistency is reached. Return the chicken to the pan along with the broccoli and the rest of the chives and mix until well combined. Season with pepper if desired (you probably won't need any salt).

Sprinkle the breadcrumb mix over the top and bake in the oven for 10–15 minutes until the chicken and broccoli are cooked and the topping is crisp.

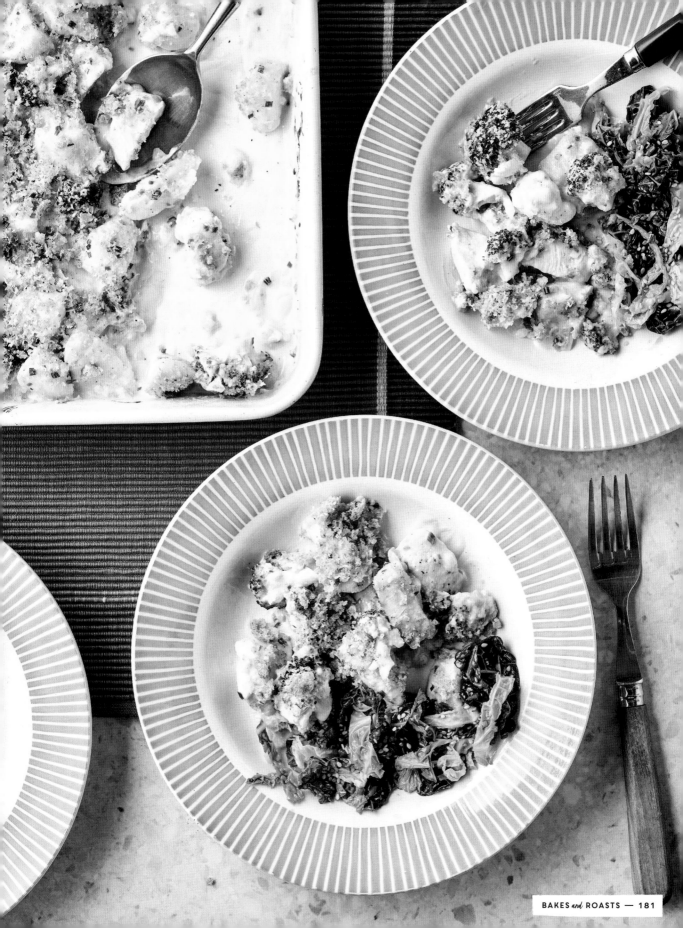

HUNTER'S CHICKEN PIE

Use GF stock cube and Henderson's relish

🕐 **20 MINS**   🗑 **1 HOUR**   ✕ **SERVES 4**

F **BF** **GF**

PER SERVING:
479 KCAL / 50G CARBS

low-calorie cooking spray
500g diced chicken breast
2 smoked bacon medallions,
   cut into 5mm (¼in) pieces
2 medium onions, peeled
   and chopped
2 tsp garlic granules
½ tsp dried oregano
1 tsp English mustard powder
2 tsp sweet smoked paprika
1 tbsp tomato puree
1 x 400g tin chopped tomatoes
200ml chicken stock
   (1 very low-salt chicken
   stock cube dissolved in
   200ml boiling water)
2 tbsp balsamic vinegar
1 tbsp Henderson's relish or
   Worcestershire sauce
2 medium carrots, peeled
   and sliced
½ tsp granulated sweetener,
   or caster sugar if you prefer
   (optional)
700g potatoes, peeled and cut
   into 4cm (1½in) chunks
80g reduced-fat mature
   Cheddar, grated
sea salt and freshly ground
   black pepper
sprinkle of finely chopped
   parsley, to serve

TO ACCOMPANY *(optional)*
80g steamed green vegetables
   (+ 35 kcal per serving)

One of our favourite things to serve alongside Hunter's Chicken is a big dollop of mash, so we thought why not combine the two into one family-friendly dish? This pie has tender chunks of chicken in a rich and smoky BBQ sauce and is topped with a cheesy, bacon mash to create the ultimate comforting meal.

Special Occasion

Spray a large saucepan with low-calorie cooking spray and place over a medium-high heat. Add the chicken, cook for 2–3 minutes to seal, then transfer to a plate and set to one side. In the same pan, fry the bacon for 2 minutes (or longer if you like it crispy). Transfer to a plate and set to one side.

Turn the heat down to medium, give the pan another spray with low-calorie cooking spray (no need to clean the pan – you want to keep the bacon flavours) and sauté the onions for 5 minutes until they are softening. Add the garlic granules, oregano, mustard powder and smoked paprika and stir well, then stir in the tomato puree, chopped tomatoes, stock, vinegar and Henderson's relish. Add the carrots and return the chicken to the pan. Reduce the heat and simmer, uncovered, for 20–25 minutes, until the carrots are cooked and the sauce is thick and rich. Taste and add the sweetener if desired.

Meanwhile, preheat the oven to 200°C (fan 180°C/ gas mark 6) and cook the potatoes in a saucepan of boiling salted water for about 15 minutes. When you can slide a knife easily through the potatoes, drain, return to the pan and mash well. Stir the bacon and three-quarters of the grated cheese into the mashed potato and season with black pepper and a little salt if you wish.

Transfer the cooked chicken to an ovenproof dish. Top it with the mash and use a fork to fluff up the top. Sprinkle with the remaining cheese and bake in the oven for 20–25 minutes until golden on the top. Remove from the oven, sprinkle with parsley and serve with your choice of accompaniment.

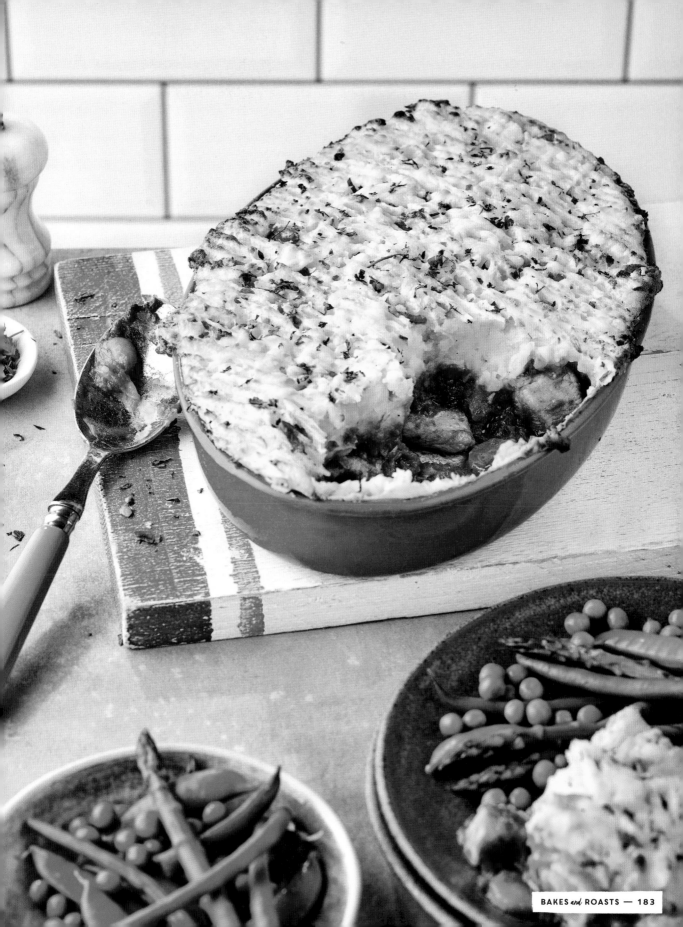

FORGOTTEN LAMB

🕐 **5 MINS***   🍲 **1 HOUR**   ✕ **SERVES 6**

*PLUS OVERNIGHT MARINATING

F **LC** **GF**

PER SERVING:
424 KCAL / 3.6G CARBS

100g reduced-fat natural
   yoghurt
1 tbsp tomato puree
juice of 1 lemon
1 tsp sweet smoked paprika
1 tsp dried oregano
½ tsp ground turmeric
1 tsp salt
1kg half leg of lamb

The name may sound mysterious but there's no big secret: this recipe was a happy accident! We forgot that we had put the lamb in its marinade the day before and it was left to marinate for a full 24 hours, meaning the spices had plenty of time to infuse the meat and develop its flavour. It turned out to be one of the most amazing lamb dishes we've ever had, and so Forgotten Lamb was born! It's great with wholemeal pittas, pickled red onion, and a 0%-fat yoghurt mixed with fresh mint.

Weekly Indulgence

To make the marinade, mix all of the ingredients except the lamb in a large non-metallic mixing bowl. Put the lamb in the bowl, coat it well in the marinade, then cover and refrigerate overnight.

Transfer the lamb to a roasting tin and cook for 1 hour, or according to the instructions indicated on the lamb packaging.

❝
"Thank you for creating such a wonderful recipe book!"

—— SOPHIE

TIP: You can slice the cooked lamb into portions and freeze.

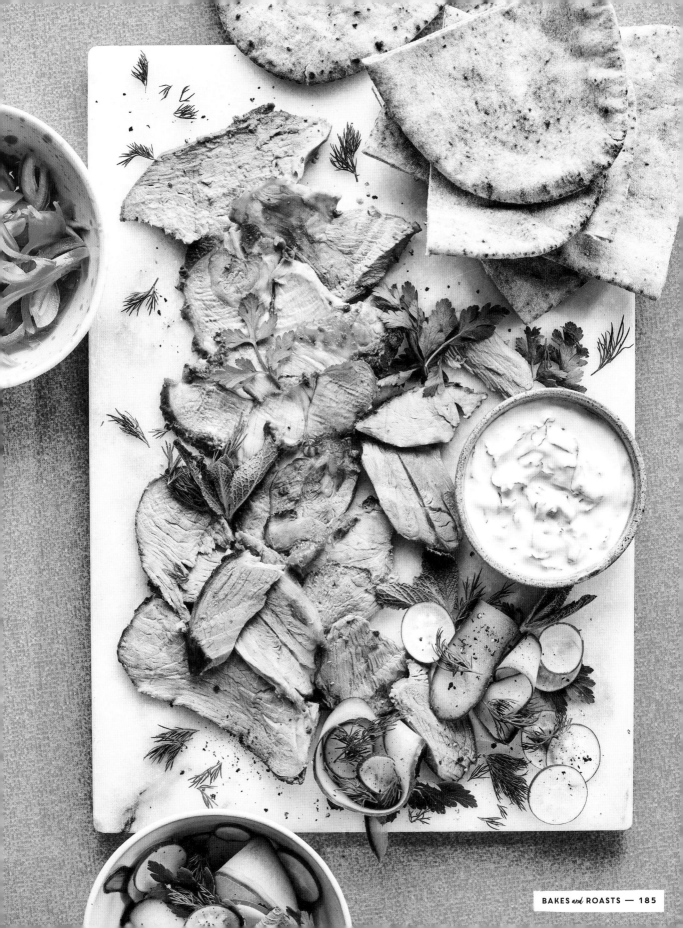

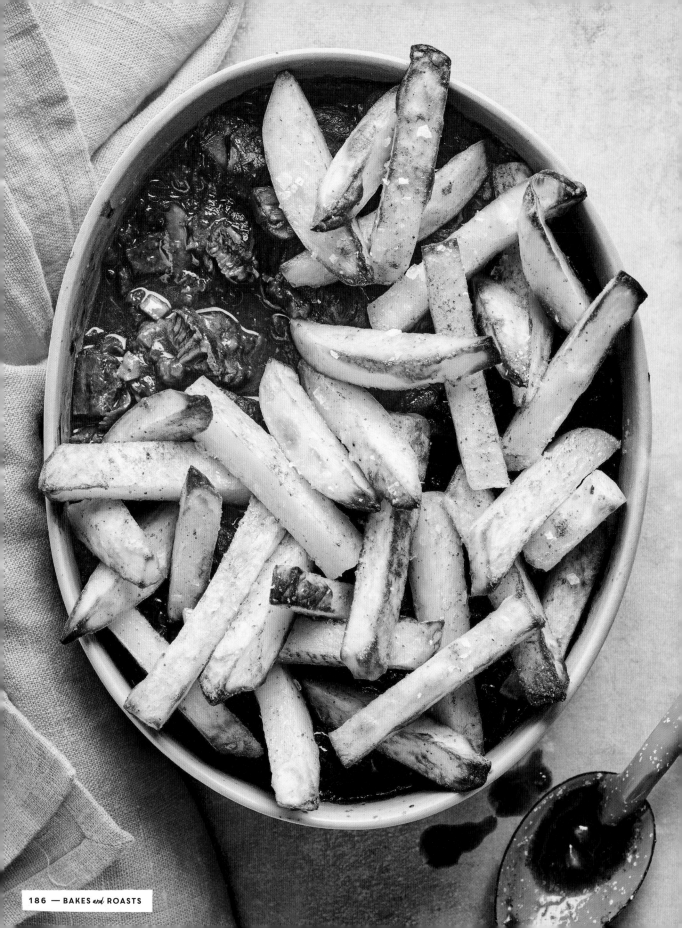

STEAK *and* CHIPS PIE

⏱ **25 MINS**   🍲 **VARIABLE** (SEE BELOW)   ✕ **SERVES 4**

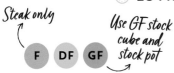

Steak only

F **DF** **GF**

Use GF stock cube and stock pot

PER SERVING:
316 KCAL / 38G CARBS

low-calorie cooking spray
1 onion, peeled and diced
400g diced stewing steak,
 all visible fat removed
300g carrots, peeled and diced
200g mushrooms, cut in half
300ml beef stock (1 stock pot
 and 1 very low-salt stock
 cube dissolved in 300ml
 boiling water) (250ml stock
 for the slow-cooker method)
15g cornflour
500g potatoes, peeled
½ tsp all-purpose seasoning
 (such as Schwartz 'Season-
 All' spice mix)

TO ACCOMPANY
80g steamed green
 vegetables (+ 35 kcal
 per serving)

Steak pie and chips is a classic pub staple, but we've given it a makeover by switching out the high-fat pastry for an even better topping: chips! We've packed it full of veggies and a savoury gravy so you can bring a taste of slimming-friendly pub grub to your kitchen without even having to leave the house.

Everyday Light

OVEN METHOD
🍲 **3 HOURS 40 MINS**

Preheat the oven to 180°C (fan 160°C/gas mark 4).

Spray an ovenproof casserole dish with low-calorie cooking spray and place over a medium heat. Add the onion and cook for 3–4 minutes until it starts to soften, then add the diced steak and cook for 5 minutes until the steak has browned on all sides. Add the carrots, mushrooms and stock to the pan, stir well, then cover with a lid and place in the preheated oven for 2–2½ hours.

When the steak is cooked and tender, mix the cornflour with a little water and stir it into the pie mix. Cover and cook for another 20–30 minutes until thickened. Remove from the heat and set aside.

Increase the oven temperature to 220°C (fan 200°C/gas mark 7).

Cut the potatoes into chips about 1cm (½in) wide and place in a bowl of cold water to rinse off the starch. Drain the chips in a colander then dry them using some kitchen towel. Place them on a baking tray, spray with low-calorie cooking spray and sprinkle over the spice mix. Pop them in the oven for 20 minutes, turning the chips once. The chips will be slightly tender at this point but not completely cooked. Remove from the oven and set aside.

Reduce the oven temperature to 180°C (fan 160°C/gas mark 4). Arrange the chips evenly over the top of the steak mix and cook in the oven uncovered for 15–20 minutes until golden.

SLOW-COOKER METHOD
🍲 HIGH: 3 HOURS 50 MINS LOW: 6 HOURS 50 MINS

SPECIAL EQUIPMENT
Slow cooker

Put the steak, onion, mushrooms, carrots and stock in the slow cooker, cover and cook on high for 3 hours or low for 6 hours.

Preheat the oven to 220°C (fan 200°C/gas mark 7).

Cut the potatoes into chips about 1cm (½in) wide and place in a bowl of cold water to rinse off the starch.

Drain the chips in a colander then dry them using some kitchen towel. Place them on a baking tray, spray with low-calorie cooking spray and sprinkle over the spice mix. Pop them in the oven for 20 minutes, turning the chips once. The chips will be slightly tender at this point but not completely cooked. Remove from the oven and set aside.

When the steak is cooked and tender, mix the cornflour with a little water and stir it into the pie mix. Cover and cook for another 20–30 minutes until thickened. Cover and set aside.

Reduce the oven temperature to 180°C (fan 160°C/gas mark 4).

Pour the pie mix into an ovenproof dish, arrange the chips evenly over the top of the pie mix and cook in the oven for 15–20 minutes until golden.

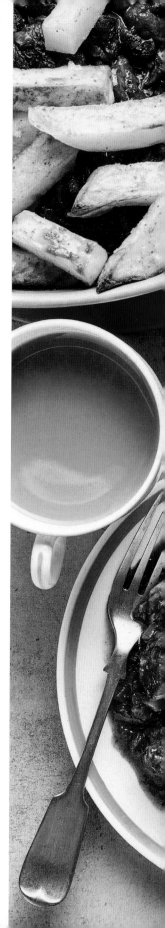

"
" Pinch of Nom's meals have been amazing and completely changed my way of thinking and my lifestyle."

—— CHRIS

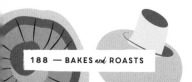

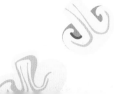

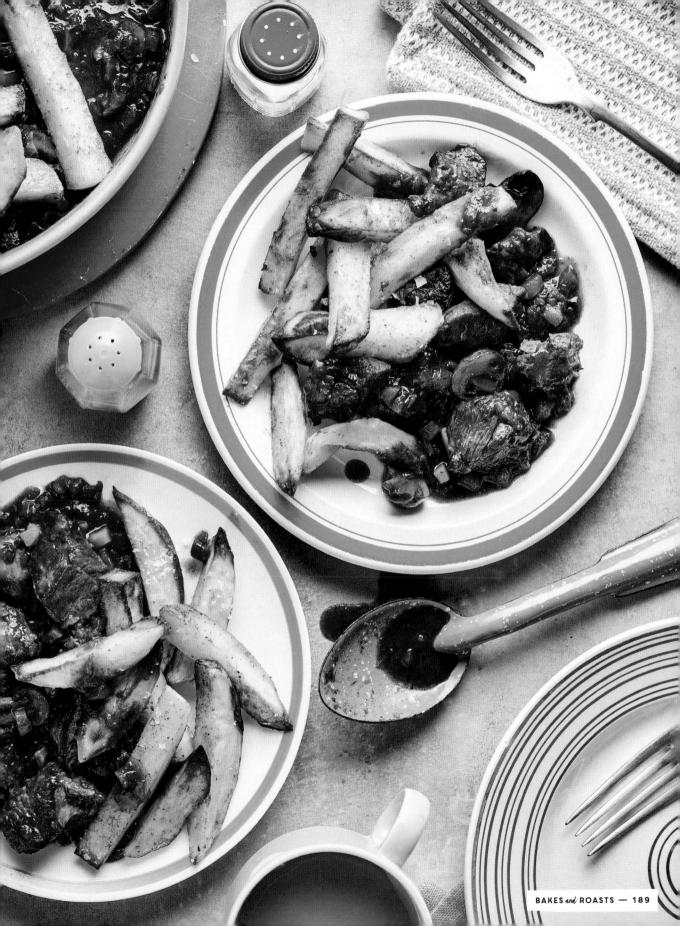

ONE-POT MEDITERRANEAN CHICKEN RICE

🕐 **20 MINS** 📦 **1 HOUR** ✕ **SERVES 4**

For rice reheating, see page 12

Use GF stock cube

F **DF** **GF**

PER SERVING:
349 KCAL / 46G CARBS

1½ tsp smoked sweet paprika
1½ tsp ground allspice
½ tsp ground turmeric
½ tsp salt
6 skinless, boneless chicken
   thighs (visible fat removed),
   about 450g in total
low-calorie cooking spray
1 onion, peeled and diced
1 carrot, peeled and diced
1 celery stick, diced
6 garlic cloves, peeled and
   left whole
4 mushrooms, thickly sliced
140g cherry tomatoes
juice of 1 lemon
500ml chicken stock
   (1 very low-salt chicken stock
   cube dissolved in 500ml
   boiling water)
200g long-grain rice, rinsed
   and drained
handful of flat-leaf parsley
   leaves, roughly chopped

Our One-pot Mediterranean Chicken Orzo recipe caused a huge stir when we published it online, and this new version uses fluffy, savoury rice instead of orzo pasta! We've made this dish naturally gluten free, and it's a real people-pleaser dinner. We love making a big batch and freezing the leftovers for another day.

Everyday Light ⎯⎯⎯⎯⎯⎯⎯⎯⎯⎯⎯⎯⎯⎯

Preheat the oven to 200°C (fan 180°C/gas mark 6).

Combine the paprika, ground allspice, turmeric and salt in a bowl, coat the chicken in the spice mixture and set aside for 10 minutes.

Spray a large casserole dish with low-calorie cooking spray and place over a medium heat. Add the seasoned chicken thighs and cook for about 2 minutes until they start to brown, then turn them over and brown on the other side for a further 2 minutes. Remove and set aside.

Add a few more sprays of low-calorie cooking spray to the dish, then add the onion, carrot, celery, garlic and mushrooms and fry for 6–8 minutes until the onion is soft. Add the tomatoes, lemon juice and 100ml of the chicken stock, return the chicken to the pan and bake in the oven with the lid on (or covered with foil) for 20 minutes.

Carefully remove the dish from the oven, add the rice, parsley and the rest of the stock, stir and return to the oven for 30 minutes with the lid off. The dish is ready when the rice has absorbed all the stock and is tender and fluffy.

TIPS: We used standard white rice, but some varieties take slightly different times to cook. If at the end of the cooking time you find the rice isn't quite cooked, pop the lid back on the dish and put it back into the oven for 5–10 minutes until it is ready. If you don't have a lidded dish suitable for both the hob and the oven, cook the first part in a saucepan, up until you need to return the chicken to the pan, and transfer to a deep roasting dish before covering with foil.

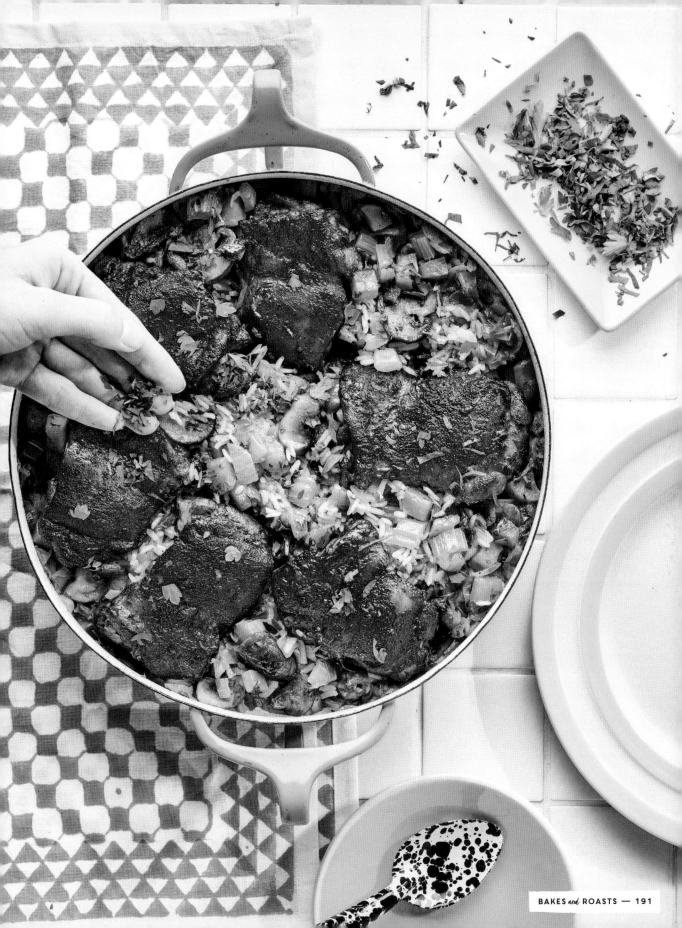

CREAMY GARLIC SALMON

If using fresh fish →

Use GF stock cube and Henderson's relish ←

(F) (BF) (LC) (GF)

🕐 **10 MINS**　📦 **30 MINS**　✕ **SERVES 4**

PER SERVING:
350 KCAL / 7.4G CARBS

low-calorie cooking spray
1 onion, peeled and thinly sliced
3 garlic cloves, peeled
  and crushed
250g button mushrooms,
  thinly sliced
1 tsp white wine vinegar
1 tbsp Henderson's relish or
  Worcestershire sauce
1 tsp Dijon mustard
400ml fish or chicken stock
  (1 fish or chicken stock
  cube dissolved in
  400ml boiling water)
4 skinless, boneless salmon
  fillets (about 125g each),
  cut into quarters
175g low-fat cream cheese
salt and pepper
a few chives, chopped,
  to garnish

TO ACCOMPANY (optional)
50g uncooked basmati
  rice per portion, cooked
  according to packet
  instructions (+ 173 kcal per
  125g cooked serving) and 80g
  steamed green vegetables
  (+ 35 kcal per serving)

This dish is a twist on our super-popular Creamy Garlic Chicken recipe and is perfect for fish lovers. Think you're not a fan of salmon? Think again, as this Creamy Garlic Salmon is so delicious and indulgent that it's sure to change your mind! Perfect for a midweek dinner, this recipe is guaranteed to be a new family favourite.

Special Occasion

Spray a large frying pan with low-calorie cooking spray and place over a medium heat. Add the onion, garlic and mushrooms and cook for 5–10 minutes until lightly golden. Add the white wine vinegar, Henderson's relish or Worcestershire sauce, Dijon mustard and stock, stir well, reduce the heat to low and simmer for about 10 minutes until reduced by half.

Add the salmon pieces and simmer over a low heat for about 10 minutes, until the salmon is opaque and flakes when tested. Carefully turn over the salmon pieces halfway through cooking, taking care not to break up the fish too much.

When the salmon is cooked, gently stir in the cream cheese until completely blended in. Again, take care not to break up the salmon too much. Season to taste with salt and pepper and serve, sprinkled with some chopped chives and with your choice of accompaniment.

TIP: You want chunks of salmon, so avoid stirring too much otherwise you will end up with flakes rather than chunks.

SWAP THIS: Garnish the dish with finely chopped spring onion instead of chives, if you prefer.

HOW TO BATCH: Cool the fish within 2 hours of cooking, then divide into individual portions and freeze immediately. Find detailed guidelines on reheating on page 12.

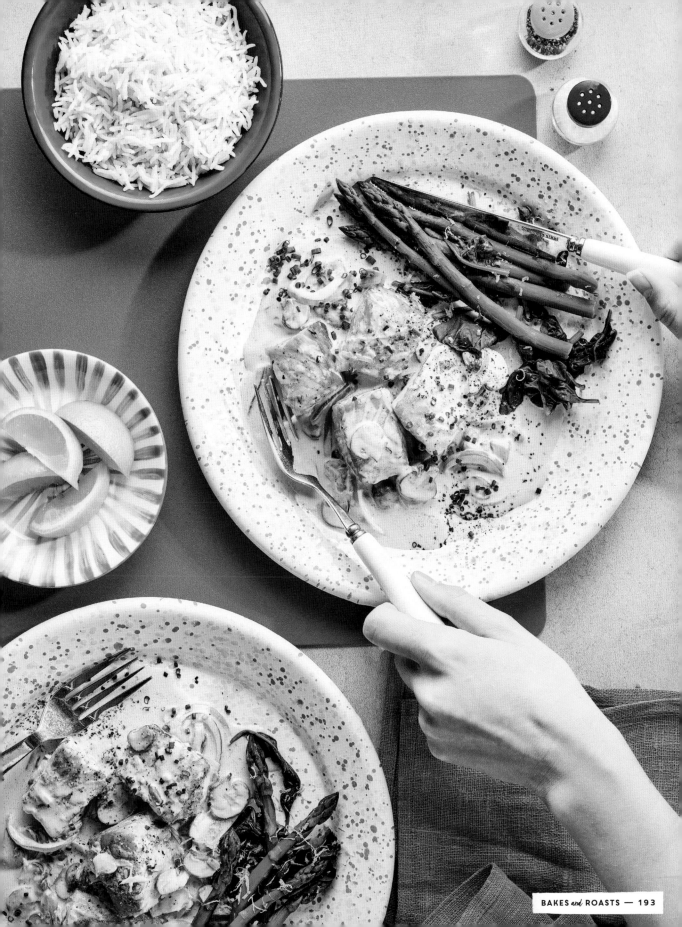

CHESTNUT ROAST

🕐 **20 MINS**   🍲 **45 MINS***   ✕ **SERVES 6**

***PLUS 10 MINUTES RESTING TIME**

PER SERVING:
184 KCAL / 31G CARBS

SPECIAL EQUIPMENT
900g (2lb) loaf tin

low-calorie cooking spray
1 onion, peeled and
    finely chopped
1 large carrot, peeled
    and grated
150g mushrooms, finely
    chopped (a food processor
    is good for this)
1 tsp garlic granules
½ tsp dried thyme
2 tbsp dark soy sauce
1 tbsp tomato puree
1 tsp white wine vinegar
60g wholemeal bread
2 x 180g bags ready-cooked
    chestnuts, roughly chopped
sea salt and freshly ground
    black pepper
1 medium egg, beaten

Chestnuts are a staple part of Christmas, with the rustic aroma filling the kitchen when they're roasting away. Did you know they're lower in fat than many other nuts, too? For a veggie-friendly main that's not only limited to the holidays, this Chestnut Roast is the ideal choice. Packed with filling mushrooms and nutritious veggies, it's a roast-dinner treat that won't stray too far from slimming plans!

Everyday Light

Preheat the oven to 200°C (fan 180°C/gas mark 6). Spray the loaf tin with low-calorie cooking spray and line it with baking parchment.

Spray a large frying pan with low-calorie cooking spray and place over a medium heat. Add the onion, carrot and mushrooms and sauté for about 10 minutes. The vegetables will release some liquid – keep sautéing until this has evaporated and you have a drier mix. Add the garlic granules, thyme and soy sauce and stir over the heat for another minute, then stir in the tomato puree and white wine vinegar. Remove from the heat.

Blitz the bread in a blender to make breadcrumbs. Place the cooked vegetables in a mixing bowl and add the breadcrumbs and chestnuts. Mix until well combined. Taste the mix and season with salt and pepper to taste. When you are happy with the seasoning, stir in the egg and press the mix into the prepared loaf tin.

Bake the chestnut roast in the preheated oven for 30–35 minutes, until golden and firm to touch.

Remove from the oven and allow to rest in the tin for 10 minutes before turning out and cutting into six slices. Serve with your choice of accompaniments.

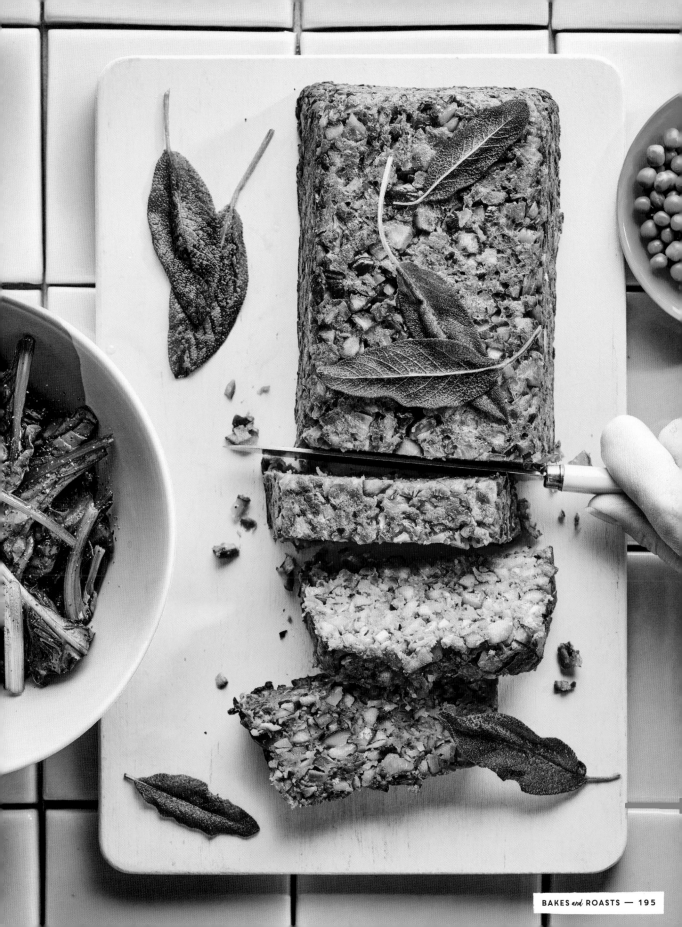

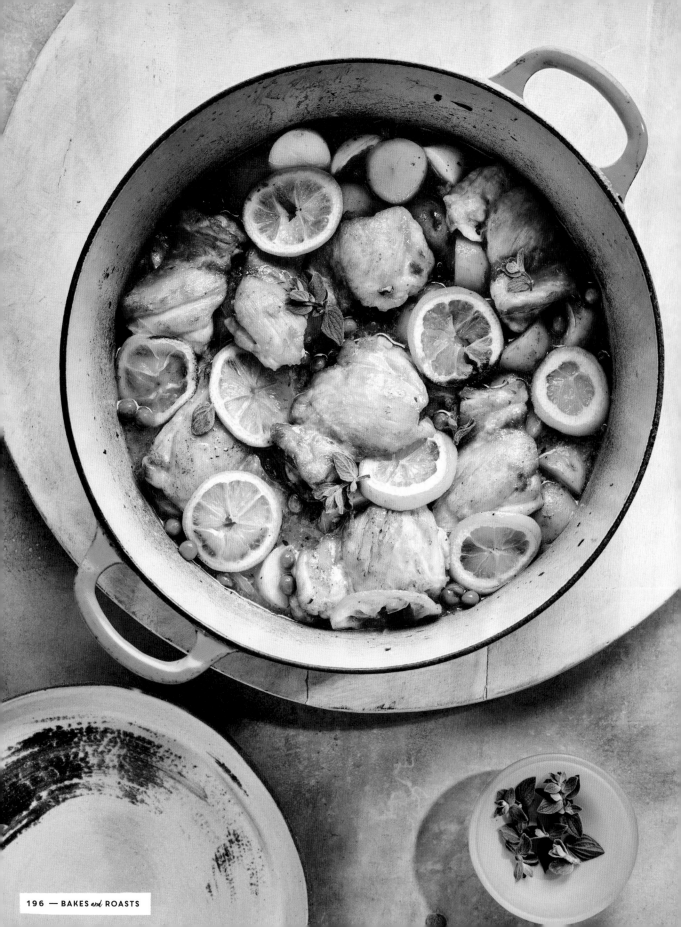

CHICKEN VESUVIO

Use GF stock cube and stock pot

🕐 **10 MINS** | 🍲 **1 HOUR** | ✕ **SERVES 4**

PER SERVING:
357 KCAL / 37G CARBS

SPECIAL EQUIPMENT
Large, shallow casserole dish (about 30cm/12in)

low-calorie cooking spray
8 skinless, boneless chicken thighs (visible fat removed), about 600g in total
sea salt and freshly ground black pepper
2 onions, peeled and thinly sliced
4 garlic cloves, peeled and crushed
1 tsp dried oregano
750g new potatoes, cut into half (or thirds if large), so they are evenly sized and no larger than 3cm (1¼in)
500ml chicken stock (1 chicken stock cube dissolved in 500ml boiling water)
1 white wine stock pot
1 lemon, sliced
100g frozen garden peas

An Italian/American dish with famous roots in Chicago, this Chicken Vesuvio has been given a Nom makeover to create a slimming-friendly, easy midweek meal. Succulent chicken thighs and golden roast potatoes soak up all the delicious flavours of the sauce, and this one-pot dish saves you time and effort as well as calories!

Everyday Light

Preheat the oven to 200°C (fan 180°C/gas mark 6).

Spray the large casserole dish with some low-calorie cooking spray and place over a medium-high heat. Season the chicken thighs with a little salt and pepper, then add them to the pan and seal for 1–2 minutes on each side. Remove and set aside.

Give the casserole dish another spray of low-calorie cooking spray and add the onions. Sauté for 5–6 minutes until soft, then add the garlic and oregano and cook for a further minute. Add the potatoes, chicken stock and white wine stock pot, bring to the boil and cook for 5 minutes on the hob.

Nestle the chicken pieces into the dish and tuck the lemon slices in between. Place in the preheated oven and cook for 30–35 minutes, until the top of the chicken is browned and the potatoes are soft.

Remove from the oven and scatter over the peas. Return to the oven and cook for a further 5 minutes.

Serve.

TIP: If you don't have a casserole dish, use a large frying pan for steps 2–3, then transfer to a 30cm (12in) ovenproof lasagne dish and continue following the instructions.

SWAP THIS: If you can't find white wine stock pots, reduce the water used to make up the stock to 400ml and add 100ml white wine instead. This will increase the calories to 401 kcal per serving.

DANGER DOGS

🕐 **10 MINS**   🍲 **20 MINS**   ✕ **SERVES 4**

Use GF sausages

GF

PER SERVING:
351 KCAL /29G CARBS

low-calorie cooking spray
8 smoked bacon medallions
8 chicken chipolatas
2 small onions, peeled and
  thinly sliced
2 peppers (any colour),
  deseeded and thinly sliced
2 tbsp balsamic vinegar
1 tsp English mustard powder
1 tsp garlic granules
4 gluten-free finger rolls
  (use regular finger rolls
  if you prefer)

These Danger Dogs are based on a Mexican street food that's also popular in the USA and they're guaranteed to be a hit! We've used chicken chipolatas for this dish, but you can use hotdogs or even your favourite low-fat sausages instead. Serve with our BBQ Beans (page 226) or our Cowboy Fries (page 212) for a delicious fakeaway feast.

Weekly Indulgence

Preheat the oven to 200°C (fan 180°C/gas mark 6), line a baking tray with foil and spray the foil with low-calorie cooking spray.

Cut the bacon medallions lengthways down the middle to create strips. Wrap them around your sausages to cover them like pigs in blankets, using two strips (one medallion) per sausage.

Place the sausages on the lined tray and spray the tops of the wrapped sausages with more low-calorie cooking spray. Cook in the preheated oven for 20 minutes, or until the sausages are cooked through.

While the sausages are cooking, heat a frying pan over a medium-low heat, add the onions and peppers with 2 tablespoons of water and the balsamic vinegar, mustard powder and garlic granules and cook for 10 minutes until they have softened and the liquid has evaporated.

When the sausages are cooked, add two to each bun and top with some onion and pepper mix. You can have them as they are, or add your favourite sauces.

SWAP THIS: Swap the gluten-free finger rolls for hotdog buns of choice – just remember to alter the calories accordingly.

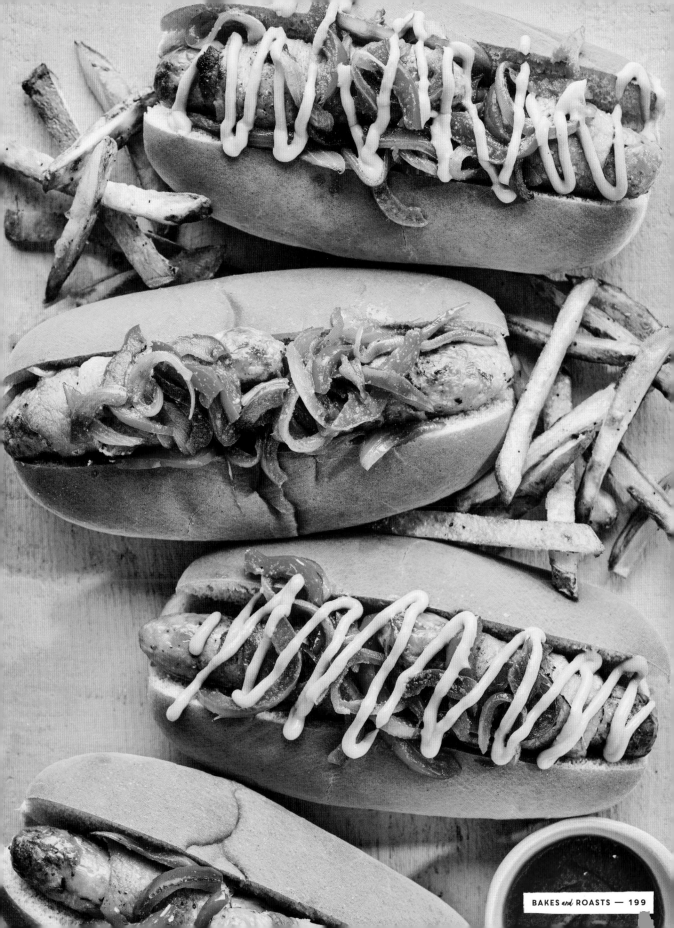

CHEESE, ONION
and POTATO PIE

🕐 **15 MINS**   🍲 **50 MINS**   ✕ **SERVES 6**

Use Henderson's relish ↗

V **F**

PER SERVING:
286 KCAL /31G CARBS

SPECIAL EQUIPMENT
Deep pie dish or ovenproof baking dish about 24 x 20 x 5cm (9½ x 8 x 2in)

600g potatoes, peeled and
  cut into small chunks
low-calorie cooking spray
300g onions, peeled and diced
240g reduced-fat mature
  Cheddar, grated
1 tsp English mustard powder
1 tsp garlic granules
2 tsp Henderson's relish or
  Worcestershire sauce
1 egg, beaten
4 sheets of filo pastry
  (about 20g per sheet)
sea salt and freshly ground
  black pepper

Our Cheese, Onion and Potato Pie is comfort food at its finest, and by replacing high-calorie shortcrust pastry with filo, this is a dish that you can enjoy even if you're counting calories. It's substantial and filling: just what you're after for an easy dinner that's full of flavour.

Everyday Light ───────────────────────

Preheat the oven to 200°C (fan 180°C/gas mark 6).

Put the diced potatoes in a saucepan of cold salted water and bring to the boil. Reduce the heat and simmer for 15 minutes, or until a fork slides easily through the potatoes.

While the potatoes are cooking, spray a frying pan with low-calorie cooking spray and place over a medium-low heat. Add the onions and sauté for up to 15 minutes until they are soft and a golden-brown colour. Don't be tempted to increase the heat to speed up this process as the slow cooking caramelises the onions and develops the flavour.

When the potatoes are cooked, drain and place in a bowl. Roughly mash them with a fork – it's fine to have some pieces remaining. Add the grated cheese (reserving a handful to top the pie), onions, mustard powder, garlic granules and the Henderson's relish or Worcestershire sauce. Add the beaten egg, season with salt and pepper and mix thoroughly.

Spray the pie dish with low-calorie cooking spray. A metal dish is best for this, as it helps to evenly cook the bottom.

Spray each sheet of filo pastry with low-calorie cooking spray and use the sheets to line the pie dish, leaving 3–4cm (1¼–1½in) over the edge of the dish. Spread the filling evenly into the pie dish and scrunch up the filo around the edge. Sprinkle the reserved grated cheese over the potato mixture, place in the preheated oven and cook for 30–35 minutes, until golden and firm. Remove from the oven, cut into six pieces and serve.

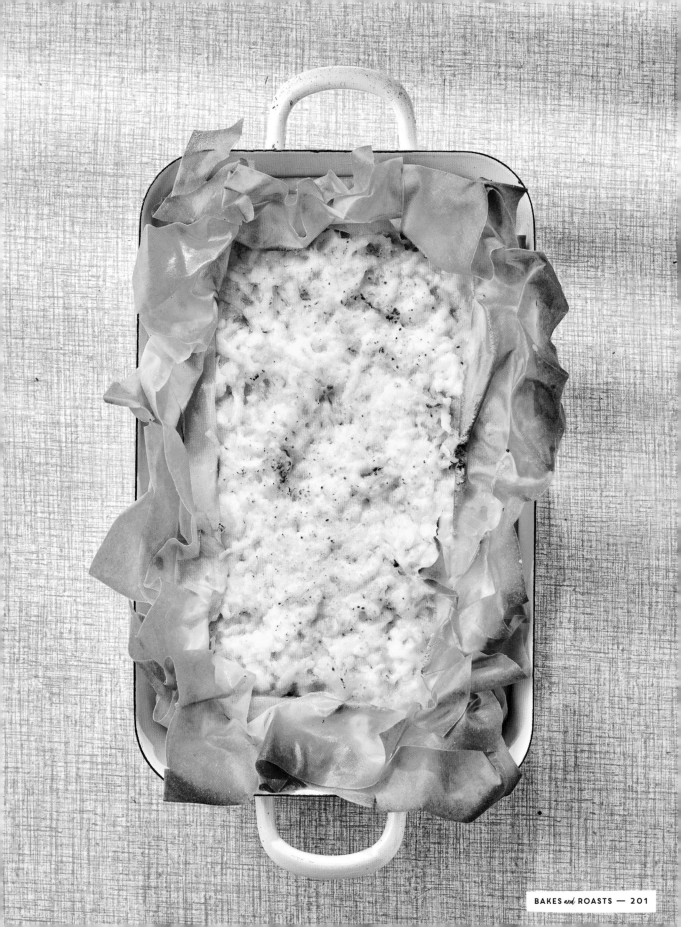

MINTED LAMB HOTPOT

🕐 **20 MINS** 🍲 **2 HOURS 30 MINS** ✕ **SERVES 4**

F **BF** **DF**

PER SERVING:
432 KCAL / 48G CARBS

SPECIAL EQUIPMENT
2.4-litre ovenproof dish

500g lean, diced leg of lamb,
   all visible fat removed
1 tbsp plain flour
1 large onion, peeled and sliced
3 carrots (about 200g), peeled
   and cut into 5mm (¼in) slices
150g swede, peeled and cut
   into 5mm (¼in) dice
2 tbsp mint sauce
½ tsp garlic granules
400ml chicken or lamb stock
   (1 chicken or lamb stock
   cube dissolved in 400ml
   boiling water)
700g potatoes, peeled and
   thinly sliced
low-calorie cooking spray
sea salt and freshly ground
   black pepper

TO ACCOMPANY
80g steamed green vegetables
   (+ 35 kcal per serving)

Using lean cuts of lamb and adding plenty of root vegetables keeps this fuss-free hotpot recipe surprisingly low in calories. The addition of a couple of spoonfuls of mint sauce elevates a simple one-pot dish to a delicious new level.

Weekly Indulgence

Preheat the oven to 170°C (fan 150°C/gas mark 3).

Toss the lamb in the flour until well coated, then put it in the ovenproof dish, along with the onion, carrots and swede, and mix together.

Stir the mint sauce and garlic granules into the stock and pour the stock into the dish.

Layer the sliced potatoes on top, so they overlap and completely cover the lamb and vegetables. Spray the potatoes with a little low-calorie cooking spray and season with salt and pepper. Cover with a lid or foil, ensuring it is as tightly sealed as possible, and place in the oven for 2 hours.

Increase the oven temperature to 190°C (fan 170°C/gas mark 5) and uncover the hotpot. Cook for a further 20–30 minutes, until the potatoes are nicely browned and soft in the middle.

Serve!

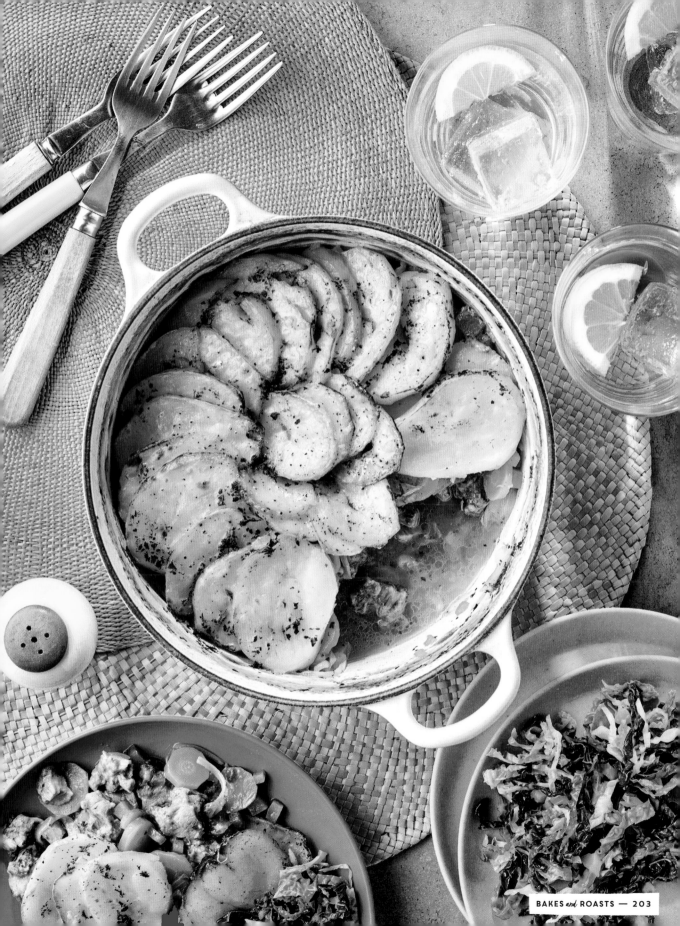

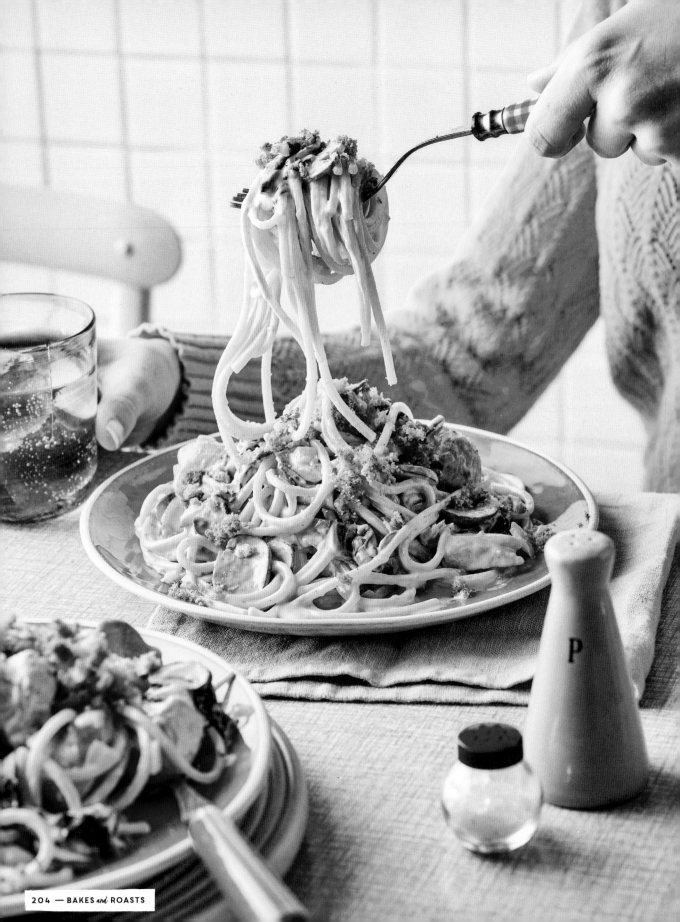

CHICKEN TETRAZZINI

🕐 **10 MINS** 🗑 **40 MINS** ✕ **SERVES 6**

F

PER SERVING:
529 KCAL / 59G CARBS

low-calorie cooking spray
4 small skinless chicken
  breasts (visible fat removed),
  about 430g in total, cut into
  2cm (¾in) chunks
2 onions, peeled and diced
1 tbsp garlic granules
200ml chicken stock
  (1 low-salt chicken stock
  cube dissolved in 200ml
  boiling water)
1 white wine stock pot or
  1 tbsp white wine vinegar
500g mushrooms, thinly sliced
170g dried spaghetti
100g fresh spinach
150g low-fat spreadable cheese
sea salt and freshly ground
  black pepper
30g wholemeal bread
15g Parmesan or strong mature
  Cheddar, finely grated
½ tsp English mustard powder

If you've never heard of Tetrazzini before, it's an American dish that is usually made with spaghetti, diced chicken or seafood and mushrooms, slathered in a buttery, creamy cheese sauce and flavoured with wine or sherry – yum! This dish doesn't exactly scream 'low calorie', but we love a challenge so we thought we'd try our hand at creating a slimming-friendly version, and it tastes amazing, even if we do say so ourselves!

Special Occasion

Preheat the oven to 240°C (fan 220°C/gas mark 9).

Spray a large saucepan with low-calorie cooking spray and place over a medium heat. Add the chicken, onions and garlic granules and cook for 5 minutes until the outside of the chicken has coloured and the onions begin to soften. Add the stock and white wine stock pot or vinegar to the saucepan, then add the mushrooms, stir and simmer for 15 minutes until the stock has reduced and the chicken is cooked through. Once done, remove from the heat.

While the chicken and mushrooms are cooking, cook the spaghetti according to the packet instructions.

Drain the spaghetti and add it to the pan with the chicken along with the spinach. Stir to combine until the spinach has wilted slightly, then add the spreadable cheese and stir to coat the pasta and chicken mix. Season to taste with salt and pepper. (Note: it may not need any salt – the saltiness of the stock and spreadable cheese may have made it salty enough.) Pour the mixture into a roasting dish and set aside while you prepare the topping.

Blitz the bread in a blender to make breadcrumbs. Stir the grated cheese and mustard powder into the breadcrumb mix. Sprinkle the breadcrumb mix on top of the spaghetti and chicken and spritz the top with low-calorie cooking spray. Place in the middle of the preheated oven and bake for 20 minutes or until the top is lightly golden.

Remove from the oven and serve.

CHEESY FAJITA ORZOTTO

🕐 **10 MINS**   🍲 **25 MINS**   ✕ **SERVES 4**

PER SERVING:
477 KCAL / 48G CARBS

low-calorie cooking spray
400g 0%-fat turkey
   breast mince
1 onion, peeled and diced
2 peppers (any colour),
   deseeded and diced
2 tsp garlic granules
2 tbsp fajita seasoning
1 tbsp tomato puree
600ml chicken stock
   (1 very low-salt chicken
   stock cube dissolved in
   600ml boiling water)
200g orzo
juice of 1 lemon
handful of fresh coriander
   leaves, chopped
120g reduced-fat mature
   Cheddar, grated
2 spring onions, trimmed and
   thinly sliced, to garnish

TO ACCOMPANY *(optional)*
2 tbsp reduced-fat sour cream
   (+ 57 kcal per tablespoon)

Experimenting with orzo instead of larger pasta shapes helped to transform this dish from a fajita pasta bake to a risotto-like bowl of creamy, indulgent deliciousness! This recipe is really versatile; you can play around with the spice level and even the type of mince you use for a flexible and filling family dinner.

Special Occasion

Spray a casserole dish with low-calorie cooking spray and place over a medium-high heat. Add the turkey mince, onion and peppers and fry for 5–6 minutes until the mince is lightly browned and the onion soft. Add the garlic granules and fajita seasoning and stir well, then stir in the tomato puree and cook for a minute, before stirring in the stock and bringing to the boil.

Add the orzo to the pan and stir well, ensuring the pasta is covered by the stock. Reduce the heat to a simmer, cover and cook for 15–20 minutes, stirring every few minutes to make sure it doesn't catch on the bottom of the pan.

When the orzo is cooked and most of the liquid has been absorbed, uncover and stir in the lemon juice and coriander. If there is still excess liquid, cook the orzo for a few minutes without the lid on – you want a consistency similar to a risotto. Stir in the cheese until it's melted, sprinkle with sliced spring onions and serve!

> " *I have never enjoyed cooking as much – and being so healthy. Every recipe is a winner for the whole family.*"
>
> —— **SUZANNA**

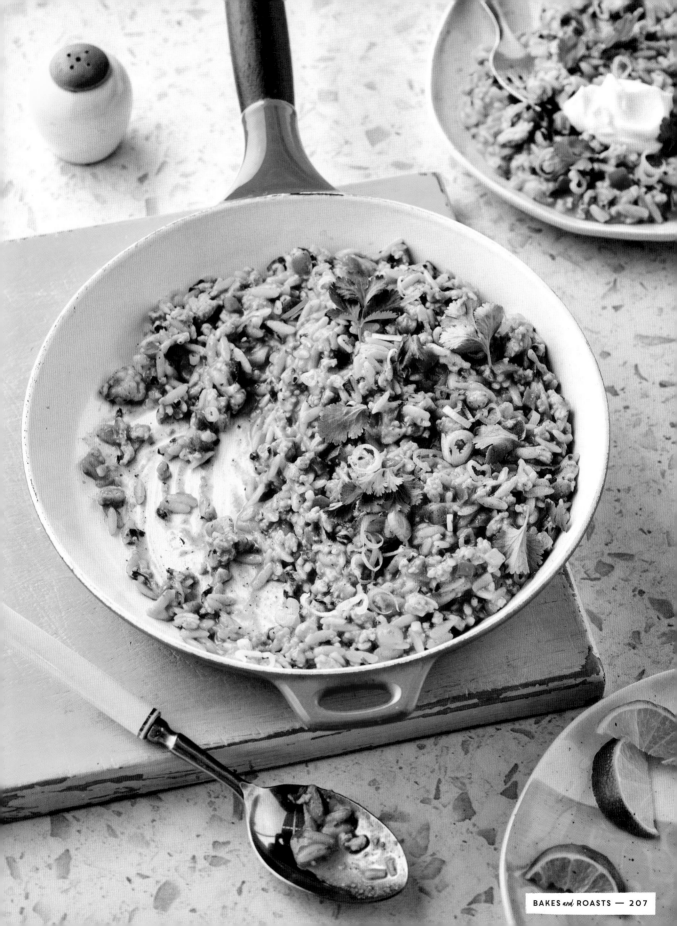

BUTTERNUT SQUASH
and BACON BAKE

🕐 **20 MINS**   🍲 **50 MINS**   ✕ **SERVES 4**

PER SERVING:
301 KCAL / 34G CARBS

SPECIAL EQUIPMENT
18 x 27cm (7 x 10½in)
ovenproof dish

600g butternut squash, peeled, deseeded and cut into 2cm (¾in) chunks
low-calorie cooking spray
2 onions, peeled and chopped
2 garlic cloves, peeled and crushed
250g chestnut mushrooms, thickly sliced
2 smoked bacon medallions, cut into 2cm (¾in) pieces
2 tsp thyme leaves, chopped
2 tsp oregano leaves, chopped
sea salt and black pepper

FOR THE CHEESE SAUCE
400ml skimmed milk
25g reduced-fat spread
2 tbsp cornflour
60g reduced-fat mature Cheddar, finely grated, plus 20g for the top
¼ tsp English mustard powder

TO ACCOMPANY *(optional)*
80g steamed green vegetables (+ 35 kcal per serving)

> **SWAP THIS:** Swap the bacon for cooked ham or chicken.

Bright and colourful, this hearty bake is perfect for dishing up on a cold autumn or winter's day! It's packed with tender vegetables and bacon, with a drizzling of light cheese sauce to keep you feeling full and satisfied.

Everyday Light ————————————————

Put the squash in a large saucepan and cover with water. Place over a high heat, cover and bring to the boil (taking care not to let the water boil over), then reduce the heat and simmer for 20 minutes, until tender. Drain well.

While the butternut squash is cooking, spray a large frying pan with low-calorie cooking spray and place over a medium heat. Add the onions and fry for 10 minutes until softened and golden, then add the garlic, mushrooms, bacon, thyme and oregano leaves, stir and cook for a further 10 minutes, until the bacon is cooked. Remove from the heat. Stir the squash into the vegetable and bacon mixture in the pan and season. Set aside while you make the sauce.

Preheat the oven to 200°C (fan 180°C/gas mark 6).

To make the cheese sauce, put the milk and reduced-fat spread in a saucepan and place over a medium heat. Heat until steaming, taking care not to let the milk boil over. Mix the cornflour in a bowl with 2 tablespoons of water until smooth, then add it to the hot milk, stirring continuously with a wooden spoon or a balloon whisk. Simmer for 4–5 minutes, until the sauce has thickened slightly. Add the 60g grated cheese and the mustard powder and stir until the cheese has melted. Season to taste with salt and pepper.

Spread out the vegetable mixture in the ovenproof dish. Pour the sauce evenly over the veg and sprinkle the remaining cheese on top. Place on a baking tray and bake in the oven for 15–20 minutes, until golden brown. Serve with your choice of accompaniment.

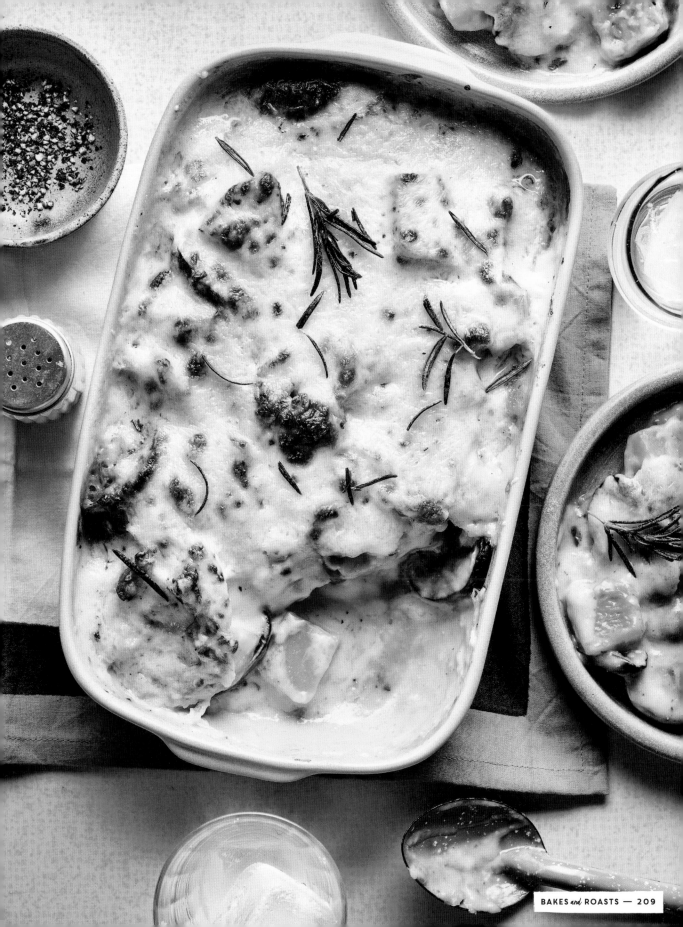

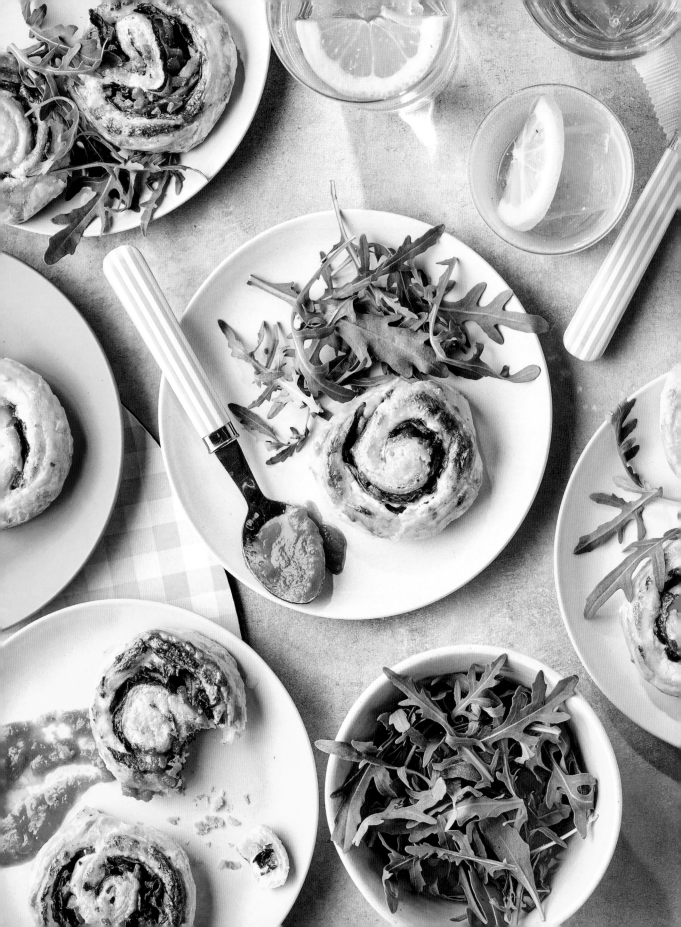

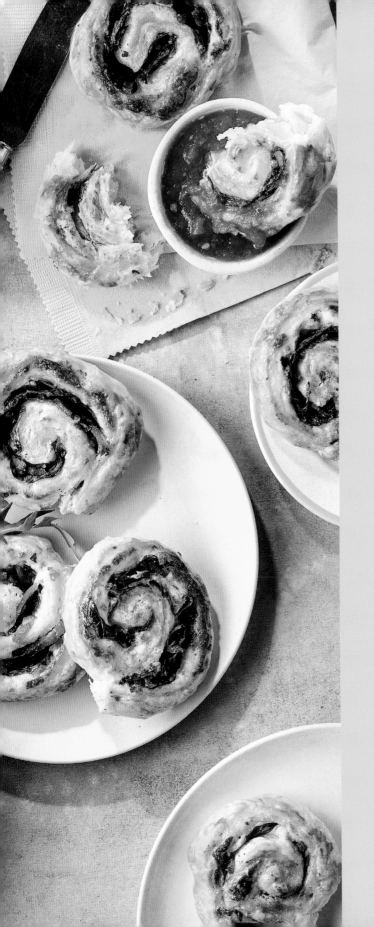

COWBOY FRIES

Bean topping only ↱

(F)

⏱ **10 MINS**   🍲 **VARIABLE** (SEE BELOW)   ✕ **SERVES 4**

PER SERVING:
364 KCAL / 50G CARBS

700g potatoes
low-calorie cooking spray
3 unsmoked bacon medallions
sea salt and freshly ground
   black pepper

FOR THE TOPPING
½ onion, peeled and diced
1 tsp garlic granules
1 tbsp BBQ seasoning
1 tsp English mustard powder
½ tsp smoked sweet paprika
1 x 400g tin chopped tomatoes
1 tbsp balsamic vinegar
2 tbsp Henderson's relish or
 Worcestershire sauce
1 tsp granulated sweetener
1 x 400g tin butter beans,
   drained and rinsed
80g reduced-fat mature
   Cheddar, grated

TO ACCOMPANY *(optional)*
75g mixed salad
   (+ 15 kcal per serving)

This dish ticks all the boxes: crispy, golden fries topped with smoky beans, crispy bacon and gooey cheese! This American-inspired dish uses a few clever swaps to keep the calories low while still packing a BBQ punch that reminds us of summer days. Serve with a crisp mixed salad for a fresh and tasty dinner, whatever the weather.

Special Occasion

OVEN METHOD
🍲 **1 HOUR**

Preheat the oven to 200°C (fan 180°C/gas mark 6).

Cut the potatoes into 1cm (½in)-thick fries (we like the skin left on, but you can peel them if you prefer). Scatter over a baking tray, spray with low-calorie cooking spray and season with a little salt and pepper, then bake in the oven for 45 minutes, turning them halfway through and giving the tray a shake.

Pop the bacon medallions on another baking tray and cook in the oven with the fries for 10–12 minutes, or longer if you like your bacon crispy. Remove and cut into small pieces. Set aside for later.

While the fries are cooking, make your topping. Spray a frying pan with low-calorie cooking spray and place over a medium heat. Add the onion and sauté for 5 minutes until soft, then add the garlic granules, BBQ seasoning, mustard powder and smoked paprika and cook for 1 minute. Add the tomatoes, balsamic vinegar, Henderson's relish or Worcestershire sauce and the sweetener, bring to a simmer and cook for 10 minutes, then stir in the butter beans and cook for a further 10 minutes.

When the fries are golden and cooked through, remove from the oven and top with the beans, grated cheese and bacon pieces.

Return to the oven for 10–15 minutes until the cheese is melted and gooey. Serve with your choice of accompaniment.

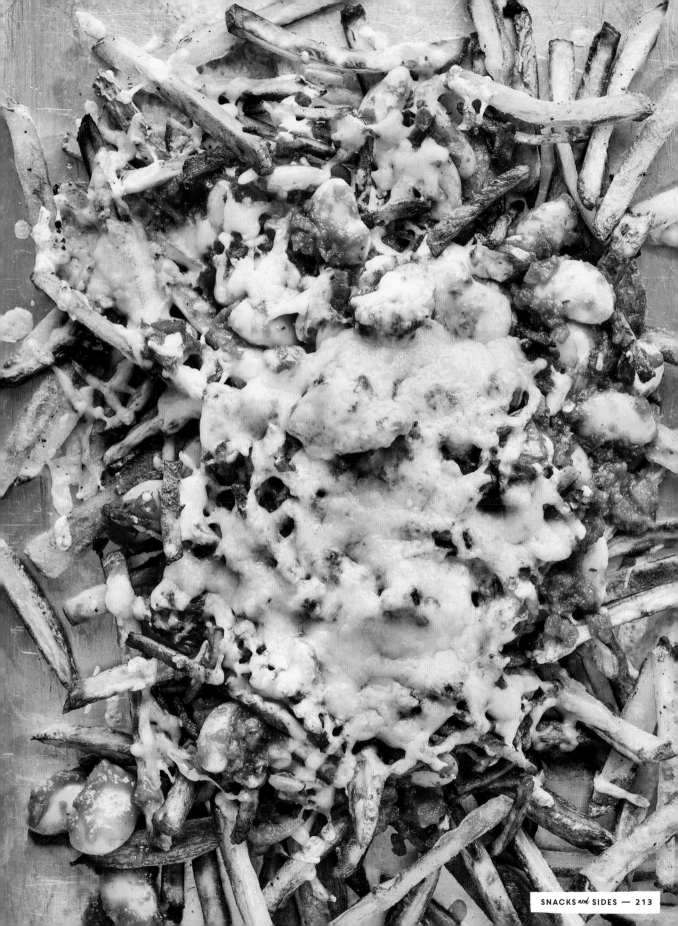

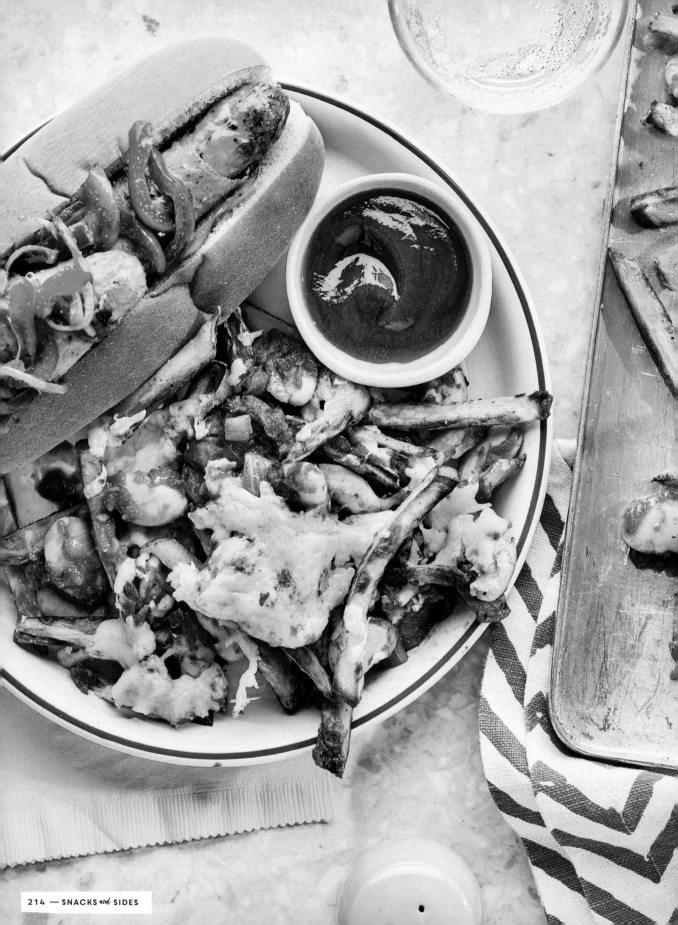

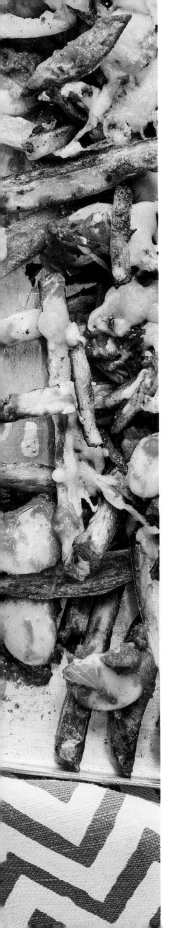

AIR-FRYER METHOD
🍲 40 MINUTES

SPECIAL EQUIPMENT
Air fryer

Preheat your air fryer to 180°C.

Spray the bacon with a little low-calorie cooking spray and place it in the air-fryer basket. Cook for 8–10 minutes, depending on how well done you like your bacon. When cooked to your liking, remove and cut into small pieces.

Cut the potatoes into 1cm (½in)-thick fries (we like the skin left on, but you can peel them if you prefer). Spray with low-calorie cooking spray and season with a little salt and pepper. Scatter over the air-fryer basket in an even layer and cook for 20–25 minutes, shaking occasionally to ensure even cooking. You may need to do this in two batches, depending on the size of your air fryer.

While the fries are cooking, make your topping. Spray a frying pan with low-calorie cooking spray and place over a medium heat. Add the onion and sauté for 5 minutes until soft, then add the garlic granules, BBQ seasoning, mustard powder and smoked paprika and cook for 1 minute. Add the tomatoes, balsamic vinegar, Henderson's relish or Worcestershire sauce and the sweetener, bring to a simmer and cook for 10 minutes, then stir in the butter beans and cook for a further 10 minutes.

Preheat the grill to medium/high.

When the fries are golden and cooked through, remove from the air fryer and place on a baking tray. Top with the beans, grated cheese and bacon pieces.

Pop under the grill for a couple of minutes until the cheese is melted and gooey.

Serve with your choice of accompaniment.

SPICED EDAMAME BEAN DIP

🕐 **5 MINS** 🍲 **5 MINS** ✕ **SERVES 6**

Use GF soy sauce ↗

VG F LC GF

PER SERVING:
80 KCAL / 5.2G CARBS

300g edamame beans,
  frozen or fresh
150g tinned cannellini beans,
  drained and rinsed
½–1 tsp Chinese 5-spice
pinch of dried chilli flakes
2 tsp lemon juice
¼ tsp soy sauce
sea salt and freshly ground
  black pepper

TO ACCOMPANY *(optional)*
100g portion of carrot sticks
  (+ 44 kcal per serving)

Shop-bought dips can be really high in calories, not to mention expensive. This tasty dip is a great alternative to traditional hummus – it's low in calories and packed full of tasty Asian flavours too! Great for a simple, quick lunch or as part of a buffet table with crunchy veggies for dipping.

Everyday Light

Cook the edamame beans according to packet instructions, then rinse in cold water and drain well.

Put all of the ingredients into a food processor and blitz until smooth. If you feel the dip is too thick, add a little boiling water and blitz again until it reaches the consistency you prefer. Season to taste with salt and pepper.

Serve with carrot sticks and other crudités if desired.

TIP: You can make this using fresh or frozen edamame beans – make sure that you buy the beans which have already been podded, or pod them yourself before weighing them.

SWAP THIS: You can make this as spicy or as mild as you like by adding more or fewer dried chilli flakes.

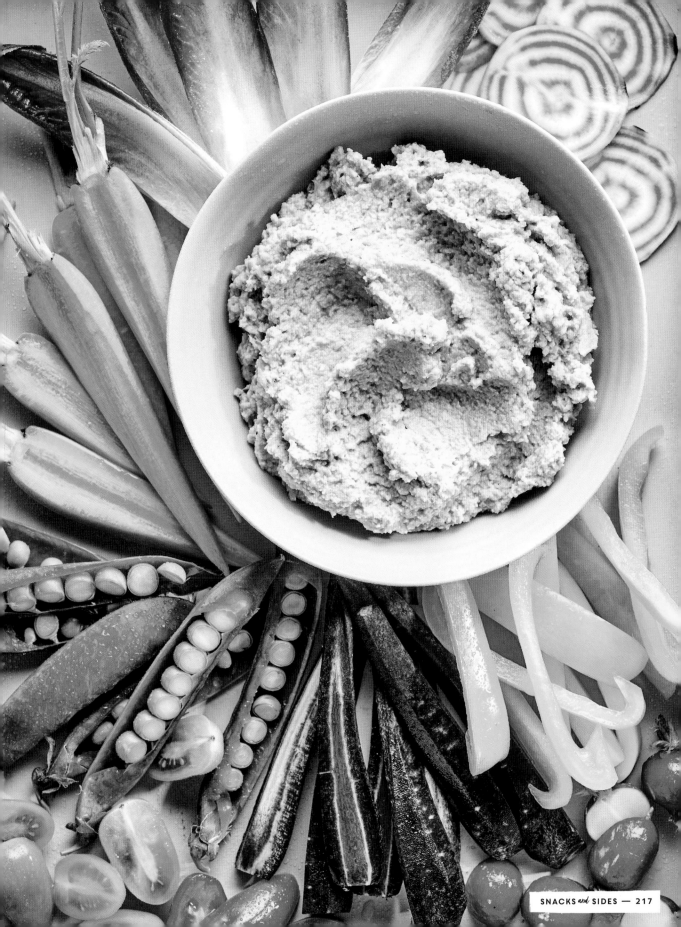

CHEESE *and* ONION MASH

🕐 **10 MINS** 🗑 **25 MINS** ✕ **SERVES 4**

PER SERVING:
252 KCAL / 40G CARBS

750g potatoes, peeled and
 cut into chunks
low-calorie cooking spray
2 red onions, peeled and
 thinly sliced
1 tsp balsamic vinegar
80g reduced-fat mature
 Cheddar, grated
sea salt and freshly ground
 black pepper

We didn't think it would be possible to improve on a bowl of classic mashed potatoes, but this Cheese and Onion Mash is a genuine pleasure! We've added caramelised onions, stirred through some reduced-fat cheese and lightly grilled the top to take this dish to the next level. Serve it with our Honey and Mustard Pork (page 179), or our Paprika Chicken (page 132), for a deliciously indulgent midweek meal.

Weekly Indulgence ——————————

Put the potatoes in a saucepan with enough water to cover, add a pinch of salt and bring to the boil. Cook for 15–20 minutes until soft.

While the potatoes are cooking, cook the onions. Spray a frying pan with low-calorie cooking spray, place over a low heat, add the onions and sauté for about 10 minutes until soft and starting to brown. Add a pinch of salt and the balsamic vinegar towards the end of cooking.

Preheat your grill.

When the potatoes are cooked, drain and mash them. Stir in the cooked onions and three-quarters of the grated cheese. Taste and season with salt and pepper.

Pile the mashed potato into an ovenproof dish and sprinkle over the rest of the cheese. Place under the hot grill for 3–4 minutes until the cheese is melted and golden.

Serve with your choice of accompaniment.

TIP: If you don't want to bother grilling the mashed potato, simply stir all the cheese through at step 4 and serve. Pick a good-quality potato for this. Yukon Gold are our favourite as they have a creamy, buttery texture, but Desiree and Maris Piper are a great choice too.

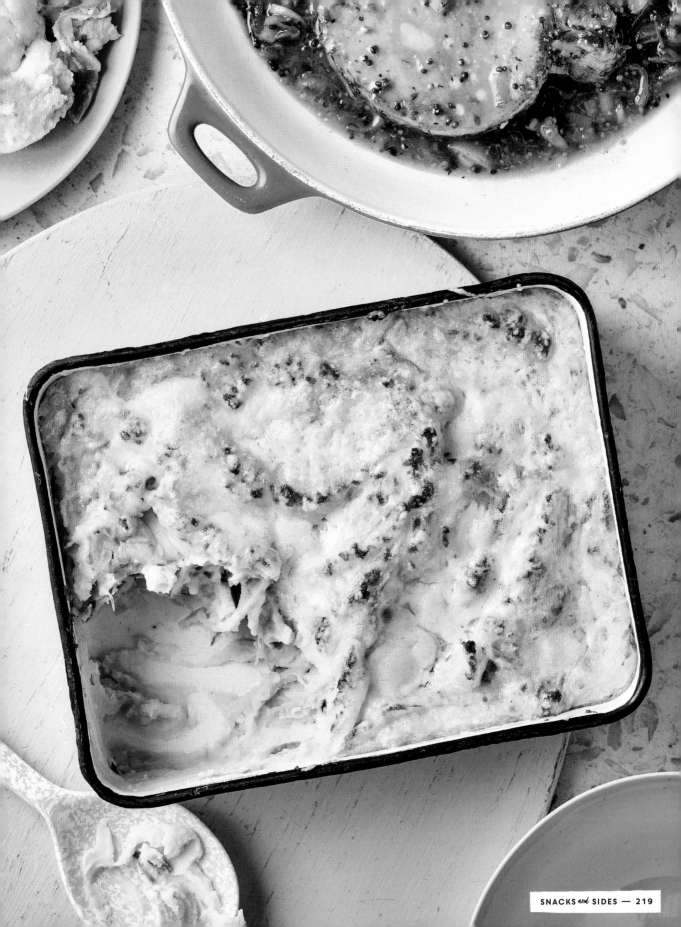

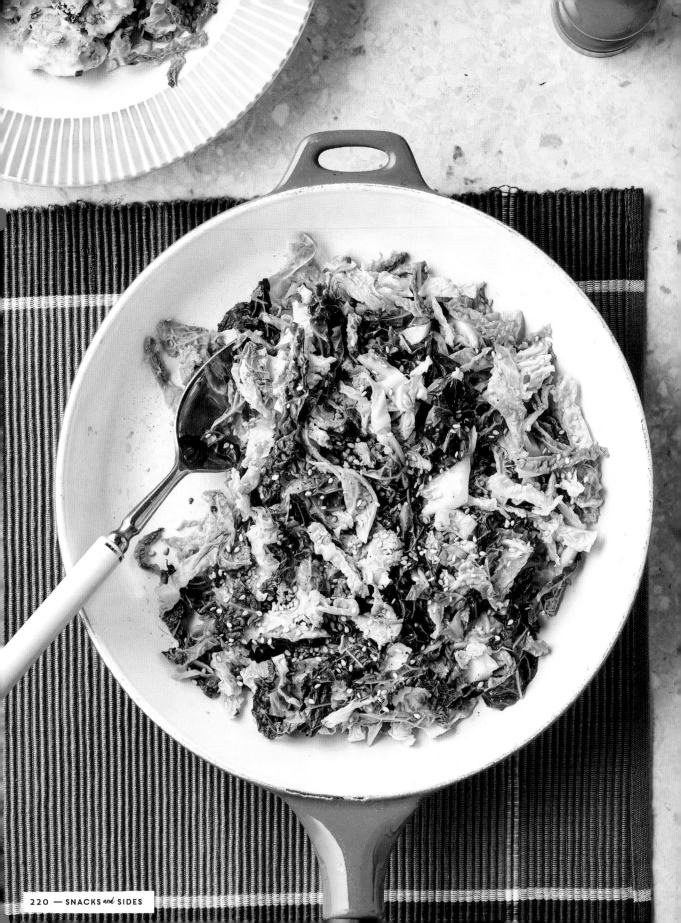

STIR-FRIED SAVOY CABBAGE

🕐 **10 MINS**   🍲 **10 MINS**   ✕ **SERVES 4**

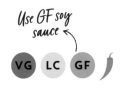

Use GF soy sauce ↖

VG **LC** **GF** 🌶

PER SERVING:
38 KCAL / 3.8G CARBS

5g sesame seeds
low-calorie cooking spray
1 small red chilli, deseeded
  and finely chopped
2 garlic cloves, peeled
  and crushed
2cm (¾in) piece of root ginger,
  peeled and finely grated
250g Savoy cabbage,
  roughly sliced
2 tbsp rice wine vinegar
2 tbsp low-sodium dark
  soy sauce
a pinch of granulated
  sweetener or caster sugar
sea salt and freshly ground
  black pepper

This quick and easy Chinese-inspired recipe uses just a few cheap ingredients to transform Savoy cabbage into a tasty, slimming-friendly side dish. This Stir-fried Savoy Cabbage would be perfect served as part of a Chinese fakeaway or even alongside other meat or fish for a midweek meal. Try it with a Chinese-style dish such as our Kung Pao Pork (page 49). If you love your food super-spicy then you can leave the seeds in the chilli to give it a bit of extra heat – you could even add another chilli to spice things up more if you like!

Everyday Light

Preheat the grill on a medium setting.

Put the sesame seeds in a small ovenproof dish and place under the hot grill to toast for 3–4 minutes until golden, taking care to watch them carefully as they can burn easily. Set aside.

Spray a large frying pan or wok with some low-calorie cooking spray and place over a medium heat. Add the chilli, garlic and ginger and fry for 1–2 minutes, until just turning lightly golden. Increase the heat to high and add the cabbage, rice wine vinegar, soy sauce and sweetener or sugar, and stir-fry for 3–4 minutes, stirring constantly. Be careful not to overcook the cabbage – it should still retain some crispness and its bright colour.

Season to taste with salt and pepper and serve at once, sprinkled with the toasted sesame seeds.

TIP: When stir-frying, use a high heat and keep moving the cabbage around the frying pan or wok to ensure it cooks quickly and stays fresh and crisp.

SWAP THIS: Swap the cabbage for roughly sliced pak choi.

BALSAMIC ROASTED ONIONS

🕐 **5 MINS** 🍲 **20 MINS** ✕ **SERVES 4**

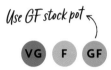

Use GF stock pot ↖

VG **F** **GF**

PER SERVING:
88 KCAL /16G CARBS

4 medium red onions
1 vegetable stock pot,
    dissolved into 1 tbsp
    boiling water
4 tbsp balsamic vinegar
2 tsp garlic granules
½ tsp dried thyme
1 tsp granulated sweetener
    or sugar
low-calorie cooking spray
freshly ground black pepper

Roasting is perfect for bringing out the sweetness in red onions. Adding tangy balsamic vinegar brings all the flavours to life, making them a great accompaniment to a traditional roast dinner or a savoury casserole! Try them with our Beef Stew and Dumplings, and Lamb Scouse (pages 162 and 165).

Everyday Light

Preheat the oven to 200°C (fan 180°C/gas mark 6).

Trim off the top of the red onions and peel away the skin. Trim off the hair-like roots, but leave the main root area intact. Cut each onion into four wedges, making sure you cut through the root (this will help keep the onion layers together).

Whisk the stock pot, balsamic vinegar, garlic granules, thyme and sweetener (or sugar) together in a small bowl.

Spray an ovenproof dish with low-calorie cooking spray and scatter in the onion wedges. Drizzle with the balsamic dressing and toss to coat thoroughly. Season with some black pepper, then cover the dish tightly with foil.

Cook the onions in the oven for 15 minutes, then remove the foil and toss the onions carefully, making sure they don't break apart. Return to the oven, uncovered, for 5 more minutes, before serving.

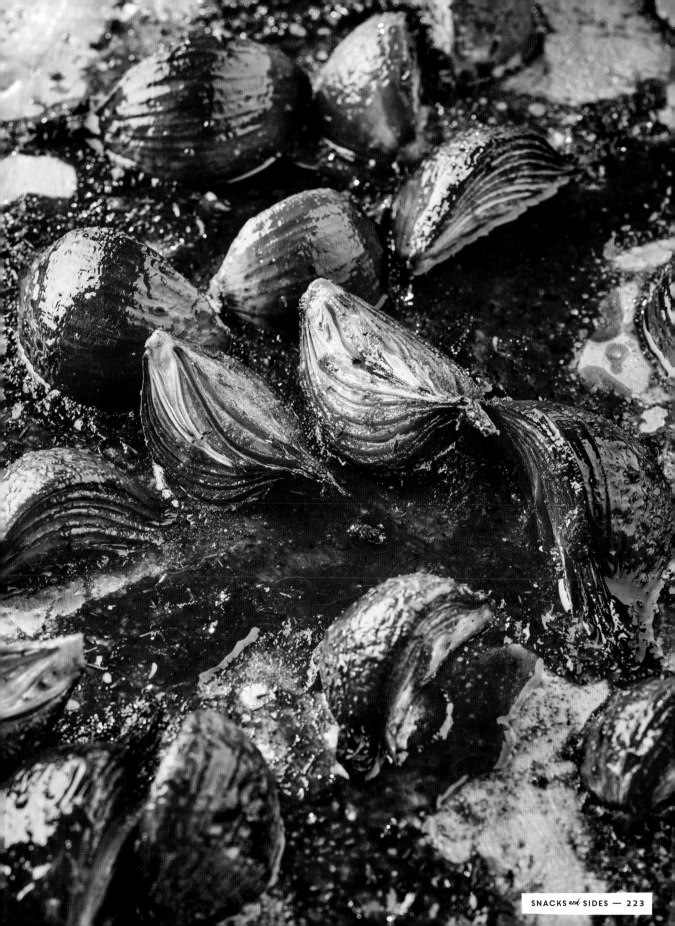

LOADED CAULIFLOWER CHEESE

 5 MINS　 **30 MINS**　✕ **SERVES 4**

Use vegetarian Italian-style hard cheese

PER SERVING:
301 KCAL / 32G CARBS

500g cauliflower, broken
　into florets
low-calorie cooking spray
1 onion, peeled and
　thinly sliced
1 garlic clove, peeled
　and crushed
3 tbsp plain flour
300ml skimmed milk
2 tsp Dijon mustard
½ tsp sriracha sauce
100g low-fat (under 5% fat)
　cream cheese
50g reduced-fat mature
　Cheddar, grated
30g Parmesan, grated
sea salt and freshly ground
　black pepper

FOR THE TOPPING
1 slice of wholemeal bread
40g reduced-fat
　Cheddar, grated
1 spring onion, trimmed
　and thinly sliced (optional)

TIP: You could add 2 bacon medallions to this recipe for an extra 23 kcal per serving. Fry until crispy in a frying pan, then slice and sprinkle on top.

SWAP THIS: Swap the skimmed milk for a non-dairy milk alternative and adjust the calories accordingly.

Just when you thought a classic cauliflower cheese couldn't get any better! We've added tender cauliflower to a silky cheese sauce and topped it with a crunchy breadcrumb mix that's exactly what you need after a day out in the cold. You can even mix it up by sprinkling it with chopped, cooked smoky bacon (as well as the spring onion) just before serving, for comfort food at its finest. Try this with our Pulled Ham in a Mustard Sauce (page 126) or One-pot Sunday Beef (page 115).

Special Occasion

Preheat the oven to 200°C (fan 180°C/gas mark 6).

Cook the cauliflower in a saucepan of boiling water for 8–10 minutes, until just soft, then drain well.

While the cauliflower is cooking, spray a frying pan with low-calorie cooking spray and place over a low heat. Add the onion and garlic and fry for 5 minutes until lightly golden and soft. Remove from the heat and set to one side.

Put the flour and 100ml of the milk in a small saucepan and place over a low heat, whisking for 1–2 minutes until it starts to thicken, then add another 100ml milk and again whisk and heat for 1–2 minutes until it starts to thicken. Add the final 100ml milk and heat for 1–2 minutes until thickened, then add the mustard and sriracha. Whisk in the cream cheese, then add the grated cheeses and whisk until melted and the sauce is creamy. Season with salt and pepper.

Place the drained cauliflower into an ovenproof dish, stir in the onion and garlic and pour over the cheese sauce.

Blitz the bread for the topping to a crumb in a food processor (or use a grater), place in a bowl and stir in the grated Cheddar. Sprinkle the crumb over the cauliflower cheese and pop in the oven for 10 minutes until the top is crispy and golden. Sprinkle with the spring onion (if using) and serve.

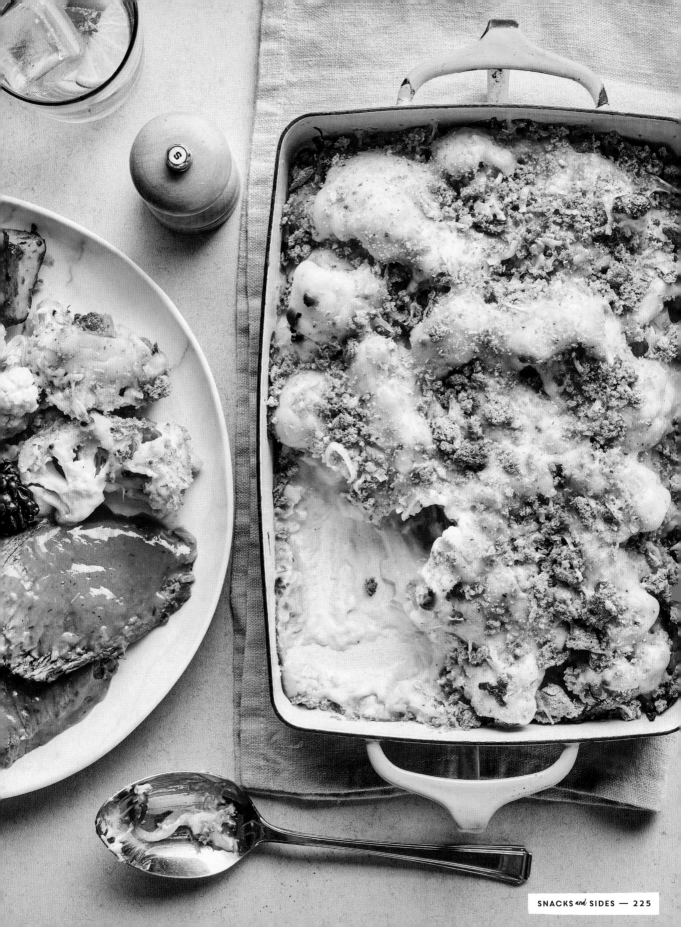

BBQ BEANS

🕐 **1 MIN**   🍲 **5 MINS**   ✕ **SERVES 4**

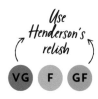

Use Henderson's relish

VG **F** **GF**

PER SERVING:
181 KCAL /24G CARBS

1 x 400g tin haricot beans,
   drained and rinsed
1 x 400g tin kidney beans,
   drained and rinsed
300g passata
1 tsp Henderson's relish or
   Worcestershire sauce
2 tbsp balsamic vinegar
1½ tsp smoked sweet paprika
1½ tsp onion granules
½ tsp garlic granules
½ tsp English mustard powder
½ tsp granulated sweetener
1 tsp ground coriander
sea salt and freshly ground
   black pepper

Baked beans are an absolute staple food for so many of us, and our homemade alternative has a smoky BBQ twist. Full of fibre to keep you feeling fuller for longer, you can use them just like regular baked beans. Try them on toast, piled on top of a baked potato or alongside your favourite fakeaway.

Everyday Light

Put all the ingredients in a saucepan and mix well. Place over a medium heat and cook for 5 minutes, stirring, or until piping hot throughout.

Serve with a main of your choice.

TIPS: Try adding a little chilli powder or hot sauce for some heat. Don't confuse onion granules for onion salt – the dish will be far too salty if you use the wrong one! The same applies to garlic granules.

SWAP THIS: You could use a regular tin of baked beans instead of haricot beans in this dish. Just reduce the passata to 250g and leave out the sweetener. Remember it will increase the calories a little, to about 204 kcal per serving.

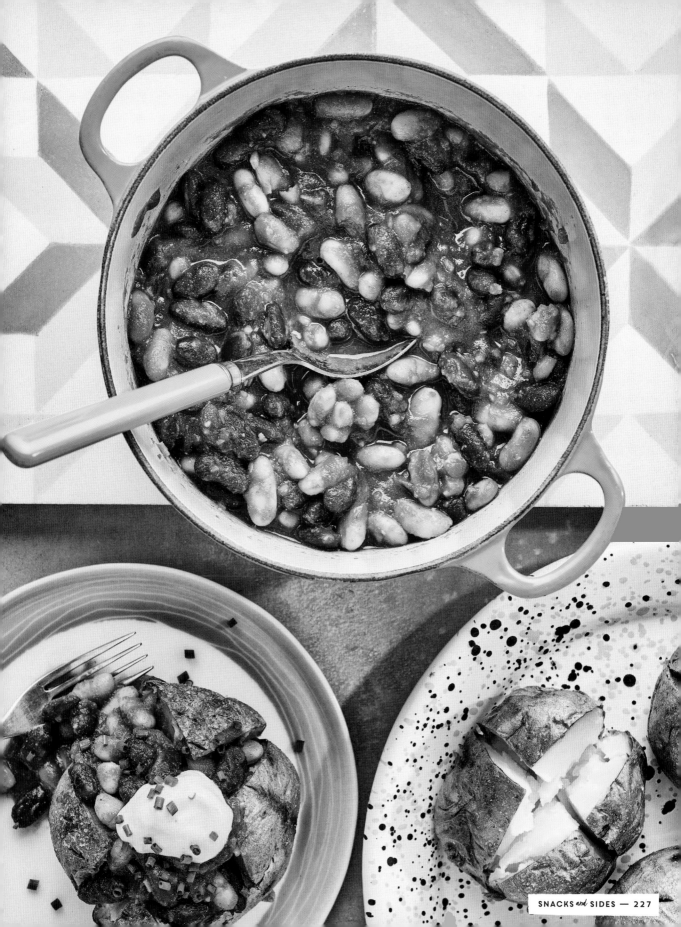

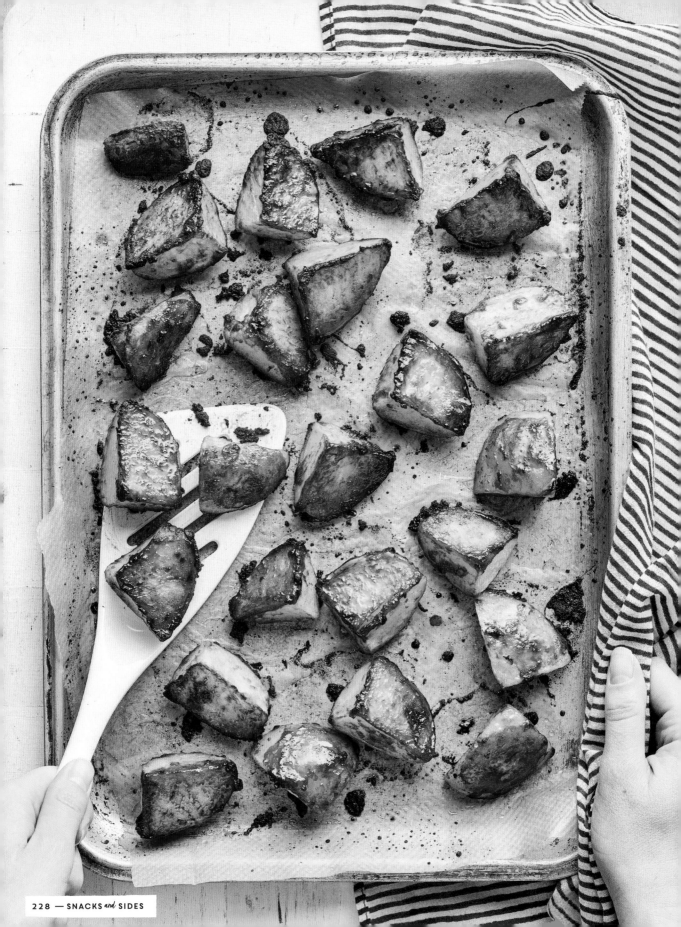

MARMITE ROASTIES

🕐 **5 MINS**　🍲 **VARIABLE** (SEE BELOW)　✕ **SERVES 2**

PER SERVING:
284 KCAL / 55G CARBS

2 large floury potatoes
　(about 600g), peeled and
　cut into 5cm (2in) chunks
1 tbsp Marmite
1 tbsp boiling water
low-calorie cooking spray

Whether you're a Marmite lover or a hater, we guarantee you'll love the savoury, distinctive flavour of these crispy roast potatoes! Elevate the humble roastie to the next level alongside your next Sunday dinner; once you've tried this simple side dish, you may never go back!

Weekly Indulgence

OVEN METHOD
🍲 **45 MINS**

Preheat the oven to 220°C (fan 200°C/gas mark 7). Put the potatoes in a saucepan of salted cold water, bring to the boil and cook for 10–15 minutes, until just soft but still holding their shape. Drain in a colander and leave for 5 minutes, then toss gently in the colander to fluff up the edges. Mix the Marmite and boiling water in a small bowl. Put the potatoes on a baking tray and spray with plenty of low-calorie cooking spray, then add the Marmite mixture and shake the tray to coat the potatoes. Roast for 15 minutes.

Remove from the oven, spray again with low-calorie cooking spray and roast for 15 more minutes until golden and crispy.

AIR-FRYER METHOD
🍲 **30 MINS**

SPECIAL EQUIPMENT
Air fryer

Put the potatoes in a saucepan of salted cold water. Place over a medium heat, bring to the boil and cook for 10–15 minutes, until just soft but still holding their shape. Drain in a colander and leave for 5 minutes, then toss gently in the colander to fluff up the edges. Mix the Marmite and boiling water in a small bowl. Preheat the air fryer to 190°C.

Put the potatoes in a bowl, add the Marmite mixture and shake until the potatoes are well coated. Add to the air fryer, spray with plenty of low-calorie cooking spray and cook for 15 minutes until golden brown and crispy.

TIP: Shake your potatoes halfway through to make sure they are crispy on all sides.

SWAP THIS: If you want a stronger Marmite flavour, add an extra tablespoon of Marmite.

HAM *and* CHEESE SPINACH SWIRLS

🕐 **10 MINS**   🍲 **20 MINS**   ✗ **MAKES 16**

After baking ↗   *Use GF puff pastry and ham* ↘

(F) (BF) (LC) (GF)

PER SWIRL:
89 KCAL / 7.1G CARBS

320g ready-rolled light puff
  pastry sheet
60g low-fat cream cheese
30g Parmesan, finely grated
40g fresh baby spinach
  leaves, stalks removed,
  leaves washed and
  completely dried
50g lean cooked ham,
  finely chopped
¼ tsp garlic granules
sea salt and freshly ground
  black pepper

TO ACCOMPANY *(optional)*
75g mixed salad (+ 15 kcal per
  serving) and 2 tbsp tomato
  ketchup (+ 15 kcal per tbsp)

TIPS: Make sure that
the spinach leaves are
completely dry before
using, otherwise they
may make the pastry
soggy, and use small baby
spinach leaves as they
will roll up well inside the
pastry. Most cooked sliced
ham is gluten free, but do
check as some isn't.

SWAP THIS: Swap the
ham for cooked bacon or
cooked chicken.

These tasty pastry swirls look so good, it's hard to believe they're so easy and quick to make! We've stuffed light puff pastry with lean ham and cheese, and added baby spinach leaves for a burst of extra nutrients. Serve them warm for a weekend breakfast treat, or with a crisp, fresh salad for a more substantial lunch.

Everyday Light

Preheat the oven to 220°C (fan 200°C/gas mark 7) and line a baking tray with non-stick baking paper.

Unroll the pastry sheet, leaving it on the greaseproof paper packing, and place it on a work surface. Spread a thin layer of low-fat cream cheese over the pastry, leaving a 1cm (½in) gap along one long edge, then sprinkle the grated Parmesan over the cream cheese, leaving the 1cm (½in) gap along the long edge. Spread the spinach leaves over the Parmesan, leaving the 1cm (½in) gap along the long edge. Place the ham over the spinach and sprinkle with the garlic granules, again leaving the gap along the long edge. Season well with salt and pepper.

Roll up the pastry, starting with the long edge without the 1cm (½in) gap and using the greaseproof paper to help you. Keep rolling it up until you have a 'Swiss roll'. When you have finished rolling up the pastry, make sure it is seam side down, then use a large serrated knife, such as a bread knife, to cut it into sixteen spiral-shaped slices.

Carefully transfer the slices to the lined baking tray, leaving gaps between each, and press the seam on each to ensure a good seal.

Bake in the preheated oven for 15–20 minutes, until golden and crisp.

These swirls are best served warm, with your choice of accompaniment.

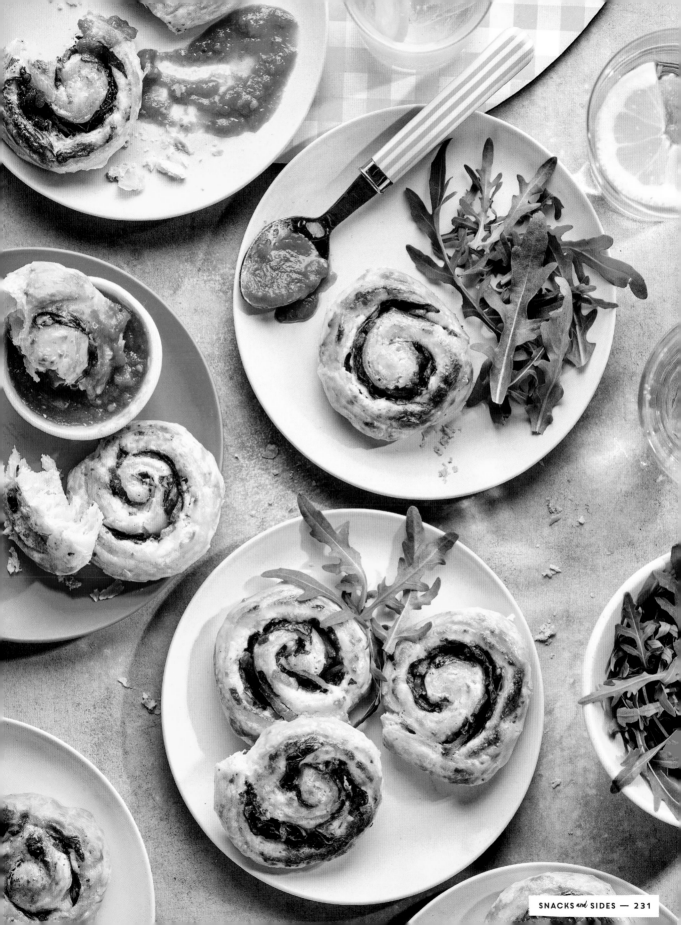

The ULTIMATE GRILLED CHEESE

🕐 **5 MINS**   🍲 **22 MINS**   ✕ **SERVES 1**

PER SERVING:
451 KCAL / 45G CARBS

low-calorie cooking spray
1 small red onion, peeled
  and sliced
3 tbsp balsamic vinegar
1 tbsp reduced-fat mayonnaise
2 medium slices of bread
  (we use wholemeal)
1½ slices gouda cheese (37.5g)

TO ACCOMPANY *(optional)*
Creamy Tomato Soup, page
  157 (+ 166 kcal per serving)

We ate the most amazing grilled cheese in Texas, and we've tried to replicate the melty deliciousness at home! You can add more gouda if you like, but be sure to adjust the calories. This is perfect paired with a piping hot bowl of Creamy Tomato Soup (page 157).

Special Occasion

HOB-TOP METHOD

Spray a frying pan with low-calorie cooking spray and place over a medium heat. Add the onion and fry gently for 2 minutes until it starts to soften. Reduce the heat to low, stir in the balsamic vinegar and cook for a further 10 minutes, stirring often.

While the onion is cooking, spread the mayonnaise on both sides of each piece of bread.

When the onion is cooked, take one of the pieces of bread and place the cheese on top. Spread the onion across the cheese and cover with the other piece of bread.

Transfer to a hot frying pan and cook over a high heat for 5 minutes on each side, keeping a close eye on it while it's cooking to make sure it doesn't burn.

Remove from the pan, slice and serve.

TIP: This is so easy to scale up and make more than 1 serving (we couldn't resist making a stack!)

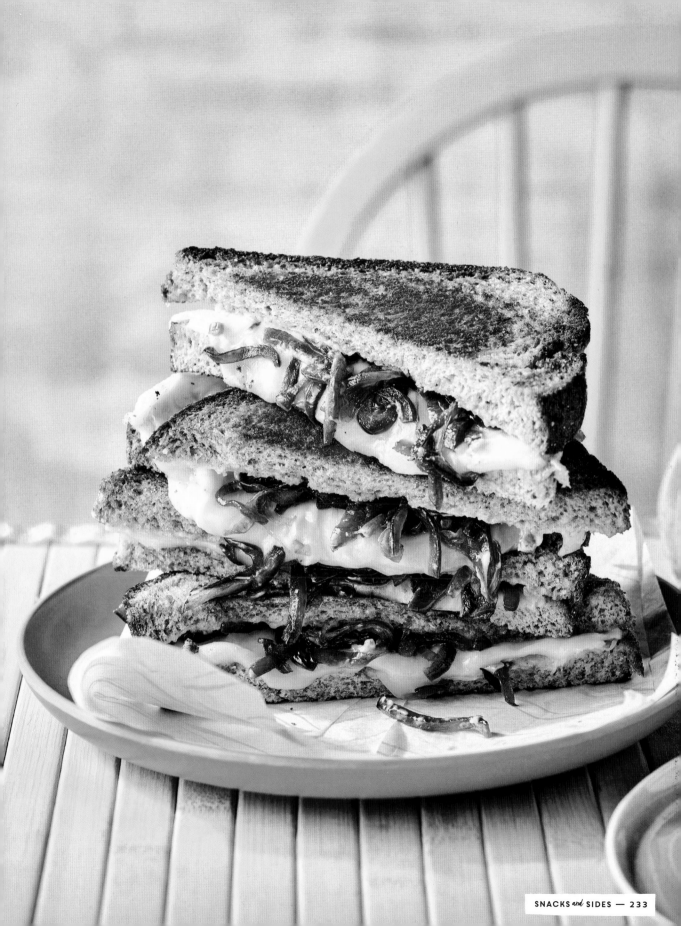

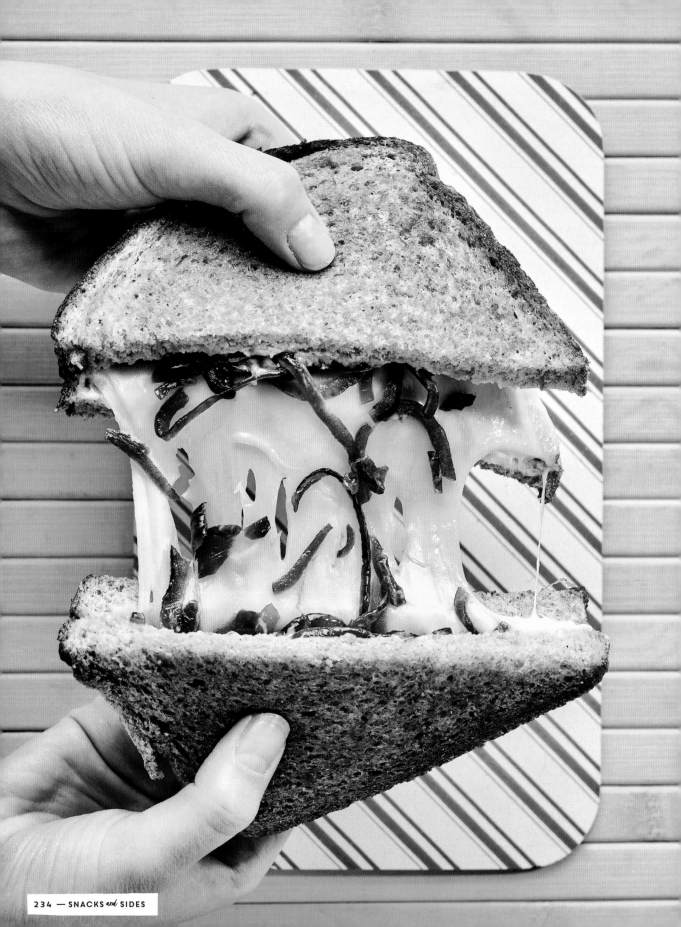

AIR-FRYER METHOD

SPECIAL EQUIPMENT
Air fryer

Preheat the air fryer to 200°C.

Spray a frying pan with low-calorie cooking spray and place over a medium heat. Add the onion and fry gently for 2 minutes until it starts to soften. Reduce the heat to low, stir in the balsamic vinegar and cook for a further 10 minutes, stirring often.

While the onion is cooking, spread the mayonnaise on both sides of each piece of bread.

When the onion is cooked, take one of the pieces of bread and place the cheese on top. Spread the onion across the cheese and cover with the other piece of bread.

Transfer to the air fryer and cook for 8–10 minutes.

Remove from the air fryer, slice and serve.

"*Just WOW. The most incredible meal. Thank you!*"

HOPE

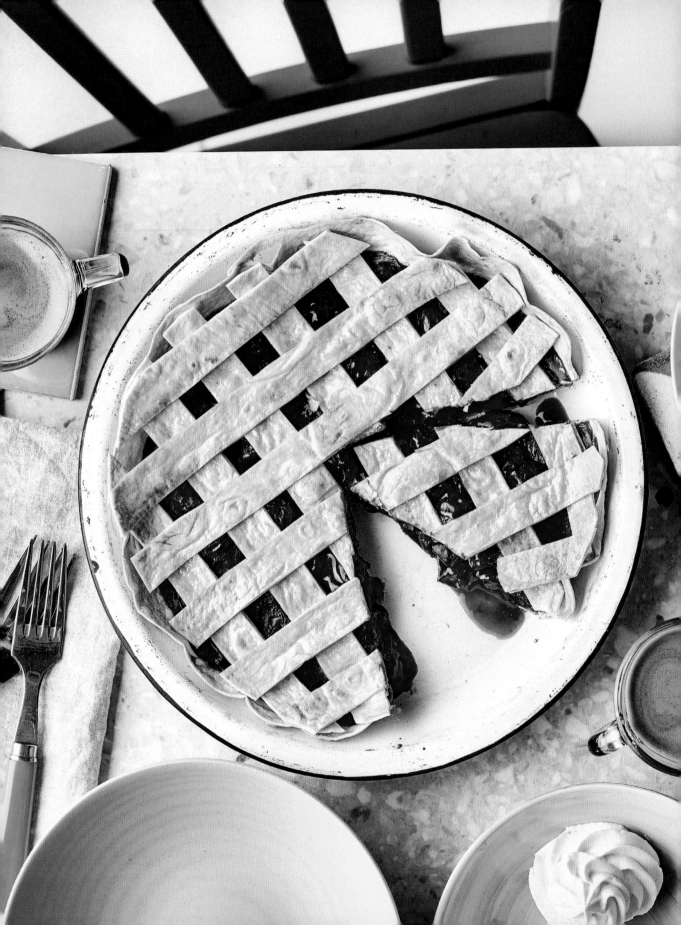

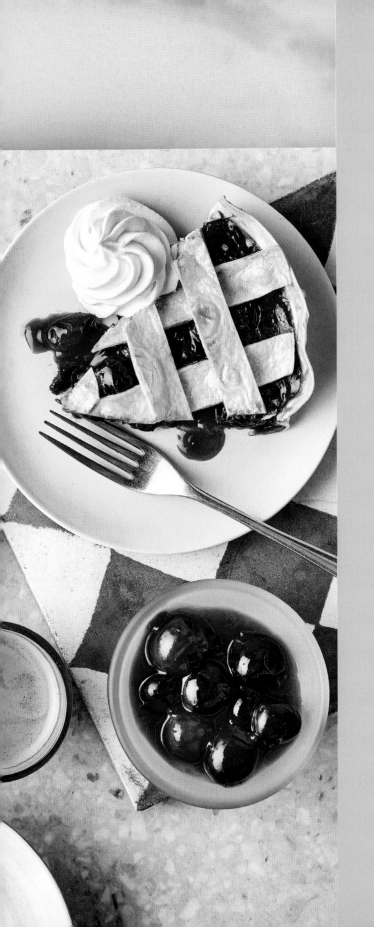

Sweet
TREATS

USING GRANULATED
SWEETENER WITH THE SAME
WEIGHT AND TEXTURE AS
SUGAR IS CRUCIAL TO THE
SUCCESS OF MANY OF
THESE RECIPES.

CHOCOLATE ESPRESSO CHEESECAKES

🕐 **10 MINS***   🍲 **NO COOK**   ✕ **SERVES 4**

*PLUS 1 HOUR CHILLING

PER SERVING:
276 KCAL /24G CARBS

FOR THE CHEESECAKE
1 tbsp cocoa powder
1 tbsp espresso powder
2 tbsp boiling water
8 Oreo biscuits
1 tbsp reduced-fat spread
100g low-fat cream cheese
100g ricotta cheese
100g fat-free Greek-style
  yoghurt
3 tsp granulated sweetener

FOR THE TOPPING
1 Oreo biscuit
1 tsp espresso powder
1 tsp cocoa powder
low-fat aerosol cream

This simple cheesecake dessert will satisfy your chocolate cravings, and it has an added hit of coffee! We've used Oreo biscuits for a chocolate-flavoured no-butter base, and a creamy cheesecake with no double cream needed. The best part about this pud is that you don't even need to turn the oven on! These are not traditional cheesecakes but more of a soft-set dessert. After chilling, the cheesecake mix will be slightly firmer.

Weekly Indulgence ────────────────

Combine the cocoa, espresso powder and boiling water in a small bowl and mix until smooth. Set to one side to cool.

Blitz the eight Oreo biscuits in a food processor to fine crumbs, or crush them in a food bag by bashing them with a rolling pin.

Melt the reduced-fat spread in a small saucepan over a very low heat or in a small bowl in the microwave, then tip in the Oreo crumbs and 1 teaspoon of the espresso and cocoa mix and stir until combined. Tip into four small serving dishes and press down firmly to make an even layer. Pop in the fridge while making the cheesecake mixture.

Combine the cream cheese, ricotta, yoghurt and sweetener in a bowl, then beat with an electric hand whisk until smooth. Pour in the remaining espresso and cocoa mixture and whisk until fully incorporated. Spoon the cheesecake mixture into each serving dish, on top of the biscuit base. Smooth the top with the back of a spoon and pop the dishes back in the fridge for an hour until chilled and set.

To make the topping, crush the Oreo biscuit to fine crumbs, stir in the espresso powder and cocoa and set to one side.

Remove the cheesecakes from the fridge and serve with a swirl of low-fat aerosol cream (about 1 tablespoon) and a sprinkling of the crushed Oreo topping.

TIP: If you don't have espresso powder, use instant coffee granules. Add them to a food bag and bash with a rolling pin until you have a fine powder.

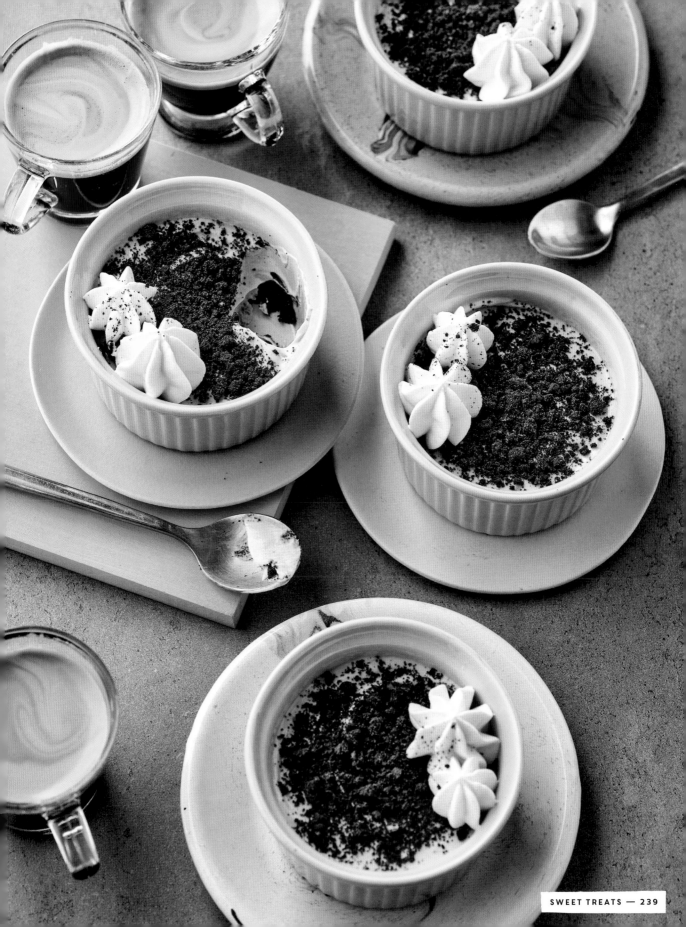

CHOCOLATE CUSTARD

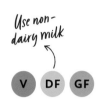

Use non-dairy milk

V **DF** **GF**

PER SERVING:
95 KCAL /15G CARBS

3 medium egg yolks
2 tbsp cornflour
1 tbsp cocoa powder
4 tbsp granulated sweetener
500ml semi-skimmed milk

🕐 **5 MINS**   🍲 **10 MINS**   ✕ **SERVES 8**

This Chocolate Custard might bring back a few childhood memories, especially if it's served over a warm chocolate sponge! We love our custard to be nice and thick, but if you prefer a thinner custard, simply add one tablespoon of cornflour instead of two. Serve with our Choco Nut Lava Cakes (page 263), Apple Brown Betty (page 245), Banana Sponge Puddings (page 242), Treacle Sponge (page 266), Jam Roly Poly (page 258) or Coconut and Jam Sponge (page 254) for a truly decadent dessert that you'd never believe is slimming friendly!

Everyday Light

Put the egg yolks, cornflour, cocoa powder and sweetener in a large heatproof jug. Add 2 tablespoons of the milk and stir to form a smooth paste.

Pour the remaining milk into a medium saucepan and place over a medium heat. Heat until steaming hot, taking care not to let it burn or boil over.

Gradually pour the steaming hot milk into the mixture in the jug, stirring with a wooden spoon or whisking with a balloon whisk until completely blended.

Pour the mixture back into the saucepan and place over a medium heat. Cook the custard, stirring constantly with a wooden spoon or balloon whisk, for about 5 minutes, until there are a few small bubbles starting to appear on the surface and the custard is starting to thicken.

As soon as the custard has thickened, remove it from the heat. Don't let the custard overheat or boil otherwise it may burn or split.

Pour into a clean heatproof jug and serve with a dessert of your choice.

TIP: If you wish to cut down on calories further, you could use skimmed milk instead of semi-skimmed, and adjust the calories accordingly.

SWAP THIS: You can use skimmed or non-dairy milk if you prefer.

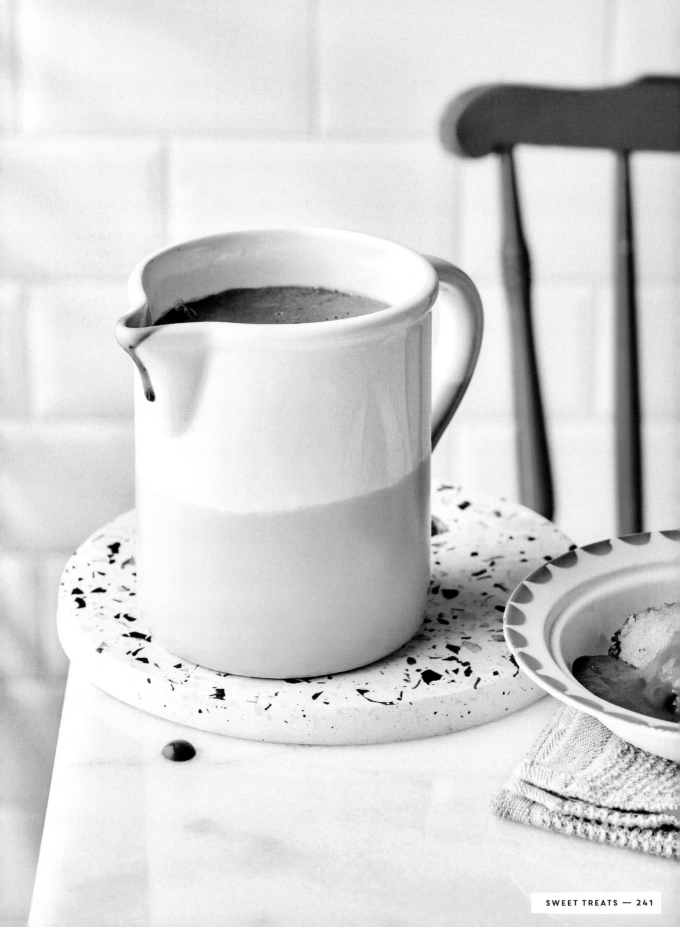

BANANA SPONGE PUDDINGS

🕐 **10 MINS** 🍲 **20–25 MINS** ✕ **SERVES 4**

Use dairy-free custard ←

Use GF flour and baking powder ↗

V **F** **BF** **DF** **GF**

PER SERVING:
177 KCAL / 29G CARBS

SPECIAL EQUIPMENT
4 x 125ml ramekin dishes

50g reduced-fat spread, plus a little extra for greasing
1 small ripe banana, peeled
4 tsp 50%-less sugar caramel dessert topping
50g brown granulated sweetener
50g self-raising flour
½ tsp baking powder
1 medium egg, beaten with a fork
¼ tsp vanilla extract

TO ACCOMPANY *(optional)*
Chocolate Custard, page 240 (+ 95 kcal per serving), or Custard from our *Quick & Easy* book (+ 58 kcal per serving)

SWAP THIS: If you prefer, swap the brown sweetener for white.

Don't throw away your leftover ripe bananas. Instead, transform them into a sweet, sticky pudding with a caramel kick! We're 'bananas' about reducing food waste, especially when it results in dishes that taste as good as this! Add a dollop of custard for a comforting pud that's ready to enjoy in just over half an hour.

Weekly Indulgence —————————————

Preheat the oven to 180°C (fan 160°C/gas mark 4). Thoroughly grease the four ramekin dishes with the little extra reduced-fat spread.

Cut eight thin round slices from one end of the banana and set aside. Mash the remaining banana in a bowl and set aside. Place 1 teaspoon of the caramel dessert topping in the bottom of each ramekin dish and spread it out. Place two banana slices on top of the caramel dessert topping in each ramekin dish.

Put the remaining 50g reduced-fat spread in a medium bowl with the sweetener, flour, baking powder, beaten egg and vanilla extract and beat with an electric hand whisk or wooden spoon for 2–3 minutes until smooth. Fold in the mashed banana until completely mixed.

Divide the sponge mixture between the four ramekin dishes, level the tops and place on a baking tray.

Place in the preheated oven and bake for 20–25 minutes, or until risen and golden brown. To test if they're ready, insert a small sharp knife into the centre of the puddings: when the sponges are cooked the knife will come out clean.

Run a round-bladed knife around the edge of the sponges in the ramekins to help release the sponges, then turn them out onto a serving plate. Alternatively, serve them in the ramekin dishes.

Serve hot with your choice of accompaniment.

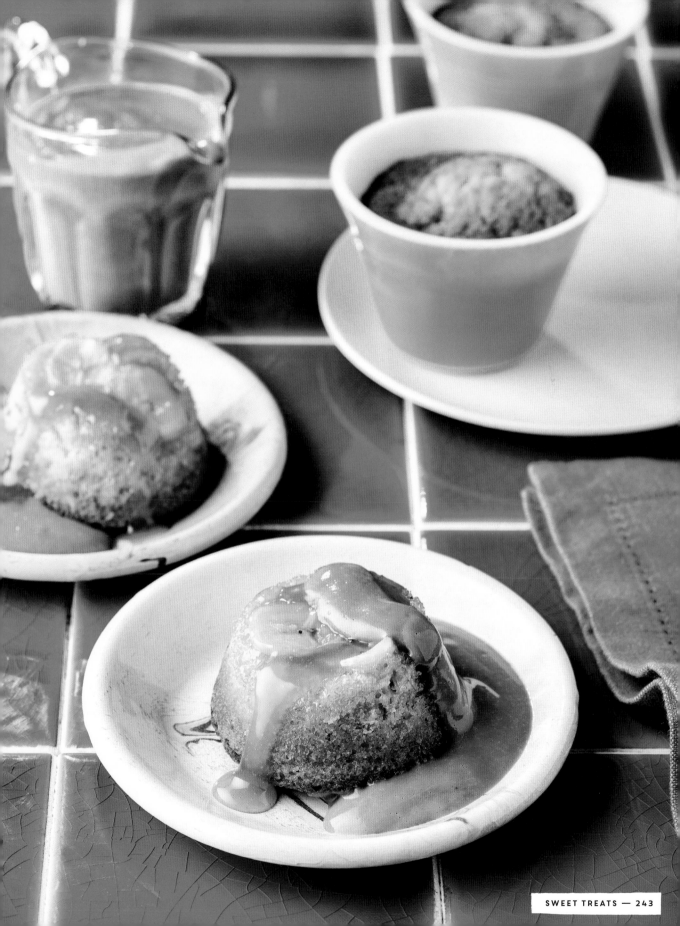

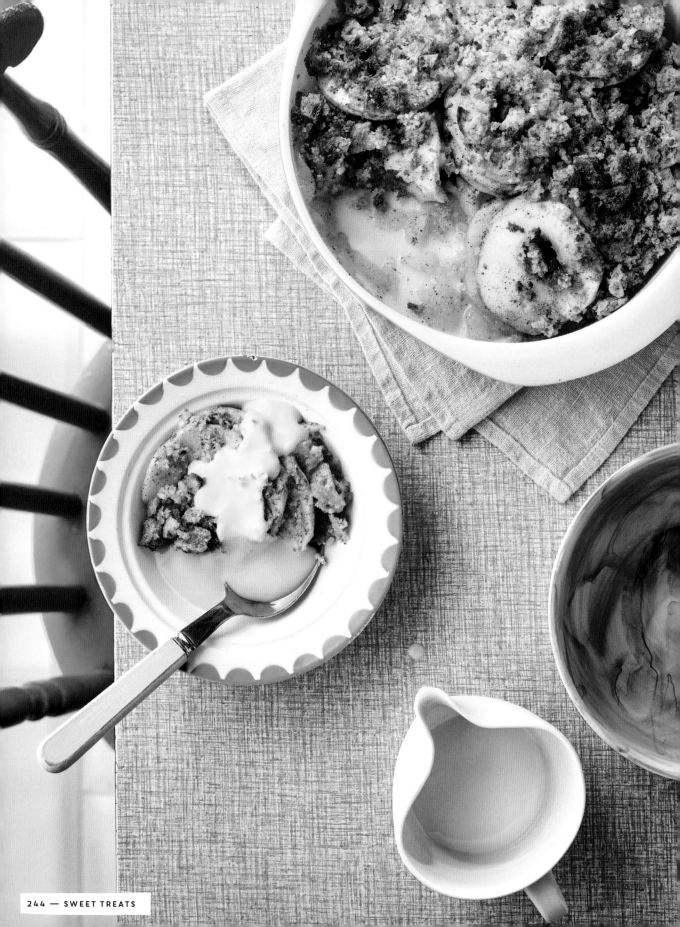

APPLE BROWN BETTY

🕐 **25 MINS**   🍲 **40 MINS**   ✕ **SERVES 4**

Use dairy-free custard →   *Use GF bread →*

(V) (F) (BF) (DF) (GF)

PER SERVING:
155 KCAL / 24G CARBS

SPECIAL EQUIPMENT
18 x 27cm (7 x 10½in)
ovenproof dish

600g Bramley cooking
  apples, peeled, cored
  and thinly sliced
2 tbsp lemon juice
50g granulated sweetener
½ tsp ground cinnamon
½ tsp ground nutmeg

FOR THE TOPPING
2 medium slices
  wholemeal bread
5g white granulated sweetener
25g reduced-fat spread, plus
  a little extra for greasing

TO ACCOMPANY
Chocolate Custard, page
  240 (+ 95 kcal per serving),
  or Custard from our
  Quick & Easy book
  (+ 58 kcal per serving)

Who says breadcrumbs are just for savoury dishes?
Our take on an American-style baked apple pudding
contains tender apples topped with crispy, sweet
breadcrumbs. It makes a delicious dessert that's
a great alternative to apple crumble. We think it's
perfect for warming you up on a chilly winter's day!

Weekly Indulgence

Preheat the oven to 200°C (fan 180°C/gas mark 6).

Tear the bread for the topping into large pieces,
place in the food processor and blitz to make coarse
breadcrumbs (alternatively, grate the bread to crumbs
using a coarse grater).

Spread the breadcrumbs out on a baking tray and place
in the oven for 4–5 minutes to dry them out. Keep an eye
on the breadcrumbs as they can burn easily, and stir them
halfway through so they dry out evenly.

Remove the breadcrumbs from the oven and set aside,
leaving them to cool on the tray. Grease the ovenproof
dish with a little reduced-fat spread.

Put the apples, lemon juice, sweetener, cinnamon and
nutmeg in a medium bowl and stir well. Place the apple
mixture in the greased dish and spread it out evenly.

Put the dried breadcrumbs in a small mixing bowl, add
the sweetener and stir in until evenly mixed.

Melt the reduced-fat spread in a small saucepan
over a low heat until just melted, then pour it into the
breadcrumbs and sweetener and stir until evenly mixed.

Sprinkle the breadcrumb topping over the apples and
place in the preheated oven for 30–35 minutes, or until the
apples are soft and the breadcrumbs are browned.

Remove from the oven and leave to stand for 10 minutes
before serving. Serve with custard.

CREAMY LIME PIE

🕐 **30 MINS***   🍲 **NO COOK**   ✕ **SERVES 4**

***PLUS 3–4 HOURS (OR OVERNIGHT) CHILLING**

Use vegetarian gelatine

(V) (GF)

→ Use GF digestive biscuits

PER SERVING:
230 KCAL /22G CARBS

SPECIAL EQUIPMENT
18cm (7in) round, loose-bottomed fluted metal flan tin

FOR THE BASE
50g reduced-fat spread,
 plus a little extra
 for greasing
10 reduced-fat digestive
 biscuits

FOR THE FILLING
150g reduced-fat
 cream cheese
200g fat-free Greek-style
 yoghurt
finely grated zest and juice
 of 2 limes (about 50ml juice)
1 tbsp granulated sweetener
3 gelatine leaves (8g)
2 tbsp hot water

TO DECORATE
lime slices, halved
finely grated zest of 1 lime

TIP: Make sure to give the pie its full chilling time – don't be tempted to cut it earlier or you risk it not being set!

This dessert really does taste as good as it looks! Tangy and sweet, with a crunchy crust, this light pie is delicious on a summer's day. We've used reduced-fat ingredients to keep the calories low while making sure it is still bursting with fresh, zingy lime flavours. Serve with a squirt of low-fat aerosol cream, if you like, bearing in mind that this will increase the calories.

Weekly Indulgence

Lightly grease the flan tin with a little reduced-fat spread.

Blitz the biscuits in a food processor to fine crumbs, or crush them in a food bag by bashing them with a rolling pin. Tip the biscuit crumbs into a small mixing bowl. Melt the reduced-fat spread in a small saucepan over a very low heat or in a small bowl in the microwave on low, then pour it into the bowl of biscuit crumbs and stir to combine.

Tip the biscuit-crumb mixture into the greased flan tin and spread it out. Using the back of a dessert spoon, press the crumbs down onto the base and up the sides of the tin to form a biscuit crumb pie case. Place in the fridge while you make the filling.

To make the filling, stir the reduced-fat cream cheese in a medium bowl with a wooden spoon until smooth and softened. Add the yoghurt, lime zest, lime juice and granulated sweetener and stir well until evenly combined.

Lay the gelatine leaves flat in a small dish and cover with about 150ml cold water. Push the leaves down to submerge them, making sure they don't stick together. Leave to soak for 5 minutes until they are like jelly, then remove and squeeze out excess water. Discard the soaking water. Place the squeezed gelatine in a cup and pour over the 2 tablespoons of hot (but not boiling) water. Stir until the gelatine has dissolved and the liquid is clear and free of lumps. You can place the cup in a bowl of hot water if you need a little more heat to dissolve the gelatine.

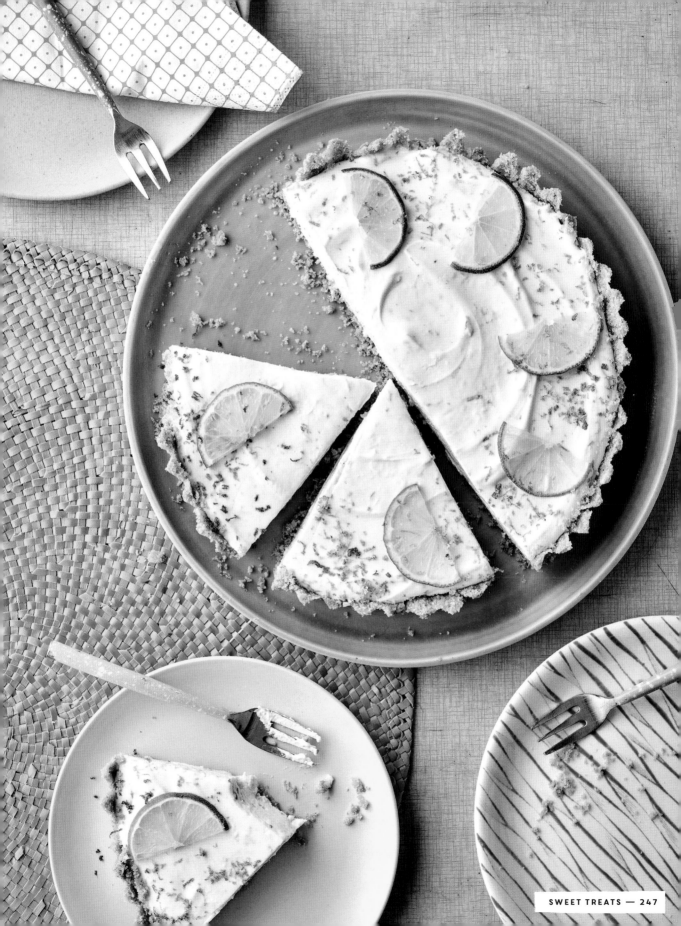

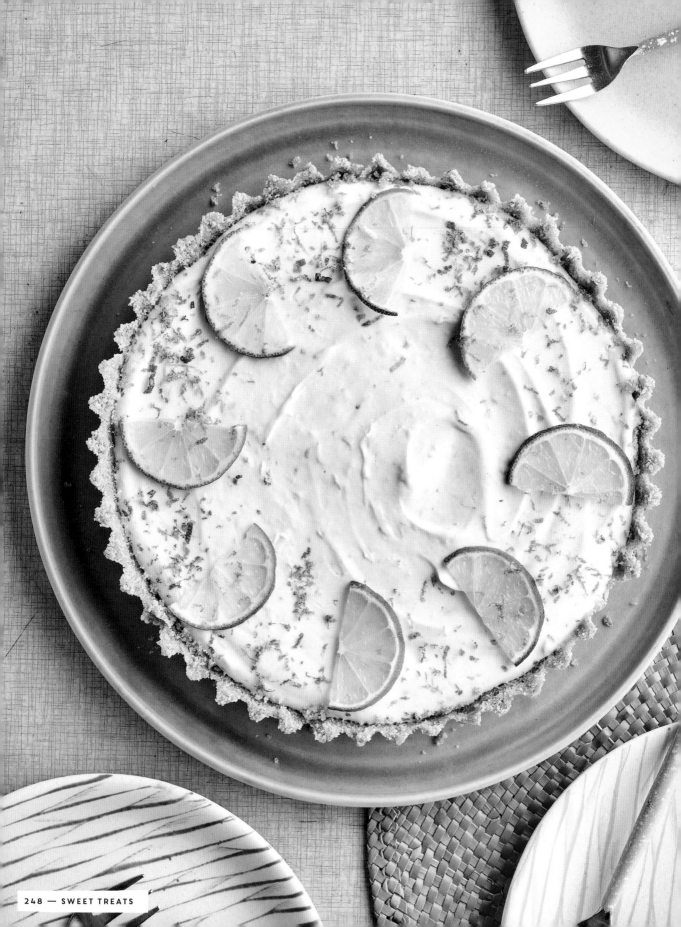

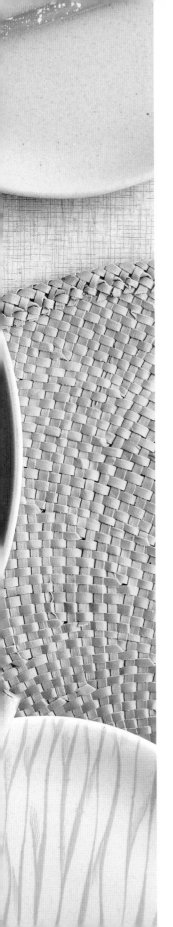

Add a couple of tablespoonfuls of the creamy lime filling to the dissolved gelatine and stir until completely blended. Pour quickly into the bowl of remaining filling and stir until well combined.

Scrape the filling mixture into the chilled pie case, spread it out evenly and place in the fridge for 3–4 hours (or overnight) to set.

After chilling, the filling should be set. Carefully remove the outer ring from the flan tin. An easy way to do this is to stand a jug with a level rim upside down on the work surface and carefully place the flan tin on top of the jug, holding the sides of the tin. Gently press the tin down and the pie will be released from the outer ring. The pie will still be on the metal base of the flan tin.

Place the lime pie on a serving plate. You can either leave the pie on the metal flan tin base or carefully slide the pie off the base and onto the plate.

To decorate, place halved lime slices around the edge of the pie and sprinkle with the grated lime zest. Serve the pie on its own or with a squirt of low-fat aerosol cream.

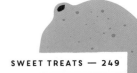

"*Thank you for all your wonderful recipes.*"

KAREN ——

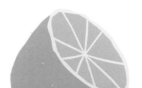

MILLIONAIRE'S SHORTBREAD

🕐 **30 MINS**   🍲 **30 MINS***   ✕ **MAKES 20 PIECES**

*****PLUS COOLING**

Use GF flour ←

V **F** **BF** **GF**

PER PIECE:
127 KCAL / 16G CARBS

SPECIAL EQUIPMENT
18 x 18cm (7 x 7in)
square cake tin

FOR THE SHORTBREAD LAYER
100g softened unsalted butter,
  plus a little extra for greasing
25g caster sugar
25g granulated sweetener
150g plain flour, sifted

FOR THE CARAMEL
160g sugar-free creamy toffees
2 tsp light double
  cream alternative

FOR THE TOP
50g milk chocolate, broken
  into pieces

TIPS: We used Werther's Original Sugar-free Creamy Toffees. Make sure you measure the light double cream alternative accurately; it must be 2 level teaspoons. This will achieve the correct consistency for the caramel layer. Using real butter instead of reduced-fat spread in the shortbread helps make it crisp.

These sticky, chocolatey treats would usually be considered off-limits if you are watching your calories, but we've used substitutions to make a lower-calorie version which is just as delicious. Usually, the caramel layer is made with calorie-packed sweetened condensed milk, sugar and butter, but here we've used sugar-free creamy toffees instead. The caramel, crisp shortbread and chocolate drizzle makes this a special treat that you can enjoy without regret!

Everyday Light ───────────────────

Preheat the oven to 180°C (fan 160°C/gas mark 4) and grease the cake tin with a little butter, then line the base and sides with non-stick baking paper.

Put the butter, sugar and sweetener in a medium bowl and beat with an electric hand whisk or wooden spoon until light and fluffy. Add the flour and stir until combined. Squeeze the mixture together with clean hands to make a smooth ball – you may need damp hands to help bring the dough together (avoid over-handling as this may make the dough tough).

Place the dough in the base of the tin and use your knuckles and fingertips to gently press it into a thin, even layer that covers the base. Prick it all over with a fork and bake for 20–25 minutes until light golden. Remove from the oven and leave in the tin to cool completely.

For the caramel, put the toffees in a small saucepan over a very low heat and stir for about 2 minutes until just melted. Remove from the heat and stir until completely melted. Stir in the cream alternative. Quickly pour the caramel over the shortbread and spread it out evenly with the back of a spoon. Leave to set for about 20 minutes or until firm.

Use the baking paper to transfer the caramel shortbread from the tin to a surface. Melt the chocolate in a small heatproof bowl over a small pan of simmering water, stirring until melted, then drizzle it over the caramel and leave to set. Use a large, sharp knife to cut the shortbread into twenty pieces, remove from the paper and serve.

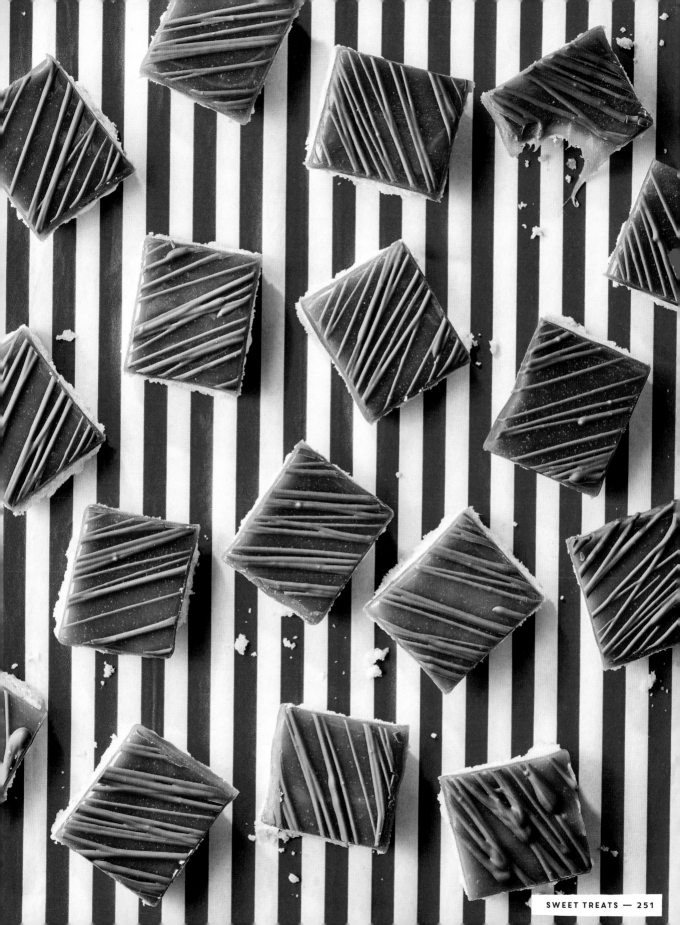

CHOCOLATE BAKED BANANAS

🕐 **5 MINS**   🍲 **20 MINS**   ✕ **SERVES 4**

Use gelatine-free marshmallows

Use dairy-free yoghurt or ice cream

(V) (DF) (GF)

PER SERVING:
110 KCAL / 21G CARBS

SPECIAL EQUIPMENT
Small ovenproof dish

a little reduced-fat spread,
  for greasing
2 medium bananas, peeled
  and sliced in half lengthways
  (or sliced in half with skin on)
60g low-calorie chocolate syrup
10g pink and white mini
  marshmallows

TO ACCOMPANY
a dollop (60g) of low-fat
  Greek-style yoghurt (+ 35 kal
  per serving) or a small scoop
  (60g) of low-calorie ice
  cream (+ 46 kcal per serving)

These Chocolate Baked Bananas are a simple and indulgent dessert that will satisfy any sweet cravings. The sweet treat only needs a handful of ingredients, and can be rustled up in a flash. It's important to make sure you're using ripe bananas for this recipe, as under-ripe ones may not cook through and over-ripe bananas can go mushy! Serve with some low-fat Greek-style yoghurt or a scoop of low-calorie ice cream for a pudding that feels much naughtier than it actually is.

Everyday Light

Preheat the oven to 200°C (fan 180°C/gas mark 6) and grease a small ovenproof dish with reduced-fat spread. Place the banana halves cut-side up in the greased dish. Drizzle the low-calorie chocolate syrup over the banana halves, cover the dish with foil and bake in the preheated oven for 10 minutes.

Remove the bananas from the oven and take off the foil. Sprinkle the mini marshmallows over the bananas and return the dish to the oven, uncovered, for a further 10 minutes, until the bananas have softened and the marshmallows are melting.

Serve at once, alone, or with a dollop of low-fat Greek-style yoghurt or a small scoop of low-calorie ice cream (scoop the banana flesh out of the skins if you've baked them skin on).

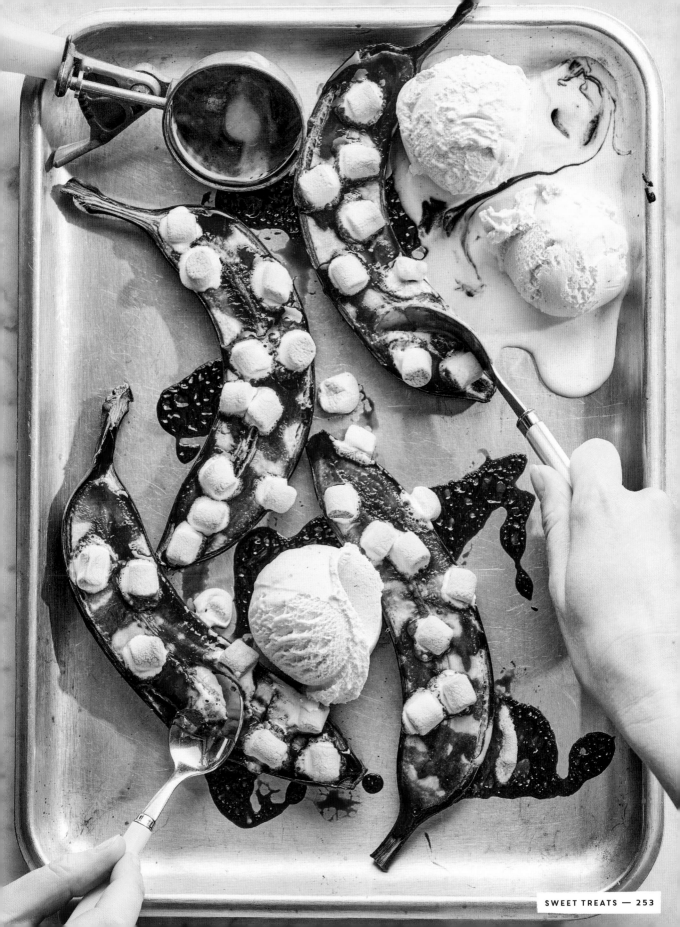

COCONUT *and* JAM SPONGE

🕐 **10 MINS**   🍲 **25 MINS**   ✕ **MAKES 16 SQUARES**

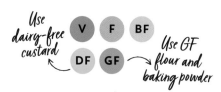

Use dairy-free custard ←

Use GF flour and baking powder

PER SERVING:
103 KCAL / 13G CARBS

SPECIAL EQUIPMENT
20 x 22cm (8 x 8½in)
ovenproof dish

100g self-raising flour
100g reduced-fat spread,
 plus a little extra
 for greasing
50g granulated sweetener
50g caster sugar
½ tsp baking powder
2 medium eggs
1 tsp vanilla extract

FOR THE TOPPING
4 tbsp reduced-sugar
 raspberry or other red jam
15g desiccated coconut

TO ACCOMPANY *(optional)*
Chocolate Custard, page
 240 (+ 95 kcal per serving)

Remember that sweet, fruity coconut and jam sponge you used to have as part of your school dinner? With our slimming-friendly take on this classic pudding, even grown-ups can enjoy it all over again! By swapping half the sugar for sweetener, this recipe brings all of the flavour without the extra calories. You'll still get that raspberry, coconutty hit and it's perfect when served with creamy custard or alongside a cuppa for an afternoon pick-me-up.

Everyday Light

Preheat the oven to 180°C (fan 160°C/gas mark 4) and grease the ovenproof dish well with the reduced-fat spread.

Put the flour, reduced-fat spread, granulated sweetener, caster sugar, baking powder, eggs and vanilla extract in a medium mixing bowl and beat together for 1–2 minutes with an electric hand whisk. Alternatively you can use a wooden spoon, but it will take more effort.

Use a rubber spatula to scrape the mixture from the mixing bowl and into the greased ovenproof dish and level the surface with a knife. Bake in the preheated oven for 20–25 minutes, until risen and golden all over. To test if it's ready, insert a small sharp knife into the centre of the sponge: when the sponge is cooked the knife will come out clean.

Put the jam in a small bowl and stir until smooth, then spread it all over the top of the warm sponge. Sprinkle the desiccated coconut all over the jam.

Cut into sixteen squares and serve alone or with your choice of accompaniment.

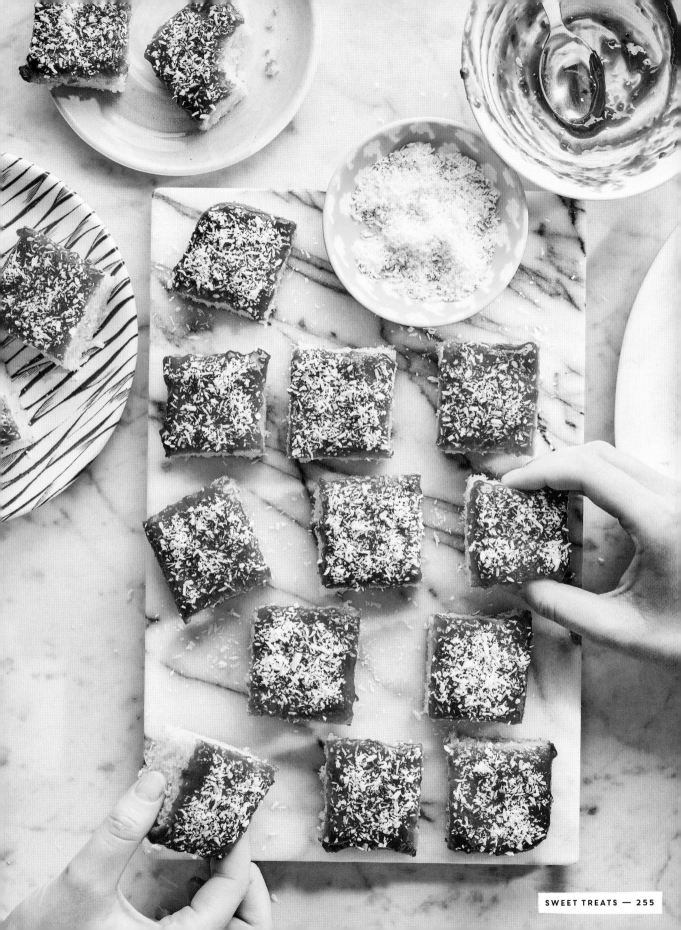

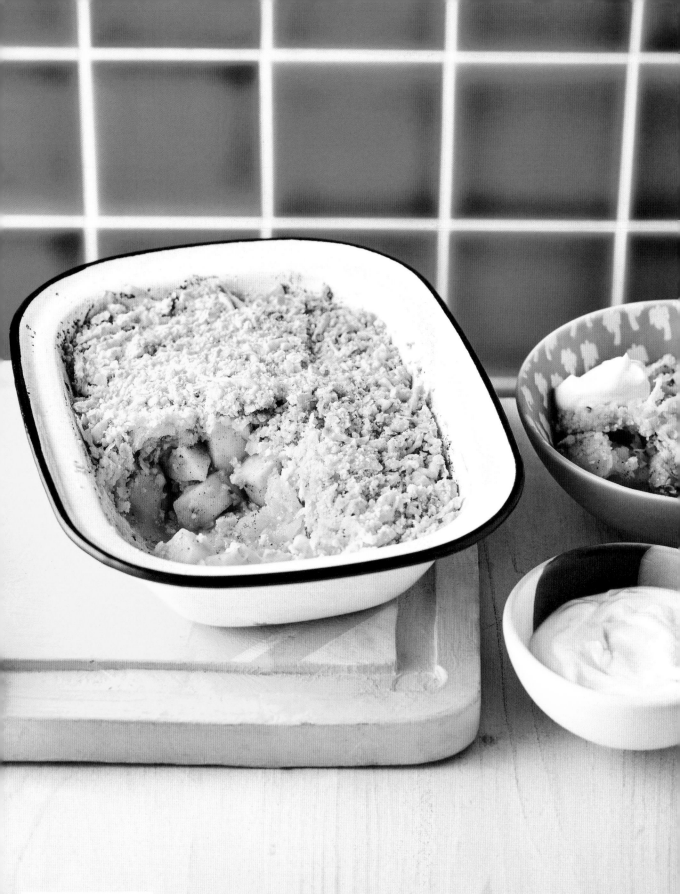

BAKED APPLE *with* A CHEESY CRUMBLE

⏱ **10–15 MINS**   🍲 **45 MINS**   ✕ **SERVES 4**

PER SERVING:
207 KCAL / 28G CARBS

SPECIAL EQUIPMENT
1-litre ovenproof dish

3–4 Bramley apples, peeled, cored and cut into 2cm (¾in) dice (about 450g peeled weight)
3 tbsp plus 1 tsp granulated sweetener (or sugar)
½ tsp ground cinnamon
juice of ½ lemon
60g plain flour
pinch of salt
30g reduced-fat spread
25g rolled oats
40g reduced-fat mild or medium Cheddar, finely grated

TO ACCOMPANY *(optional)*
60g fat-free Greek-style yoghurt (+ 35 kcal per serving)

This comforting pudding is inspired by one of our childhood food memories of snacking on sliced cheese and apples on top of buttered crackers. We've combined that with a classic crumble with a twist: it might sound unusual, but the sweet and tangy apples go really well with a slightly savoury topping!

Weekly Indulgence ──────────

Preheat the oven to 200°C (fan 180°C/gas mark 6).

Place the diced apples in the ovenproof dish, sprinkle over the 3 tablespoons of granulated sweetener (or sugar), cinnamon and lemon juice and toss everything around until well combined.

Put the flour in a bowl with the pinch of salt. Rub the reduced-fat spread into the flour with your fingertips until the mixture resembles breadcrumbs, then stir in the rolled oats and remaining 1 teaspoon of granulated sweetener. Add the grated Cheddar and rub through lightly.

Scatter the crumble on top of the apples and bake in the preheated oven for 40–45 minutes until the topping is golden and the apples are soft.

Serve each portion with your choice of accompaniment.

TIP: Swapping the sweetener for sugar will increase the sugar and calorie content of the dish, so bear this in mind if you're opting for sugar.

SWAP THIS: Cheshire cheese makes a great swap for Cheddar.

JAM ROLY POLY

🕐 **30 MINS** 🫕 **VARIABLE** (SEE BELOW) ✕ **SERVES 6**

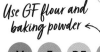

Use GF flour and baking powder ←

V F BF GF

PER SERVING:
210 KCAL / 37G CARBS

40g reduced-fat spread, plus
   a little extra for greasing
200g self-raising flour, plus
   a little extra for dusting
1 tsp baking powder
35g granulated sweetener
100ml skimmed milk
4 tbsp reduced-sugar
   raspberry jam or other
   red jam

TO ACCOMPANY *(optional)*
Chocolate Custard, page
   240 (+ 95 kcal per serving),
   or Custard from our
   Quick & Easy book
   (+ 58 kcal per serving)

Take a trip down memory lane with this old-school pud! We've skipped the traditional sugar and suet and used some slimming-friendly alternatives for a satisfying, warming dessert that comes in at only 210 calories per slice. You can even create this Roly Poly in three different ways! With sweet jam and a golden sponge, serve with a jug of hot custard for the ultimate nostalgic treat.

Weekly Indulgence ─────────────

OVEN METHOD
🫕 **40 MINS**

Preheat the oven to 180°C (fan 160°C/gas mark 4).

Cut out a large rectangle of foil and a large rectangle of non-stick baking paper, each about 30 x 38cm (12 x 15in), and place the non-stick baking paper sheet on top of the foil sheet. Grease the non-stick baking paper sheet all over with a little reduced-fat spread and place the double-layered sheet on a baking tray.

Sift the flour and baking powder into a medium mixing bowl, add the reduced-fat spread and, using clean hands, rub the fat into the flour using your fingertips until it resembles fine breadcrumbs. Stir in the granulated sweetener until evenly mixed.

Pour the milk into the dry ingredients and use a round-bladed table knife to mix until the mixture just comes together to form a soft ball of dough. Don't over-mix or handle the dough too much as this may make it tough – there is no need to knead it. Turn the dough out onto a well-floured work surface and pat it out into a 14 x 30cm (5½ x 12in) rectangle, using well-floured hands, rolling it lightly with a well-floured rolling pin. The dough will be soft, so dust the rolling pin and your hands with flour again as needed.

Mix the jam to loosen it a little, then spread it over the rectangle of dough, right to the edges, leaving a gap of about 2cm (¾in) along the narrow edge furthest away

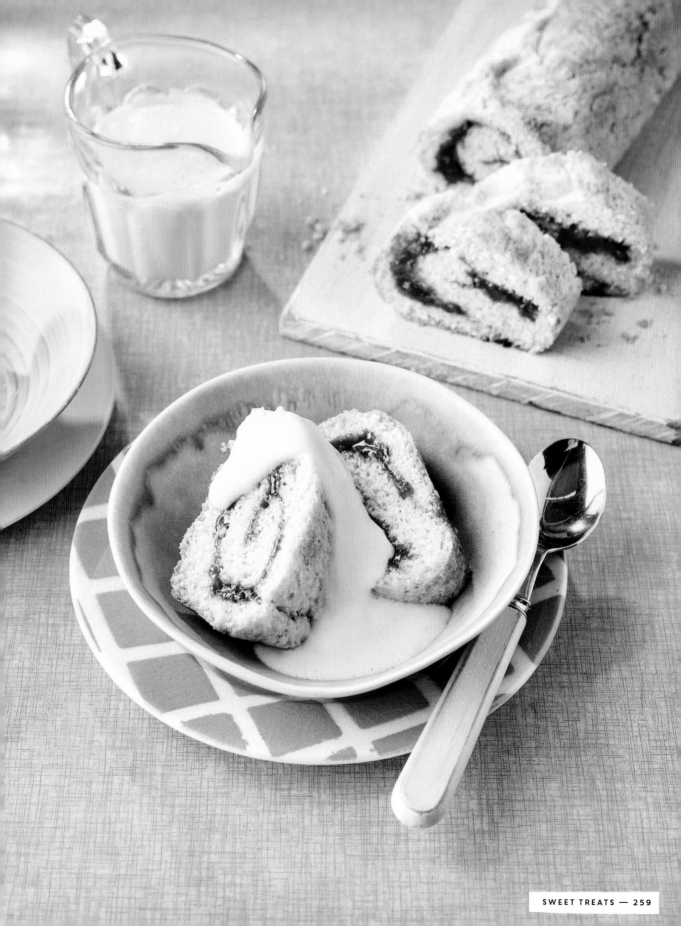

from you. Fold in the narrow edge nearest to you by about 2cm (¾in) and then start gently rolling the dough up away from you to make the spiral Roly Poly shape. You can use the long edge of a floured palette knife to help ease the Roly Poly off the work surface as you roll it up, if needed.

Carefully lift the Roly Poly onto the greased non-stick baking paper and foil sheet, placing it seam side down in the centre of the sheet. You can use a couple of fish slices at each end to help you lift the Roly Poly if needed.

Bring the two long sides of foil and non-stick baking paper up over the Roly Poly and make a couple of narrow but tight folds to seal along the top. You need to make a loose parcel with room for the Roly Poly to rise and expand lengthways and widthways, so don't wrap it tightly. Seal both ends of the parcel by making a couple of narrow but tight folds. Again,

make sure you make it a loose parcel with room for the Roly Poly to expand. Place a roasting tin or large ovenproof dish on the bottom shelf of the preheated oven. Carefully pull it out a little and fill it with boiling water from a kettle, to a depth of about 3cm (1¼in). Very carefully slide the tray of hot water back onto the oven shelf. Place the Roly Poly on the baking tray into the oven on the shelf above the water bath and bake for 40 minutes.

Remove from the oven and leave the Roly Poly to stand for 5 minutes before carefully unwrapping the foil parcel, taking care as it will still be hot. The Roly Poly should be risen, increased in size and golden brown on the outside. It should also be cooked right through and not doughy. If it is still doughy, wrap it up again and put it back in the oven for a little longer.

Cut into slices with a large serrated knife and serve with an accompaniment of choice.

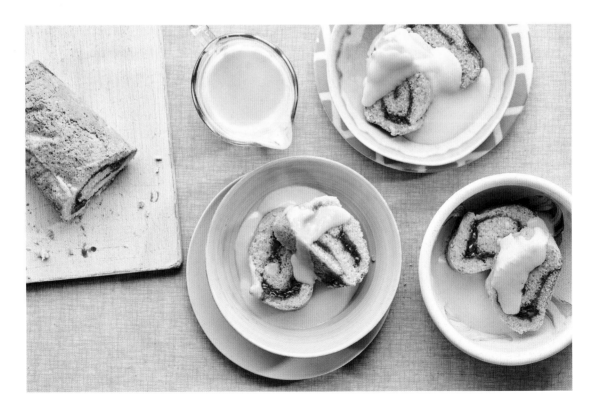

SLOW-COOKER METHOD
🍲 HIGH: 2 HOURS

SPECIAL EQUIPMENT
Slow cooker, 2 small ovenproof ramekin dishes or similar

Cut out a large rectangle of foil and a large rectangle of non-stick baking paper, each about 30 x 38cm (12 x 15in), and place the non-stick baking paper sheet on top of the foil sheet. Grease the non-stick baking paper sheet all over with a little reduced-fat spread.

Sift the flour and baking powder into a medium bowl, add the reduced-fat spread and, using clean hands, rub the fat into the flour using your fingertips until it resembles fine breadcrumbs. Stir in the granulated sweetener until evenly mixed.

Pour the milk into the dry ingredients and use a round-bladed table knife to mix until the mixture just comes together to form a soft ball of dough. Don't over-mix or handle the dough too much as this may make it tough – there is no need to knead it. Turn the dough out onto a well-floured work surface and gently roll out into a 14 x 30cm (5½ x 12in) rectangle, using a well-floured rolling pin and well-floured hands. The length of the Roly Poly will be 14cm (5½in) before cooking, so measure the internal dimensions of your slow cooker to make sure it will fit in. If it doesn't fit, make the dough rectangle a bit narrower to fit. The dough will be soft, so dust the rolling pin and your hands with flour again as needed.

Spread the jam over the rectangle of dough, right to the edges, but leave a gap of about 2cm (¾in) along the narrow edge furthest away from you. Fold in the narrow edge nearest to you by about 2cm (¾in) and then start gently rolling the dough up away from you to make the spiral Roly Poly shape. You can use the long edge of a floured palette knife to help ease the Roly Poly off the work surface as you roll it up, if needed.

Carefully lift the Roly Poly onto the greased baking paper and foil sheet, placing it seam side down in the centre of the sheet. You can use a couple of fish slices at each end to help you lift the Roly Poly if needed.

Bring the two long sides of foil and non-stick baking paper up over the Roly Poly and make a couple of narrow but tight folds to seal along the top. You need to make a loose parcel with room for the Roly Poly to rise and expand lengthways and widthways, so don't wrap it tightly. Seal both ends of the parcel by making a couple of narrow but tight folds. Again, make sure you make it a loose parcel with room for the Roly Poly to expand.

Place two small ramekin dishes (or similar) upside down in the bottom of the slow-cooker pot. This will keep the Roly Poly up above the water while it's cooking. Pour in boiling water to come halfway up the sides of the ramekins. Lay the foil-wrapped Roly Poly across the top of the ramekins, making sure it's not touching the water. If it is touching the water, remove a little water.

Place the lid on the slow cooker and turn it to the high setting. Cook for 2 hours, checking once, halfway through, that there is still enough water in the slow cooker. Don't lift the lid more than this as each time you do will add on another 30 minutes to the cooking time.

Carefully remove the Roly Poly from the slow cooker using oven gloves. Allow to sit for 5 minutes, then carefully unwrap. The Roly Poly should have risen, increased in size and be very lightly golden on the outside. It should be cooked right through and not doughy. If it is still doughy, wrap it up again and cook it for a little longer.

Cut into slices using a large serrated knife and serve with an accompaniment of choice.

ELECTRIC PRESSURE-COOKER METHOD
🍲 25 MINS

SPECIAL EQUIPMENT
Electric pressure cooker and trivet

Cut out a large rectangle of foil and a large rectangle of non-stick baking paper, each about 30 x 38cm (12 x 15in), and place the non-stick baking paper sheet on top of the foil sheet. Grease the non-stick baking paper sheet all over with a little reduced-fat spread.

Sift the flour and baking powder into a medium mixing bowl, add the reduced-fat spread and, using clean hands, rub the fat into the flour using your fingertips until it resembles fine breadcrumbs. Stir in the granulated sweetener until evenly mixed.

Pour the milk into the dry ingredients and use a round-bladed table knife to mix until the mixture just comes together to form a soft ball of dough. Don't over-mix or handle the dough too much as this may make it tough – there is no need to knead it. Turn the dough out onto a well-floured work surface and gently roll out into a 14 x 30cm (5½ x 12in) rectangle, using a well-floured rolling pin and well-floured hands. The dough will be soft, so dust the rolling pin and your hands with flour again as needed.

Carefully lift the Roly Poly onto the greased non-stick baking paper and foil sheet, placing it seam side down in the centre of the sheet. You can use a couple of fish slices at each end to help you lift the Roly Poly if needed.

Spread the jam over the rectangle of dough, right to the edges, but leave a gap of about 2cm (¾in) along the narrow edge furthest away from you. Fold in the narrow edge nearest to you by about 2cm (¾in) and then start gently rolling the dough up away from you to make the spiral Roly Poly shape. You can use the long edge of a floured palette knife to help ease the Roly Poly off the work surface as you roll it up, if needed.

Carefully lift the Roly Poly onto the greased non-stick baking paper and foil sheet, placing it seam side down in the centre of the sheet. You can use a couple of fish slices at each end to help you lift the Roly Poly if needed.

Bring the two long sides of foil and non-stick baking paper up over the Roly Poly and make a couple of narrow but tight folds to seal along the top. You need to make a loose parcel with room for the Roly Poly to rise and expand lengthways and widthways, so don't wrap it tightly. Seal both ends of the parcel by making a couple of narrow but tight folds. Again, make sure you make it a loose parcel with room for the Roly Poly to expand.

Place 500ml cold water in the bottom of the pressure cooker. Place the wrapped Roly Poly on the trivet and use the handles to lower the Roly Poly into the pressure cooker. Cover with the lid and set the valve to 'sealing'. Pressure-cook on high for 25 minutes, then set the valve to 'venting', taking extreme care not to place yourself anywhere near the escaping steam. Wait for the float valve to drop before opening the lid.

Use oven gloves to lift the Roly Poly out on the trivet. Leave to stand for 5 minutes before unwrapping.

The Roly Poly should have risen, increased in size and should be very lightly golden. It should be cooked right through and no longer doughy. If it is, wrap it up and cook for a few minutes longer.

Cut into slices using a large serrated knife and serve with an accompaniment of choice.

CHOCO NUT LAVA CAKES

Use GF self-raising flour

🕐 **30 MINS**   ▦ **VARIABLE** (SEE BELOW)   ✕ **SERVES 6**

PER SERVING:
181 KCAL / 20G CARBS

SPECIAL EQUIPMENT
4 x 125ml ramekin dishes

45g reduced-fat spread,
 plus a little extra for greasing
45g self-raising flour
25g granulated sweetener
15g cocoa powder
2 medium eggs
1 tsp vanilla extract
4 tsp chocolate hazelnut spread
5g hazelnuts, roughly chopped
¼ tsp icing sugar, for dusting

TO ACCOMPANY *(optional)*
Chocolate Custard, page 240
 (+ 95 kcal per serving)

These hot spongy desserts with an oozing chocolate and hazelnut centre are so rich and fudgy, it's hard to believe they're only 181 calories! They're delicious fresh from the oven but if you're pressed for time, pop them in the microwave for a chocolate fix on the table in minutes. Top with Chocolate Custard for the ultimate indulgence!

Weekly Indulgence ─────────────────────

OVEN METHOD
▦ **10 MINS**

Preheat the oven to 180°C (fan 160°C/gas mark 4) and lightly grease the ramekin dishes with reduced-fat spread.

Put the self-raising flour, granulated sweetener, cocoa powder, reduced-fat spread, eggs and vanilla extract in a medium mixing bowl and beat together for 1–2 minutes with an electric hand whisk or a wooden spoon.

Divide the mixture evenly among the four ramekin dishes. Drop a teaspoonful of chocolate hazelnut spread into the centre of each and sprinkle with a few chopped hazelnuts.

Place the ramekins on a baking tray and bake in the preheated oven for 8–10 minutes, until risen and spongy but still runny in the centre.

Remove from the oven and leave to stand for 5 minutes.

Dust with the icing sugar and serve at once, with an accompaniment of choice.

SWAP THIS: Swap the chocolate hazelnut spread for regular chocolate spread.

MICROWAVE METHOD
🍲 1½–2 MINS

Put the self-raising flour, granulated sweetener, cocoa powder, reduced-fat spread, eggs and vanilla extract in a medium mixing bowl and beat together for 1–2 minutes with an electric hand whisk or a wooden spoon.

Divide the mixture evenly among the four ramekin dishes. Drop a teaspoonful of chocolate hazelnut spread into the centre of each and sprinkle with a few chopped hazelnuts.

Place all four ramekins on the microwave turntable, evenly spaced apart. Cover loosely with vented cling film (to allow steam to escape they shouldn't be completely covered) and cook on high for 1½–2 minutes. Check on the cakes after about a minute and continue cooking if needed. The cakes should still be runny in the middle when you take them out of the microwave. Leave the cakes to stand for 5 minutes, then remove the cling film.

Dust with the icing sugar and serve at once, with an accompaniment of choice.

> **TIP:** Take care not to overcook the cakes, otherwise they won't have a gooey chocolate centre. Follow the timings carefully and remove them from the oven or microwave while they are still runny in the middle. Leave to stand for 5 minutes then you should have the perfect gooey centre.

" *This is the most I have ever used cookbooks in my life! I really, really love them!* "

—— CLAIRE

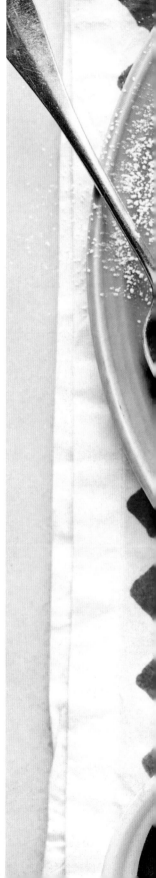

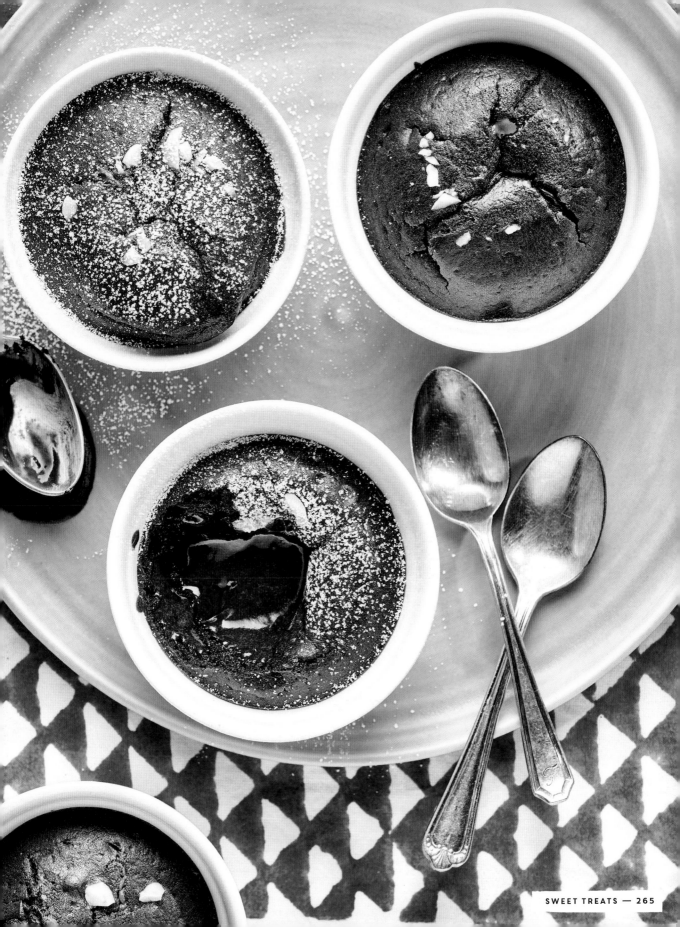

TREACLE SPONGE

🕐 **20 MINS**   🍲 **1 HOUR**   ✕ **SERVES 8**

Use dairy-free custard ↖

V F BF DF

PER SERVING:
335 KCAL / 49G CARBS

SPECIAL EQUIPMENT
1.2-litre ovenproof
pudding basin

170g reduced-fat spread, plus
 a little extra for greasing
4 tbsp golden-syrup-
 alternative fruit syrup
 (we use one made by
 Sweet Freedom)
170g self-raising flour
85g granulated sweetener
85g golden caster sugar
1 tsp baking powder
3 medium eggs
1 tsp vanilla extract

TO ACCOMPANY *(optional)*
Chocolate Custard, page
 240 (+ 95 kcal per serving),
 or Custard from our *Quick
 & Easy* book (+ 58 kcal per
 serving)

> **TIPS:** We used a golden
> syrup alternative fruit
> syrup made by Sweet
> Freedom as it contains
> fewer calories than golden
> syrup. You can find it in
> most larger supermarkets.
> Be sure to use a white
> granulated sweetener that
> has the same texture and
> weight as sugar.

This oven-baked sponge pudding soaked with sweet,
sticky syrup is delicious served with hot custard. What
could be better than a slimming-friendly pud that's just as
good as the one we enjoyed as children? Using a golden
syrup alternative reduces the calories significantly, but you
still get that recognisable texture and treacle flavour!

Special Occasion

Preheat the oven to 200°C (fan 180°C/gas mark 6) and
place a baking tray in the oven. Grease the pudding basin
thoroughly with reduced-fat spread. Cut out an 8cm (3in)
disc of non-stick baking paper. Grease the disc and place
it, greased side up, in the base of the basin. Place the
golden-syrup-alternative fruit syrup on top of the disc.

Make a lid for the basin by cutting out a 28cm (11in) disc of
foil and a 28cm (11in) disc of non-stick baking paper. Place
the foil disc on top of the paper disc to make a double
layer, then make a double pleat (about 2cm/¾in wide)
across the width of the double-layered lid. Set aside.

To make the sponge, put the flour, reduced-fat spread,
sweetener, sugar, baking powder, eggs and vanilla in a
medium bowl and beat for 1–2 minutes with an electric
hand whisk until pale and fluffy. Scrape the mixture into the
pudding basin using a rubber spatula, level the surface with
a round-bladed knife and put the pleated lid on top. Fold the
edges down over the bowl rim and tie cooking string tightly
around the basin, just under the rim, to hold the lid in place.

Bake on the hot tray in the oven for about 1 hour, until the
pudding is risen and golden. To check if it's cooked, snip off
the string, remove the lid and insert a knife: if it comes out
clean, it's cooked. If it needs longer, put the lid back on (no
need to re-tie the string) and bake for a few more minutes.

Remove the lid, run a round-bladed knife around the
pudding and carefully turn it out onto a serving plate using
oven gloves or a tea towel – it will be very hot. Remove
the paper disc, trying not to touch the pudding. Cut into
eight and serve hot with an accompaniment of choice.

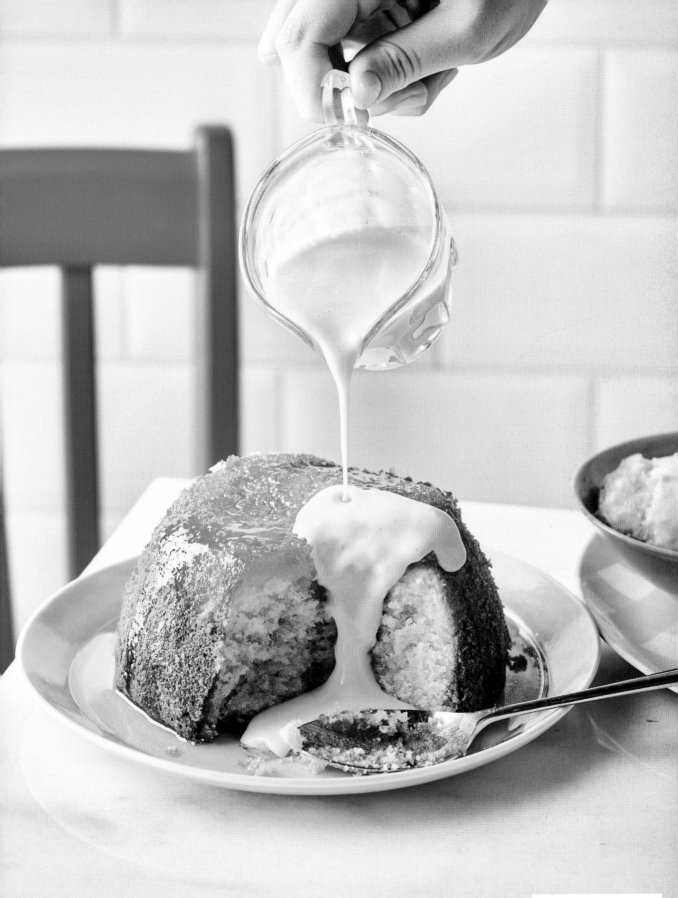

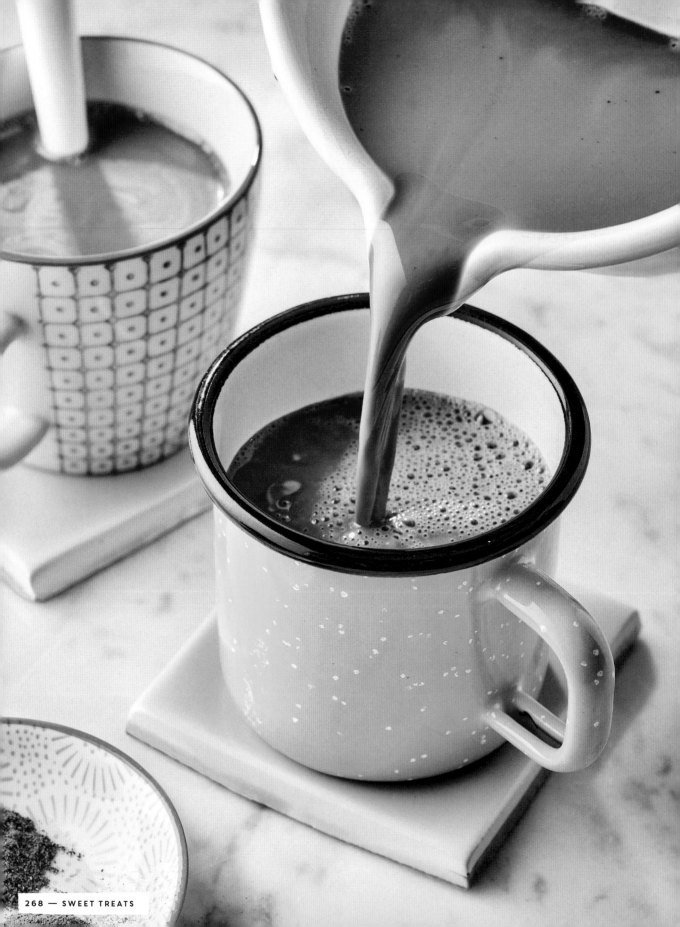

MEXICAN HOT CHOCOLATE

⏱ **1 MIN**   🍲 **4 MINS**   ✕ **SERVES 1**

PER SERVING:
94 KCAL / 12G CARBS

250ml unsweetened
  almond milk
1½ tsp cocoa powder
1–2 tsp granulated sweetener,
  to taste
½ tsp vanilla extract
¼ tsp ground cinnamon
pinch of chilli powder
pinch of salt

Our version of a Mexican Hot Chocolate is a tasty blend of sweet and savoury with a mellow kick. If it's not something you've tried before it may sound a little odd, but trust us, it works so well! If you're a fan of a chai latte or spiced teas, this will be right up your street.

Everyday Light

Place your saucepan over a medium heat and add all the ingredients.

While the milk is heating up, gently whisk the mixture continuously and cook for 3–4 minutes, or until smooth and piping hot throughout.

Pour into your favourite mug and serve.

TIP: We've kept the flavours mellow in this drink, but feel free to add extra chilli or cinnamon if you want more of a kick!

SWAP THIS: We've used unsweetened almond milk to keep the calories down, but you can use whichever milk or milk alternative you prefer. Using semi-skimmed milk will increase the calories to 167 kcal per serving.

BAKEWELL RICE PUDDING

🕐 **5 MINS**　🍲 **VARIABLE** (SEE BELOW)　✕ **SERVES 4**

PER SERVING:
188 KCAL / 28G CARBS

100g short-grain pudding rice
1 litre unsweetened
　almond milk
1 tsp almond essence
2 tbsp granulated sweetener
　or sugar
15g toasted flaked almonds

FOR THE CHERRY COMPOTE
200g frozen cherries,
　defrosted
3 tbsp orange juice
1 tbsp granulated sweetener

With its cherry and almond flavours, this is a deliciously creamy rice pudding with a Bakewell twist! Perfect for cooking on the hob, you can also pop everything in the slow cooker if you prefer. Top with the simple cherry compote and a few flaked almonds for added crunch. Psst... if you have any leftovers, pop them in the fridge and it's just as delicious when enjoyed cold for breakfast the next day.

Everyday Light

HOB-TOP METHOD
🍲 **1 HOUR**

Put the rice and unsweetened almond milk in a saucepan and bring to the boil, stirring occasionally, then turn the heat down to the lowest setting, cover loosely with a lid and simmer gently for 50 minutes, stirring frequently.

While the rice pudding cooks, prepare the compote topping. Put the defrosted cherries (including any juices that have been released) in a small saucepan, along with the orange juice and sweetener. Bring to the boil and cook rapidly for about 10 minutes or until the juices become syrupy. Remove from the heat.

When the rice pudding is cooked, take it off the heat and stir in the almond essence and sweetener (or sugar). Leave it in the pan for 10 minutes before spooning into bowls. Top with the cherry compote (warm or cold) and a sprinkle of flaked almonds. Serve!

SLOW-COOKER METHOD
🍲 **LOW: 6 HOURS**

SPECIAL EQUIPMENT
Slow cooker

Put the rice and almond milk in the slow cooker and cook on low for 6 hours.

SWAP THIS:
Swap the almond milk for skimmed/ semi-skimmed cow's milk if you prefer.

Prepare the compote ahead of time, or just before serving. Put the defrosted cherries (including any juices that have been released) in a small saucepan, along with the orange juice and sweetener. Bring to the boil and cook rapidly for about 10 minutes or until the juices become syrupy. Remove from the heat.

When the rice pudding is cooked, stir in the almond essence and sweetener (or sugar).

Spoon into bowls and top with the cherry compote (warm or cold) and a sprinkle of flaked almonds. Serve!

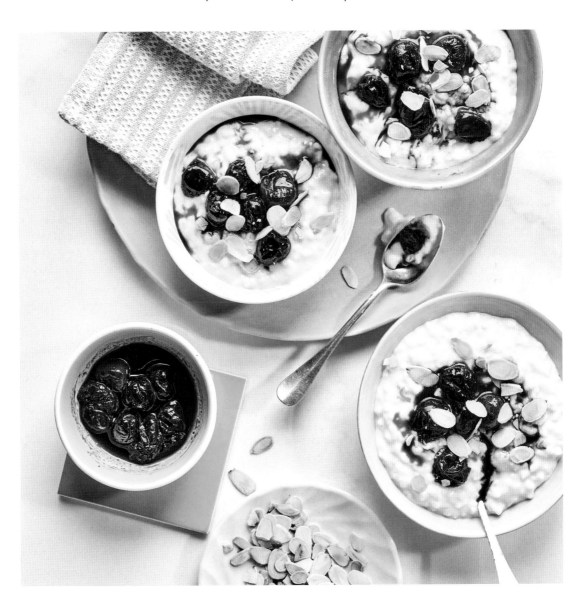

CHERRY PIE

Use GF tortilla wraps

(V) (DF) (GF)

PER SERVING:
139 KCAL / 25G CARBS

SPECIAL EQUIPMENT
20cm (8in) pie dish

low-calorie cooking spray
2 large white tortilla wraps
   (25cm/10in in diameter)
400g frozen, stoned, dark
   sweet cherries, defrosted
   (juices kept)
10g granulated sweetener,
   or to taste
1 tablespoon cornflour,
   mixed with 1 tbsp water
   until smooth
½ medium egg, beaten

🕐 **25 MINS**   🍲 **25 MINS**   ✕ **SERVES 6**

With a crunchy crust and stuffed with juicy cherries, it's no wonder that cherry pie is one of the nation's favourites! We've used a surprising ingredient instead of shortcrust pastry to make the pie case, keeping the calories low while making sure it looks amazing on the table.

Everyday Light ——————————————

Preheat the oven to 180°C (fan 160°C/gas mark 4) and grease the pie dish well with low-calorie cooking spray. Place a wrap in the dish and press it in so the edges form a shallow rim around the dish. Make three or four small snips around the edge to help mould the sides of the pie case into the dish if you need to. Press any snipped sections firmly together to seal. Part-bake the pie case for 12–15 minutes. Only the middle should be crisp and the whole case should be white.

Meanwhile, make the cherry filling. Place a sieve over a measuring jug. Pour the defrosted cherries and juice into the sieve and let the juice drain into the jug. Place the drained cherries in a small saucepan. Measure the juice in the jug and if you have less than 150ml, make it up to 150ml with water. If you have more than 150ml juice, drain some off until you are left with 150ml juice. Pour the juice (or juice and water) into the saucepan with the cherries and taste: frozen cherries can vary in sweetness, so add sweetener to taste, stirring it into the fruit. Place over a medium heat, stir in the cornflour mixture and simmer gently for 3–5 minutes, until thickened and glossy. Set aside.

Place the remaining wrap on a work surface and cut out 12 x 1cm (½in)-wide strips across the width of the wrap. Brush the strips with beaten egg. Spread the filling out evenly in the part-baked case. Brush beaten egg around the case edge. Place six strips across the top of the pie at equal intervals, glazed-side up, trimming to fit by snipping off any excess with scissors. Gently press into place on the egg-washed pie edge. Repeat with the six remaining strips, placing them over the first six strips in criss-cross formation to make a lattice. Bake for 8–10 minutes or until golden. Remove from the heat and leave to stand for 5 minutes, then serve alone or with a swirl of aerosol cream.

TIPS: Sometimes the odd stone makes it into a bag of frozen pitted cherries – keep an eye out and remove if you see them. Use fresh cherries if you prefer. Before you start, make sure your wraps are large enough to fit your pie dish, with the edges coming up the side of the dish to make a shallow edge.

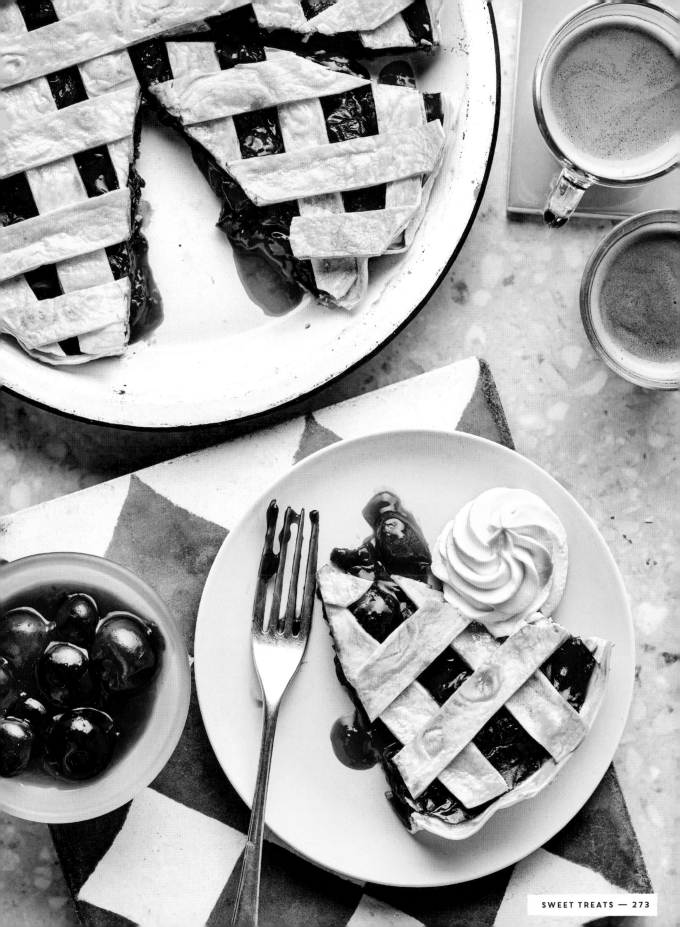

BISCOFF BLONDIES

⏱ **10 MINS** 🍲 **40 MINS** ✕ **MAKES 16 BLONDIES**

PER BLONDIE:
148 KCAL / 16G CARBS

SPECIAL EQUIPMENT
18 x 18cm (7 x 7in)
square cake tin

100g reduced-fat spread, plus
   a little extra for greasing
200g sweet potatoes, peeled
   and cut into small chunks
100g plain flour
50g golden caster sugar
50g granulated sweetener
½ tsp baking powder
1 tsp vanilla extract
2 medium eggs
100g crunchy Biscoff spread,
   plus 20g for the topping
40g white chocolate,
   roughly chopped

We've used a surprising hidden ingredient to keep these super-indulgent Biscoff Blondies beautifully moist. They have a delicious, caramelly, biscuit flavour and are full of white chocolate chunks to make them extra special. A little melted Biscoff spread drizzled over the top really helps to take these blondies to the next level – you'd never guess that they're slimming friendly!

Everyday Light ————————————————

Preheat the oven to 180°C (fan 160°C/gas mark 4). Grease the cake tin with a little reduced-fat spread and line the base and sides with non-stick baking paper.

Put the sweet potatoes in a small saucepan of boiling water, reduce the heat, cover and simmer for 10–15 minutes or until tender. Drain well and mash with a fork. Leave to cool completely.

Place the cooled sweet potato in a medium bowl. Add the flour, reduced-fat spread, sugar, granulated sweetener, baking powder, vanilla, eggs and 100g Biscoff spread and beat with an electric hand whisk for 1–2 minutes or until just combined. Fold in the white chocolate, then scrape the mixture into the lined tin. Level the surface with a knife. Bake in the oven for 20–25 minutes, until lightly golden. To test if it's ready, insert a small sharp knife into the centre: when it's cooked the knife will come out clean.

Remove from the oven and leave to cool in the tin on a wire rack (the residual heat from the tin will help them set and create the desired texture). When it's completely cool, use the baking paper to lift the blondies out of the tin and place them on the work surface.

Place the remaining Biscoff spread for the topping in a small cup and melt until runny, either by heating it in the microwave on low for 30–40 seconds, stirring occasionally until runny, or placing the cup in a bowl of boiling water and stirring until runny. Drizzle the melted Biscoff spread over the Blondies. Leave to set, then cut into sixteen squares using a large sharp knife. Remove from the baking paper and serve.

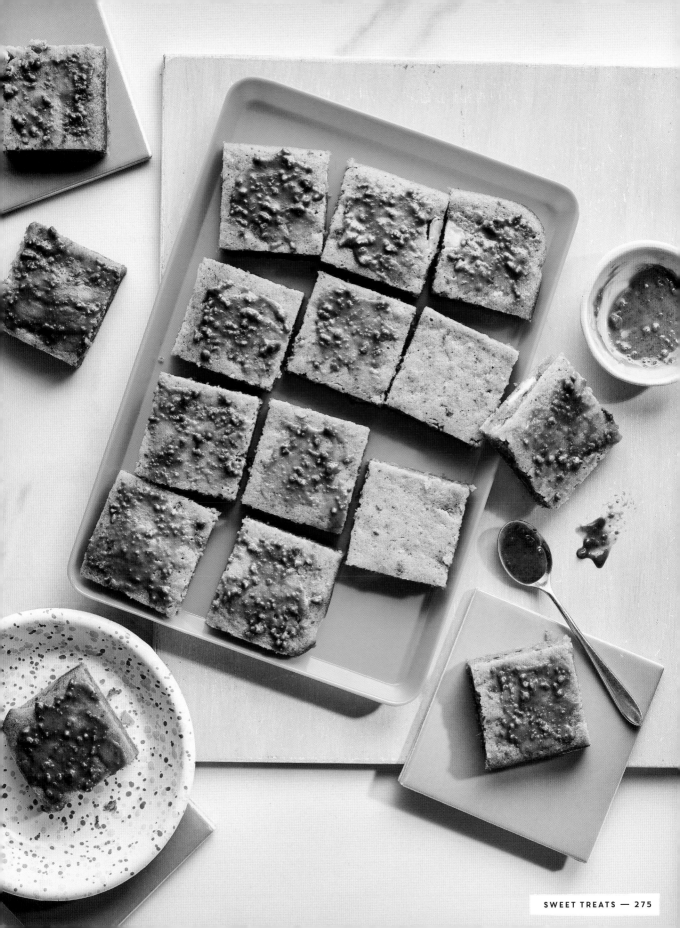

NUTRITIONAL INFO PER SERVING

Breakfast	ENERGY KJ/KCAL	FAT (G)	SATURATED FAT (G)	CARBS (G)	SUGAR (G)	FIBRE (G)	PROTEIN (G)
MARMITE MUSHROOMS ON TOAST	783/187	5.8	3.2	20	3.6	3.5	13
SLOW-COOKER OATS	460/109	1.9	0.4	17	4.1	1.6	5.3
BLUEBERRY AND APPLE OATS	713/169	2.3	0.4	30	9.5	4.3	5.8
PEANUT BUTTER AND BANANA OATS	1122/267	7.5	0.7	37	18	4.4	11
NUTELLA BAKED OATS	2274/542	19	5.5	65	23	3.6	29
CHOCOLATE PANCAKES	1211/289	8.9	3	34	8.4	4.8	20
BREAKFAST CALZONES	727/173	4.8	2.3	19	3.4	4.6	11
PIZZA-TOPPED OMELETTE	1548/370	18	7.6	18	14	5.4	29

FAKEAWAYS	ENERGY KJ/KCAL	FAT (G)	SATURATED FAT (G)	CARBS (G)	SUGAR (G)	FIBRE (G)	PROTEIN (G)
VODKA PASTA	2162/512	5.1	1.7	84	17	8.6	20
HALLOUMI COUSCOUS BURGERS WITH SALSA	1689/401	9.2	4.2	57	11	8.3	17
OVEN-BAKED PASANDA CURRY	803/191	4.8	0.8	4	2.3	1.2	33
CREAMY LEMON CHICKEN	812/192	2.9	0.9	2.3	1.9	0.5	39
KUNG PAO PORK	1257/298	5.5	0.3	38	17	5.6	25
SWEET AND SPICY MEATBALLS	1326/315	8.1	2.8	28	24	2	31
MARGHERITA CHICKEN	1017/241	5.8	3	6.1	5.3	1.3	39
PEANUT BUTTER CHICKEN CURRY	1442/342	5.8	1.3	18	13	6.7	49
CARIBBEAN LAMB CURRY	1348/321	13	6.7	25	7	4.6	25
SCRUNCHILADAS	1339/318	6	2.8	36	12	9.2	24
RAINBOW SOUP	292/69	1.2	0.5	10	6.3	3.2	2.4

FAKEAWAYS	ENERGY KJ/KCAL	FAT (G)	SATURATED FAT (G)	CARBS (G)	SUGAR (G)	FIBRE (G)	PROTEIN (G)
TANDOORI CHICKEN	971/233	14	3.8	4.4	3	1.2	22
CRISPY CHICKEN WITH SWEET AND SOUR SAUCE	1457/345	3.8	1.1	36	18	7	37
STICKY CHICKEN AND PINEAPPLE SALAD	1355/320	3.6	0.8	28	26	5.7	39
GARLIC MUSHROOM BIRYANI	1710/404	2.7	0.7	78	13	5.8	15
CHICKEN AND CHEESE CURRY	1488/353	9.2	4.9	12	8.5	2.9	4
KATSU CHICKEN NUGGETS AND CURRY DIP	1264/299	4.4	1	27	7.1	4.4	37
CHEESY CHIPS AND GRAVY	960/228	4.9	3	34	4.5	4.4	10
TAMARIND AND COCONUT FISH	1240/295	11	7.1	21	9.3	4.6	27
SPAGHETTI CARBONARA	2167/516	18	6.4	47	5.6	5.1	39
COCONUT PAD THAI NOODLES	1292/308	11	2.2	35	11	7.4	14
BOLOGNESE CHEESE FRIES	1598/379	6.7	3.3	49	17	8.4	24
CHILLI CHEESY 'NACHOS'	2201/522	8.1	3.7	64	22	18	38
TACHOS	1372/326	9.4	3.7	35	6.9	6.1	21
I CAN'T BELIEVE IT'S NOT BUTTER CHICKEN	1344/320	12	2.5	18	14	6	32

BATCH COOK	ENERGY KJ/KCAL	FAT (G)	SATURATED FAT (G)	CARBS (G)	SUGAR (G)	FIBRE (G)	PROTEIN (G)
CREAMY ROASTED RED PEPPER AND CHICKEN PASTA	1257/297	3.1	1.1	38	9.8	4.8	25
CURRIED SAUSAGES	1663/394	4.3	1	61	24	13	21
BANGERS AND MASH PIE	1655/392	4.9	1.4	54	15	10	26
SWEET POTATO CHILLI	1460/346	2.7	0.4	57	23	14	14
BACON AND LEEK MAC 'N' CHEESE	1933/459	15	5.8	50	8.2	3.1	31
SLOW-COOKER STROGANOFF	1096/261	8.6	3	8.5	5.1	1.4	37
ONE-POT SUNDAY BEEF	1948/462	8.8	3.1	29	12	6.7	62

BATCH COOK *Continued*	ENERGY KJ/KCAL	FAT (G)	SATURATED FAT (G)	CARBS (G)	SUGAR (G)	FIBRE (G)	PROTEIN (G)
SPANISH RICE	1617/383	7	2.2	65	6.5	3.8	12
STUFFED PASTA BOLOGNESE	1753/417	14	7.9	34	13	4.8	34
PULLED HAM IN A MUSTARD SAUCE	808/191	3.8	1.6	1.9	1.9	0.9	37
CHEESY AUBERGINE BAKE	790/188	5.8	3.2	19	17	6.4	9.5
PAPRIKA CHICKEN	1150/273	5	2.1	13	11	5.5	40
CREAMY, CHEESY GARLIC MUSHROOM RISOTTO	1713/406	6.4	3.2	69	5.6	4.9	16
HOMITY PIE	1214/288	7.3	3.2	40	6.5	4.4	13

STEWS *and* SOUPS	ENERGY KJ/KCAL	FAT (G)	SATURATED FAT (G)	CARBS (G)	SUGAR (G)	FIBRE (G)	PROTEIN (G)
MATZO BALL SOUP	721/171	3.3	0.9	17	6.1	3.5	17
BEEF AND BAKED BEAN STEW	1320/313	5	1.8	35	9	9	27
GERMAN POTATO SOUP	678/161	2.1	0.5	25	5.8	4.5	8.1
CURRIED CHICKEN AND RICE SOUP	1157/274	2.7	1	35	14	5.3	24
GREEK POTATO STEW	909/215	3	1.3	34	12	6.3	8.9
CREAMY CHICKEN SOUP	725/172	1.7	0.4	26	6.7	4.4	12
CREAMY TOMATO SOUP	704/166	1.2	0.4	26	17	5.9	6.5
FISH CHOWDER	1140/270	2.6	0.7	30	6.9	3.9	30
SMOKY CHICKPEA STEW	1068/253	3	0.3	42	11	9.9	8.9
BEEF STEW AND DUMPLINGS	1951/463	8	2.7	57	18	12	35
LAMB SCOUSE	1665/396	12	5.5	44	9.9	7	24
KATE'S TAGINE	1938/460	7.9	1.7	45	29	17	42

BAKES & ROASTS	ENERGY KJ/KCAL	FAT (G)	SATURATED FAT (G)	CARBS (G)	SUGAR (G)	FIBRE (G)	PROTEIN (G)
CHICKEN, BACON AND LEEK COTTAGE PIE	1704/403	6.1	2.2	39	5.9	5.3	46
TIPSY BBQ CHICKEN	801/190	3.4	0.9	15	13	0.6	22
VEGETARIAN COTTAGE PIE JACKETS	1919/454	4.2	1	77	8.9	14	20
HONEY AND MUSTARD PORK	1062/252	6.7	1.6	22	21	2.5	25
CREAMY GARLIC AND PARMESAN CHICKEN	1085/258	8.1	4.5	4.7	3.5	1.9	41
HUNTER'S CHICKEN PIE	2022/479	7.8	3.5	50	16	8.8	46
FORGOTTEN LAMB	1761/424	31	16	3.6	3.3	1.5	30
STEAK AND CHIPS PIE	1332/316	4.8	1.8	38	9.3	6.8	27
ONE-POT MEDITERRANEAN CHICKEN RICE	1478/349	4.9	1.2	46	5.4	3.3	29
CREAMY GARLIC SALMON	1462/350	21	4.6	7.4	4.8	1.5	33
CHESTNUT ROAST	774/184	2.4	0.6	31	11	6.2	6.4
CHICKEN VESUVIO	1506/357	5.3	1.4	37	8.5	6.6	37
DANGER DOGS	1479/351	8	1.6	29	7.7	9.9	35
CHEESE, ONION AND POTATO PIE	1201/286	10	5.9	31	4.9	3.4	16
MINTED LAMB HOTPOT	1819/432	11	4.5	48	13	7.9	31
CHICKEN TETRAZZINI	2231/529	8.8	0.7	59	8.9	6.6	51
CHEESY FAJITA ORZOTTO	2012/477	12	5.6	48	10	4.2	41
BUTTERNUT SQUASH AND BACON BAKE	1265/301	10	4	34	16	5.5	17

Snacks and SIDES	ENERGY KJ/KCAL	FAT (G)	SATURATED FAT (G)	CARBS (G)	SUGAR (G)	FIBRE (G)	PROTEIN (G)
COWBOY FRIES	1534/364	6.8	3.1	50	7.8	9	21
SPICED EDAMAME BEAN DIP	334/80	2.5	0	5.2	1.3	4	7

Snacks and SIDES Continued	ENERGY KJ/KCAL	FAT (G)	SATURATED FAT (G)	CARBS (G)	SUGAR (G)	FIBRE (G)	PROTEIN (G)
CHEESE AND ONION MASH	1062/252	4.9	2.9	40	5.8	4.4	9.9
STIR-FRIED SAVOY CABBAGE	161/38	1.3	0.2	3.8	3.3	2.2	1.8
BALSAMIC ROASTED ONIONS	370/88	1.1	0.4	16	10	1.7	2.3
LOADED CAULIFLOWER CHEESE	1265/301	9.7	5.3	32	11	4.5	21
BBQ BEANS	762/181	1.3	0.2	24	6	10	12
MARMITE ROASTIES	1202/284	0.8	0.2	55	3	6	12
HAM AND CHEESE SPINACH SWIRLS	373/89	5.5	3	7.1	0.5	0.5	2.8
THE ULTIMATE GRILLED CHEESE	1887/451	20	8.5	45	14	6.2	19

Sweet TREATS	ENERGY KJ/KCAL	FAT (G)	SATURATED FAT (G)	CARBS (G)	SUGAR (G)	FIBRE (G)	PROTEIN (G)
CHOCOLATE ESPRESSO CHEESECAKES	1154/276	15	7.9	24	14	3.2	11
CHOCOLATE CUSTARD	398/95	3.6	1.5	15	2.8	0.5	3.7
BANANA SPONGE PUDDINGS	741/177	7.1	1.8	29	6	2.5	3.3
APPLE BROWN BETTY	649/155	4.8	1.1	24	15	3	2.7
CREAMY LIME PIE	964/230	11	3.5	22	7.9	1.1	11
MILLIONAIRE'S SHORTBREAD	533/127	6.6	4.1	16	2.8	0.5	1
CHOCOLATE BAKED BANANAS	463/110	2.2	0.7	21	17	1.9	1.1
COCONUT AND JAM SPONGE	429/103	5.4	1.6	13	5.1	0.6	1.6
BAKED APPLE WITH A CHEESY CRUMBLE	866/207	7.7	2.6	28	11	3.3	5.4
JAM ROLY POLY	883/210	5.5	1.3	37	6	1.7	4.1
CHOCO NUT LAVA CAKES	755/181	11	2.8	20	4.8	1.2	2.7
TREACLE SPONGE	1402/335	16	3.8	49	19	1.8	4.8
MEXICAN HOT CHOCOLATE	392/94	4.4	1.2	12	0.5	1.3	4

Sweet TREATS	ENERGY KJ/KCAL	FAT (G)	SATURATED FAT (G)	CARBS (G)	SUGAR (G)	FIBRE (G)	PROTEIN (G)
BAKEWELL RICE PUDDING	792/188	5.3	0.5	28	7.7	1.8	5.3
CHERRY PIE	588/139	2.5	0.9	25	9	2.3	3.7
BISCOFF BLONDIES	620/148	8.4	2.2	16	7.9	0.6	2.1

ACCOMPANIMENTS	ENERGY KJ/KCAL	FAT (G)	SATURATED FAT (G)	CARBS (G)	SUGAR (G)	FIBRE (G)	PROTEIN (G)
LOW-CALORIE TORTILLA WRAP (40G)	441/104	0.5	0.3	21	1.4	2.8	3
100G CARROT STICKS	184/44	0.5	0.1	7.7	7.2	3.9	0.5
50G NEST OF EGG NOODLES	727/171	1	0.2	33	0.8	2	6.6
60G LOW KCAL ICE CREAM (HALO VANILLA BEAN)	194/46	1	0.5	7.2	2.9	1.5	2.3
75G MIXED SALAD	64/15	0	0	2	2	0.5	1.1
80G STEAMED GREEN VEGETABLES	145/35	0.5	0	3	1.6	3	3.3
50G BASMATI RICE (RAW)	733/173	0.5	0	38	0	0.6	4.3
60G WHOLEMEAL BREAD ROLL	644/152	2	0.5	25	1.5	3.3	6.8
60G FAT-FREE GREEK-STYLE YOGHURT	148/35	0	0	2.3	2.3	0	6.3
165G BAKED POTATO	697/165	0.5	0.2	34	2.3	4.3	4.1
225G BAKED POTATO	951/225	0.5	0.2	47	3.1	5.9	5.6
50G GLUTEN FREE CIABATTA ROLL (SCHÄR)	463/110	1.3	0.3	21	2.5	4.4	1.8

INDEX

Page numbers in *italics* refer to illustrations

ACKNOWLEDGEMENTS

We owe a million thank yous to so many people for all their support throughout the creation of this book.

We want to say a huge thank you, firstly, to all of our followers on social media and all those who continue to make our recipes and let us know what you want next! We're so proud that Pinch of Nom has helped, and continues to help, so many people.

Thank you to our publisher Carole Tonkinson. To Martha Burley, Bríd Enright, Jodie Mullish, Sian Gardiner, Katy Denny, Laura Nickoll, Jess Duffy, Zainab Dawood and the rest of the team at Bluebird for helping us create this book and believing in Pinch of Nom throughout this journey. Major thanks also to our agent Clare Hulton for your unwavering support and guidance.

To Mike English for the amazing photos and to Kate Wesson for making our food look so, so good and to Octavia Squire for all your assistance. Big thanks go out to Emma Wells and the team at Nic&Lou for making this book so beautiful! A special shout-out to Mel Four at Bluebird for creating the beautiful cover.

We also want to thank our friends and family who have made this book possible.

Special thanks go to Laura Davis and Katie Mitchell for the endless hours you've put into this and for working so hard to get things right!

A huge thank you to our wonderful team of recipe developers who work tirelessly to help us bring these recipes to life: Lisa Allinson, Cate Meadows, Sharon Fitzpatrick and Holly Levell.

Massive thanks also go to Sophie Fryer, Nicola Dales and Hannah Cutting for your writing and marketing support.

Additional thanks to Matthew Maney, Rubi Bourne, Vince Bourne and Cheryl Lloyd for supporting us and the business – we are so proud to work alongside you all.

To our wonderful moderators and online support team: thank you for all your hard work keeping the peace and for all your support.

Furry thanks to Mildred, Ginger Cat, Freda and Brandi for the daily moments of joy.

And finally... Huge thanks go to Paul Allinson for your implicit support. And to Cath Allinson who is never forgotten.

ABOUT THE AUTHORS
KATE *and* KAY

Founders of Pinch of Nom
www.pinchofnom.com

Kate Allinson and Kay Featherstone owned a restaurant together on the Wirral, where Kate was head chef. Together they created the Pinch of Nom blog with the aim of teaching people how to cook. They began sharing healthy, slimming recipes and today Pinch of Nom is the UK's most visited food blog with an active and engaged online community of over 3 million followers.

Keep on track with the new

PINCH OF NOM FOOD PLANNER: COMFORT FOOD

PUBLISHING 2022